Advances in Predictive, Preventive and Personalised Medicine

Volume 17

Halina Podbielska, Wrocław University of Science and Technology
Wrocław, Poland

R. Andrew Tasker, University of Prince Edward Island, Charlottetown, PE, Canada

Christine Nardini, University of Bologna and Verona, Cryolab and Diatheva, Italy/
Laboratory Medicine, Karolinska Institute, Stockholm, Sweden

Lotfi Chaari, Higher Institute of Computer Science and Multimedia of Sfax
Sakiet Ezzit, Tunisia

Jiri Polivka Jr., Department of Histology and Embryology, Biomedical Centre
Faculty of Medicine in Plzeň, Plzeň, Czech Republic

Silvia Mandel, University of Haifa, Haifa, Israel

Carl Erb, Private Institute of Applied Ophthalmology, Berlin, Germany

Wei Wang, School of Medical and Health Sciences, Edith Cowan University
Perth, WA, Australia

What this book series is about… Current healthcare: What is behind the issue? For many acute and chronic disorders, the current healthcare outcomes are considered as being inadequate: global figures cry for preventive measures and personalised treatments. In fact, severe chronic pathologies such as cardiovascular disorders, diabetes and cancer are treated after onset of the disease, frequently at near end-stages. Pessimistic prognosis considers pandemic scenario for type 2 diabetes mellitus, neurodegenerative disorders and some types of cancer over the next 10-20 years followed by the economic disaster of healthcare systems in a global scale. Advanced healthcare tailored to the person: What is beyond the issue? Advanced healthcare promotes the paradigm change from delayed interventional to predictive medicine tailored to the person, from reactive to preventive medicine and from disease to wellness. The innovative Predictive, Preventive and Personalised Medicine (PPPM) is emerging as the focal point of efforts in healthcare aimed at curbing the prevalence of both communicable and non-communicable diseases such as diabetes, cardiovascular diseases, chronic respiratory diseases, cancer and dental pathologies. The cost-effective management of diseases and the critical role of PPPM in modernisation of healthcare have been acknowledged as priorities by global and regional organizations and health-related institutions such as the Organisation of United Nations, the European Union and The National Institutes of Health. Why integrative medical approach by PPPM as the medicine of the future? PPPM is the new integrative concept in healthcare sector that enables to predict individual predisposition before onset of the disease, to provide targeted preventive measures and create personalised treatment algorithms tailored to the person. The expected outcomes are conducive to more effective population screening, prevention early in childhood, identification of persons at-risk, stratification of patients for the optimal therapy planning, prediction and reduction of adverse drug-drug or drug-disease interactions relying on emerging technologies, such as pharmacogenetics, pathology-specific molecular patters, sub/cellular imaging, disease modelling, individual patient profiles, etc. Integrative approach by PPPM is considered as the medicine of the future. Being at the forefront of the global efforts, The European Association for Predictive, Preventive and Personalised Medicine (EPMA, http://www.epmanet.eu/) promotes the integrative concept of PPPM among healthcare stakeholders, governmental institutions, educators, funding bodies, patient organisations and in the public domain. Current Book Series, published by Springer in collaboration with EPMA, overview multidisciplinary aspects of advanced bio/medical approaches and innovative technologies. Integration of individual professional groups into the overall concept of PPPM is a particular advantage of this book series. Expert recommendations focus on the cost-effective management tailored to the person in health and disease. Innovative strategies are considered for standardisation of healthcare services. New guidelines are proposed for medical ethics, treatment of rare diseases, innovative approaches to early and predictive diagnostics, patient stratification and targeted prevention in healthy individuals, persons at-risk, individual patient groups, sub/populations, institutions, healthcare economy and marketing.

Springer and the Series Editors welcome book ideas from authors. Potential authors who wish to submit a book proposal should contact Nathalie L'horset-Poulain, Executive Editor (e-mail: nathalie.lhorset-poulain@springer.com)

Halina Podbielska • Marko Kapalla
Editors

Predictive, Preventive, and Personalised Medicine: From Bench to Bedside

Springer

Editors
Halina Podbielska
Department of Biomedical Engineering
Wrocław University of Science & Technology
Wroclaw, Poland

Marko Kapalla
F.D. Roosevelt University General Hospital of Banská Bystrica
Banská Bystrica, Slovakia

ISSN 2211-3495 ISSN 2211-3509 (electronic)
Advances in Predictive, Preventive and Personalised Medicine
ISBN 978-3-031-34883-9 ISBN 978-3-031-34884-6 (eBook)
https://doi.org/10.1007/978-3-031-34884-6

This Springer imprint is published by the registered company Springer Nature Switzerland AG
The registered company address is: Gewerbestrasse 11, 6330 Cham, Switzerland

Preface

Dear Reader

We are very glad to present to you the newest book volume in our long-term series of books dedicated to Advances in Predictive, Preventive and Personalized Medicine (PPPM/3PM) [https://www.springer.com/series/10051]. This book is a joint effort of contributors from 12 countries. Altogether, there are 19 chapters dedicated to specific fields related to the fundamental research, technology applications, and practical use of PPPM/3PM principia in healthcare and medicine. The chapters are ordered on the basis of the content and the relation to the neighboring chapters. The logical structure starts with introductory chapter on PPPM innovation in primary, secondary, and tertiary care, then continues with suboptimal health, which we find fundamental for prediction and prevention, further highlighting mitochondrial health as another basic perspective in health and suboptimal health. Further, you will find PPPM issue in prehabilitation processes in concert with protocols for early recovery after surgery, pain chronification prediction, and pain management. Next chapters are focused on particular diseases like assessing and managing unproper body postures in preschool children, using multiomics methods in pituitary adenomas, use of thermal imaging for prediction and prevention in diabetic patients, computer-assisted diagnostics in breast cancer, role of microbiome in liver diseases, telemedicine and COVID-19 lessons in diabetes care, continuing with sleep disorders highlighting the importance of good sleep for good health. Further, an interesting chapter on modern psychiatry and mental health is presented, followed by wound healing stimulation technologies, artificial intelligence algorithms to analyze weather conditions for predictions of cerebrovascular accidents, electrophysiology in cardiac care, periodontal health, eye health as an essential attribute of good health, implementation of artificial intelligence in data analysis, and completing with wearable devices as the practical example for PPPM implementation and help in monitoring lifestyle changes. We hope that in this book you will find important and useful information for practical application and for personal and population education and that you realize that the predictive, preventive, and personalized medicine is undoubtedly the future of healthcare, a future we have the opportunity to observe it becoming a present reality.

As editors, here we also want to express our cordial thanks to all contributors for their great work done to make this book volume a valuable contribution to the whole series. Thank You.

Wroclaw, Poland
Banská Bystrica, Slovakia

Halina Podbielska
Marko Kapalla

Contents

About the Editors

Halina Podbielska, D.Sc. Eng. M.D. is Professor Ordinarius in the Biomedical Engineering Department at the Wrocław University of Science and Technology (WUST). She received her M.Sc. and Engineering Degree in Applied Physics/Optics from the Faculty of Fundamental Problems of Technology of Wroclaw University of Technology WrUT (now WUST) and her Ph.D. degree in Physics from the Institute of Physics, both awarded by a special Award for Excellence. She also received her M.D. degree from the Faculty of Medicine of Medical Academy Wrocław (now Medical University). She completed her postgraduate study in business and management at the Faculty of Informatics and Managing conducted by the Central State University of Connecticut/USA.

Halina was a founder of the Biomedical Engineering Institute at the Faculty of Fundamental Problems of Technology WruST in 2007, and served for years as a Director and the Head of the Biomedical Engineering Department. Additionally, in 2007–2014 she was appointed as a full professor in the Department of Physical Therapy at the Faculty of Physiotherapy of the Wroclaw University School of Physical Education for teaching students of Physiotherapy and Cosmetology on modern aspects of physical medicine with special emphasis on modern aspects of biophotoelectronics and personalized medicine. She was visiting scientist in several scientific institutions worldwide: at the University of Frankfurt/Main (1984–85), University of Muenster (1985–86) as an A. v. Humboldt Foundation fellow, and at the Weizmann Institute of Science, Israel (1989–1990).

In 2002–2005 she was a visiting professor at the Institute of Optics of Technical University in Berlin. She was also visiting scientist at the Charite Medizin University of Berlin (2005) conducting research at the Medical Laser Technology Center LMTB, Germany. Her professional experiences include biomedical engineering with emphasis on medical application of optics, nanomaterials, and physical and personalized medicine. She is an author or coauthor of over 400 publications and holds 13 registered patents related to biomedical technologies and personalized approaches. She is a Board Member of Polish Society of Biomedical Engineering and member of many internationally recognized bodies (OSA, SPIE, OWLS, EPMA). She holds a distinction of OSA Senior Member. She is a member of the Scientific Council of the Institute of Biocybernetics and Biomedical Engineering of Polish Academy of Science in Warsaw and a member of the Committee of Biocybernetics Biomedical Engineering of Polish Academy of Science and of

Board of the International Centre for Biocybernetics, Warsaw. She is a member of the Editorial Board of the journal *Biocybernetics and Biomedical Engineering*. She is/was acting as an expert for grant evaluation in the sixth and seventh Framework Program and Horizon 2020 of EC. She has been a grants reviewer for the National Institutes of Health, USA, Ministry of Science, Latvia, and Polish authorities.

From 2008 she has been a member of the Academic Advisory Board and Representative of Biomedical Engineering of EPMA (European Association for Predictive, Preventive and Personalized Medicine) and Editorial Board member of *EPMA Journal*. In 2021 she received a prestigious EPMA Highest Recognition of Exceptional Achievements in International Networking in the field of biomedical sciences.

Marko Kapalla, RNDr. PhD. graduated in 1994 at the Faculty of Natural Sciences of Comenius University in Bratislava, Slovakia, where he received his M.Sc. degree in Biochemistry. In 1996 he wrote a scientific philosophical book *Complexity of Information* where he discusses a wide range of stimulating topics related to science, philosophy, physics, information, entropy, life phenomenon, consciousness, universe, and other topics. In 1999 his book was published by Veda, the publishing house of Slovak Academy of Sciences. In 2014, he presented and defended, in the field of Normal and Pathological Physiology, his dissertation on "The Role of Laboratory Diagnostics and Modern Information Systems in the Development of the Concept of Predictive, Preventive and Personalized Medicine" which became the pioneering work on predictive, preventive, and personalized medicine (PPPM) awarded by Ph.D. at the Faculty of Medicine of Comenius University in Bratislava, Slovakia. He acquired practical experience in the advanced techniques of molecular biology during his study at the University of Vienna, Austria, as well as during his study stays at the University Hospital Bonn, Germany. Since 1998, he has been working in the field of clinical laboratory diagnostics where he acquired his professional experience and expertise at several positions as specialized clinical biochemist, head of the clinical laboratory, manager for consolidation and integration of the clinical laboratory complex at the FDRH University Hospital in Banská Bystrica, Slovakia, and the corporate quality manager in one of the largest networks of accredited clinical laboratories in Slovakia. Since 2007 he has also been the CEO of Negentropic Systems, Ltd., the company that is developing progressive laboratory information systems. Since 2018 he has served as the CEO of PPPM Centre, Ltd., a private company that was founded in Slovakia in order to fulfill EPMA visions of practical application of PPPM. Since 1997 he has been a member of the Slovak Society of Clinical Biochemistry; from 2015 to 2019 he was also a member of the Executive board of SSKB. In 2008 he became one of five founding members of the European Association for Predictive, Preventive and Personalized Medicine (EPMA) and since then he has been a member of the EPMA Board of Directors as well as EPMA National Representative in Slovakia. Since 2022 he has been EPMA Vice-president for European Affairs. He is also an Associate editor of *The EPMA*

Journal (IF (2021) 8.836 by Clarivate; CiteScoreTracker (2022) 11.2 by Scopus) and a regular reviewer for *The EPMA Journal* with well over 100 reviewed articles, 69 of which are peer reviews verified by Clarivate. He authored and coauthored over 65 publications and scientific contributions, including one book and five book chapters, and gave over 45 invited lectures at numerous international and national conferences on laboratory diagnostics and predictive, preventive, and personalized medicine. His professional interests are mainly focused on PPPM, clinical laboratory diagnostics, vitamins, nutrition, innovation in healthcare, complex factors influencing health, clinical data analysis, and the development of clinical information systems and information technology in healthcare.

PPPM Innovation in Primary, Secondary and Tertiary Care

Olga Golubnitschaja, Marko Kapalla, Halina Podbielska, and Vincenzo Costigliola

1 Health-to-Disease Transition in Focus of Advanced Bio/Medical Sciences and Healthcare Services

Reactive medicine has reached its ethical, economic and technological limits as demonstrated by pandemic spread of acute infections such as COVID-19 [1–3] as well as pandemics of chronic disorders. To this end, currently, more than half of billion patients are diagnosed with diabetes type 2, over 70 million of glaucoma

O. Golubnitschaja (✉)
European Association for Predictive, Preventive and Personalised Medicine, EPMA, Brussels, Belgium

3P Medicine Research Unit, University Hospital, Rheinische Friedrich-Wilhelms Universität Bonn, Bonn, Germany
e-mail: olga.golubnitschaja@ukbonn.de

M. Kapalla
European Association for Predictive, Preventive and Personalised Medicine, EPMA, Brussels, Belgium

F.D. Roosevelt University General Hospital of Banská Bystrica, Banská Bystrica, Slovakia

H. Podbielska
European Association for Predictive, Preventive and Personalised Medicine, EPMA, Brussels, Belgium

Department of Biomedical Engineering, Wrocław University of Science and Technology, Wrocław, Poland
e-mail: info@halinapodbielska.pl

V. Costigliola
European Association for Predictive, Preventive and Personalised Medicine, EPMA, Brussels, Belgium

European Medical Association, EMA, Brussels, Belgium

H. Podbielska, M. Kapalla (eds.), *Predictive, Preventive, and Personalised Medicine: From Bench to Bedside*, Advances in Predictive, Preventive and Personalised Medicine 17, https://doi.org/10.1007/978-3-031-34884-6_1

patients are predisposed to blindness, breast and prostate cancers together reached a pandemic scale, whereby prostate cancer management costs increase more rapidly than for any other cancer [4–7]. Therefore, the paradigm change promoted by the European Association for Predictive, Preventive and Personalised Medicine (EPMA, Brussels, www.epmanet.eu), namely from reactive medical services to predictive approach, cost-effective targeted prevention and personalisation of treatment algorithms is essential to advance healthcare, to increase life quality of population and to improve health economy in a short- and long-term way [8–10].

In a long-term manner, the most cost-effective strategy is to focus scientific and healthcare effort on the health-to-disease transition, in order to the reverse current pandemic trends [11]. Internationally accumulated knowledge about sub-optimal health conditions is of pivotal importance to apply PPPM strategies protecting affected population against health adverse effects of internal and external risk factors. Health risk assessment and cost-effective targeted prevention is detailed in this book and can be well exemplified by sub-optimal health of individuals with the Flammer syndrome phenotype [12] amongst others.

2 A Holistic Approach by 3P Medicine Is the Clue

Systemic effects are characteristic for sub-optimal health conditions, transition from health-to-diseases as well as progression of multi-factorial disorders such as metabolic syndrome, malignancies and neurodegenerative processes. Therefore, a holistic approach by 3P medicine is the clue in disease prediction, prevention and treatment. To this end, mitochondrial health is considered instrumental to monitor stability of the health condition, to detect systemic reactions towards multi-factorial stressors and to assess adequacy of the stress response towards environmental changes, redox balance, the innate and acquired immunity as well as severity of the acute and chronic disorders. Well-known mitochondrial burnout-associated pathologies include chronic fatigue, accelerated ageing, auto/immune disorders, hormonal dysregulation and infertility, eye pathologies, metabolic and mood disorders, severe respiratory diseases, impaired healing, neurodegenerative and cancerous alterations [13]. Contextually, mitochondrial health quality control is considered in the book for the holistic predictive diagnostic approach in PPPM framework.

3 Technological Innovation

Health protection, life quality and robustness of diagnostic and treatment approaches are the main criteria of quality considered in the framework of the PPPM-relevant technological developments. Consequently, non-invasive, user-friendly, reliable and cost-effective diagnostic approaches, PPPM-relevant products and medical services are highly prioritised. Technological solutions adapted to these criteria are detailed in the book such as diagnostic approaches utilising tear fluid as the non-invasive source of biomarkers specific for ocular and systemic diseases [14], telemedical approach utilising wearable sensors for permanent monitoring individuals at risk and in chronic medical conditions, and application of artificial intelligence, amongst others.

4 Conclusion

In conclusion, the **anticipated progress beyond the state of the art in primary, secondary and tertiary care**, and PPPM benefits are summarised below:

- Primary healthcare.
  - Whole-body health quality check-up.
  - Pre-pregnancy check-up.
  - Accompanying diagnostics in sport medicine and supervised physical activities.
  - Accompanying diagnostics in physiotherapeutic and well-being services.
  - Health-to-disease transition check-up and targeted protection amongst others.
- Secondary healthcare.
  - Early-stage disease detection and targeted prevention of the disease progression.
  - Treatment algorithms tailored to the individualised multi-parametric patient profile.
  - Therapy efficacy monitoring and improved individual outcomes.

The accents will get shifted towards stabilised medical conditions.

- Tertiary healthcare.
- In the tertiary healthcare the accents will get shifted from palliative care to the care of chronic medical conditions with significantly improved life quality of patients under treatment.

References

1. Radanliev P, De Roure D, Walton R, Van Kleek M, Montalvo RM, Santos O, Maddox L, Cannady S (2020) COVID-19 what have we learned? The rise of social machines and connected devices in pandemic management following the concepts of predictive, preventive and personalized medicine. EPMA J 11(3):311–332. https://doi.org/10.1007/s13167-020-00218-x
2. Richter K, Kellner S, Hillemacher T, Golubnitschaja O (2021) Sleep quality and COVID-19 outcomes: the evidence-based lessons in the framework of predictive, preventive and personalised (3P) medicine. EPMA J 12(2):221–241. https://doi.org/10.1007/s13167-021-00245-2
3. Skladany L, Koller T, Adamcova Selcanova S, Vnencakova J, Jancekova D, Durajova V, Laffers L, Svac J, Janickova K, Palkovič M, Kohout P, Golubnitschaja O (2021) Challenging management of severe chronic disorders in acute pandemic situation: chronic liver disease under COVID-19 pandemic as the proof-of-principle model to orchestrate the measures in 3PM context. EPMA J 12(1):1–14. https://doi.org/10.1007/s13167-021-00231-8
4. Kropp M, Golubnitschaja O, Mazurakova A, Koklesova L, Sargheini N, Vo TKS, de Clerck E, Polivka J Jr, Potuznik P, Polivka J, Stetkarova I, Kubatka P (2023) Thumann G diabetic reti-

nopathy as the leading cause of blindness and early predictor of cascading complications-risks and mitigation. EPMA J 14(1):21–42. https://doi.org/10.1007/s13167-023-00314-8
5. Koklesova L, Samec M, Liskova A, Zhai K, Büsselberg D, Giordano FA, Kubatka P, Golunitschaja O (2021) Mitochondrial impairments in aetiopathology of multifactorial diseases: common origin but individual outcomes in context of 3P medicine. EPMA J 12(1):27–40. https://doi.org/10.1007/s13167-021-00237-2
6. Mazurakova A, Koklesova L, Samec M, Kudela E, Kajo K, Skuciova V, Csizmár SH, Mestanova V, Pec M, Adamkov M, Al-Ishaq RK, Smejkal K, Giordano FA, Büsselberg D, Biringer K, Golubnitschaja O, Kubatka P (2022) Anti-breast cancer effects of phytochemicals: primary, secondary, and tertiary care. EPMA J 13(2):315–334. https://doi.org/10.1007/s13167-022-00277-2
7. Ellinger J, Alajati A, Kubatka P, Giordano FA, Ritter M, Costigliola V, Golubnitschaja O (2022) Prostate cancer treatment costs increase more rapidly than for any other cancer-how to reverse the trend? EPMA J 13(1):1–7. https://doi.org/10.1007/s13167-022-00276-3
8. Golubnitschaja O, Costigliola V, EPMA (2012) General report & recommendations in predictive, preventive and personalised medicine 2012: white paper of the European Association for predictive, preventive and personalised medicine. EPMA J 3(1):14. https://doi.org/10.1186/1878-5085-3-14
9. Golubnitschaja O, Baban B, Boniolo G, Wang W, Bubnov R, Kapalla M, Krapfenbauer K, Mozaffari M, Costigliola V (2016) Medicine in the early twenty-first century: paradigm and anticipation—EPMA position paper 2016. EPMA J 7:23. https://doi.org/10.1186/s13167-016-0072-4
10. Golubnitschaja O (ed) Book series "Advances in predictive, preventive and personalised medicine". Springer, Dordrecht, Heidelberg, New York, London. https://www.springer.com/series/10051
11. Wang W, Yan Y, Guo Z, Hou H, Garcia M, Tan X, Anto EO, Mahara G, Zheng Y, Li B, Wang Y, Guo X, Golubnitschaja O (2021) All around suboptimal health. A joint position paper of the suboptimal health study consortium and European Association for predictive, preventive and personalised medicine. EPMA J 12(4):1–31. https://doi.org/10.1007/s13167-021-00253-2
12. Golubnitschaja O (ed) (2019., ISBN 978-3-030-13549-2 ISBN 978-3-030-13550-8 (eBook)) Flammer Syndrome—From Phenotype to Associated Pathologies, Prediction, Prevention and Personalisation V.11. https://doi.org/10.1007/978-3-030-13550-8
13. Koklesova L, Mazurakova A, Samec M, Kudela E, Biringer K, Kubatka P, Golubnitschaja O (2022) Mitochondrial health quality control: measurements and interpretation in the framework of predictive, preventive, and personalized medicine. EPMA J 13:177–193. https://doi.org/10.1007/s13167-022-00281-6
14. Zhan X, Li J, Guo Y, Golubnitschaja O (2021) Mass spectrometry analysis of human tear fluid biomarkers specific for ocular and systemic diseases in the context of 3P medicine. EPMA J 12(4):449–475. https://doi.org/10.1007/s13167-021-00265-y

Suboptimal Health Innovation: From Bench to Bedside

Fangli Hu and Wei Wang

Abbreviations

COACS	China Suboptimal Health Cohort Study
mRNA	Messenger RNA
NCDs	Non-communicable Chronic Diseases
PPPM	Predictive, Preventive, and Personalized Medicine
SHS	Suboptimal Health Status
SHSC	Suboptimal Health Study Consortium
SHSQ-25	Suboptimal Health Status Suestionnaire-25
WHO	World Health Organization

F. Hu
The First Affiliated Hospital, Shantou University Medical College, Shantou, China

W. Wang (✉)
The First Affiliated Hospital, Shantou University Medical College, Shantou, China

School of Public Health, Shandong First Medical University and Shandong Academy of Medical Sciences, Tai'an, China

Beijing Municipal Key Laboratory of Clinical Epidemiology, Capital Medical University, Beijing, China

Centre for Precision Health, Edith Cowan University, Perth, Australia
e-mail: wei.wang@ecu.edu.au

H. Podbielska, M. Kapalla (eds.), *Predictive, Preventive, and Personalised Medicine: From Bench to Bedside*, Advances in Predictive, Preventive and Personalised Medicine 17, https://doi.org/10.1007/978-3-031-34884-6_2

1 Introduction

Non-communicable chronic diseases (NCDs) have increased in prevalence and have become the one of the top health threats of the twenty-first century [1]. As one of the biggest challenges to life quality and longevity, NCDs affect up to 20% of the global population and lead to 41 million deaths a year, contributing to 71% of all global deaths [2]. There is increasing concern over the growing number of young people who suffer from chronic diseases. For example, adolescents are a group of concern with rising numbers of new cases of type 2 diabetes mellitus [3]. Mental disorders, suicide, stroke, and cancer are also prevalent in young people [4]. These chronic diseases severely reduce the life quality of both patients and their families, resulting in a huge socio-economic burden. Unprecedented medical resources have been invested globally to curb the epidemic of chronic diseases, but with little success. However, from the viewpoint of predictive, preventive, and personalized medicine (PPPM), many NCDs can be delayed or even prevented, thus effectively reducing their incidence [5].

NCDs have a multifactorial etiology resulting from the interaction of genetic, environmental, and behavioral factors. In other words, age, genes, home and work environments, lifestyle, and dietary habits all contribute to the manifestation of NCDs [6]. Early detection and appropriate intervention are important for disease prevention and treatment. Suboptimal health status, an intermediate state between health and a diagnosable illness, emphasizes the idea that NCDs can be predicted and even prevented from further advancing of the clinical manifestations of severe pathologies [7]. Hence, defining suboptimal health and developing reliable subjective and objective measurement tools for suboptimal health allows for effective predictive diagnosis and cost-efficient prevention and treatment strategies tailored to patients with chronic health conditions. This chapter focuses on SHS, highlights its health innovation from bench to bedside, in line with the tenets of translational medicine and PPPM, and showcases leading-edge advancement in the medical and healthcare field.

2 Suboptimal Health Status

Health is "a state of complete physical, mental, and social well-being and not merely the absence of disease or infirmity" [8]. It is a challenge to assess an individual's health level. An increasing number of people around the world complain of a general malaise even without a diagnosable disease. This intermediate state between health and a diagnosable illness has been ignored by modern medicine for a long time due to the lack of systematic evidence; however, Traditional Chinese Medicine has recognized this intermediate state since ancient times, originating from the preventive treatment theory in *The Emperor' s Classic of Internal Medicine* [7]. In an effort to bridge modern Western Medicine and Traditional Chinese Medicine, the English term "suboptimal health status" was coined to describe "an overall physical status between health and illness characterized by the perception of health complaints, chronic fatigue, and a constellation of physical symptoms such as the cardiovascular system, the digestive system, the immune system, and mental status; lasting for at least 3 months" [9]. SHS is caused by a combination of environmental factors (e.g., pollution, social stresses) and unhealthy lifestyles or behaviors (e.g., lack of exercise, unhealthy dietary habits, smoking, and alcohol abuse). As a widespread public health issue, suboptimal health affects up to 75% of the global population, covering people in almost all age groups, regions, and countries, and can lead to short- or long-term adverse health outcomes [10]. People in SHS are prone to anxiety, depression, headaches, fatigue, insomnia, and other conditions. Frequent hospital visits due to suboptimal health place economic and mental burdens on people and reduce their quality of life. More seriously, if SHS status becomes chronic, it can even shorten a person's life expectancy, thus imposing a significant medical burden on society [11]. Unfortunately, SHS and its negative outcomes are still underappreciated because there are no obvious identifiable symptoms.

SHS has been well accepted as a risk factor for chronic diseases, such as cardiovascular diseases, cancers, respiratory diseases, diabetes, and stroke [12]. Unlike infectious diseases, NCDs, whose symptoms usually persist for more than 3 months, do not directly spread from person to person [13, 14], however, they are the top cause of global death, especially premature deaths in low- and middle-income countries. More importantly, this dire situation will worsen as the global aging population increases [15, 16]. Most NCDs develop from reversible suboptimal health conditions to irreversible pathology with associated complications within a few years. Therefore, as a subclinical, reversible stage of chronic diseases, SHS usually precedes the occurrence of chronic diseases [17]. Treatments for chronic diseases are usually not started until after specific clinical symptoms appear, which is considerably delayed from a PPPM perspective. SHS is a key window of opportunity in predicting chronic diseases prior to the clinical manifestations of severe pathologies and is therefore believed as a potential preventive barometer for the control and management of chronic diseases [12]. As an emerging insight into translational medicine, SHS thus deserves close attention.

3 Diagnostic Tools for SHS

SHS is ubiquitous, but hard to detect due to individual heterogeneity and the inconsistency of people's perceptions related to health [18]. Given that SHS typically predates chronic diseases, the time between the onset of suboptimal health and the clinical manifestation of the associated disease is a good opportunity to make reliable risk assessments and predictive diagnoses [9]. Hence, reliable, and valid diagnostic tools are essential to accurately identify SHS so that targeted prevention and treatment of chronic diseases can occur. What is more, under-diagnosis (the failure to identify or accurately diagnose a disease or disorder, notably in a considerable proportion of patients) and over-diagnosis (the diagnosis of a medical condition that would not otherwise cause any symptoms or problems) of NCDs has wasted a lot of medical resources and seriously increase the economic burden of health care [19, 20]. Accordingly, from the perspective of PPPM, powerful predictive instruments of SHS can not only help identify both high-risk and low-risk populations to avoid under- and over-diagnosis, but also give clinicians the chance to apply tailored preventative measures before the incidence of actual diseases. To get a more holistic picture of SHS and facilitate clinical practice of suboptimal health innovation, our team, the Suboptimal Health Study Consortium (SHSC), has developed and validated a subjective suboptimal health status questionnaire-25 (SHSQ-25) and explored verified SHSQ-25 in three major ethnic groups African, Asian, and Caucasian [9], combined with laboratory-based biochemistry health measures with a laboratory bench to clinical bed approach.

3.1 Subjective Measure

Based on the rigorous procedure of questionnaire development and assessment of reliability and validity, we created a comprehensive SHS measure tool, SHSQ-25, in 2009 [5]. As shown in Fig. 1, the SHSQ-25 covers five dimensions of suboptimal

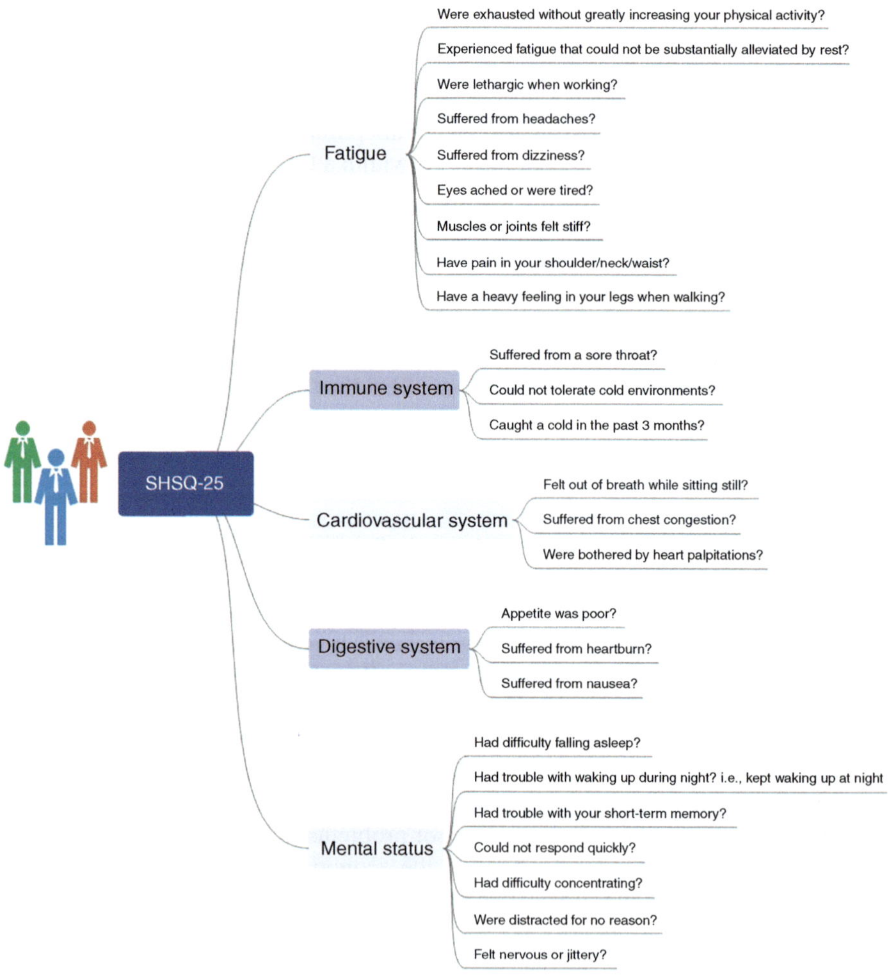

Fig. 1 Five factors and 25 components of SHSQ-25

health status: fatigue, the cardiovascular system, the digestive system, the immune system, and mental status. With the support of 25 components, SHSQ-25 is a time-efficient and cost-effective instrument to be applied for health measures. When administered, each participant is tasked with rating how often he or she undergone a specific complaint in the last 3 months. The questionnaire adopts a 5-point Likert-type scale: (1) never or almost never, (2) occasionally, (3) often, (4) very often, and (5) always. This questionnaire is suitable for extensive investigations of the general population at real-word clinical or community settings. It serves as a practical and valid predictive tool of health status to provide a perfect chance for early detection of and timely intervention for chronic diseases, thus helping to mitigate negative consequences of NCDs [21].

The SHSQ-25 is a freely available health measure instrument to evaluate health conditions and support higher precisive health measure in primary PPPM-oriented health care practice (Table 1). This simple, reliable, and valid tool is available in multiple language versions, e.g., Chinese, English, Korean, and Russian [5, 22–24], and has been applied and validated through health surveys among these major populations (Asian, African, and Caucasian) to explore the associations between SHS and NCDs risks [25]. For example, the China suboptimal health cohort study (COACS) found that SHSQ-25 can be used for routine detection and screening for cardiovascular and metabolic diseases [9, 11, 26]. Moreover, multiple cross-sectional studies conducted in Ghana reported that SHS is an important risk factor contributing to type 2 diabetes mellitus [27]. As a self-reported indicator of health condition and subclinical status, suboptimal health not only promotes the concept of PPPM, but also provides unprecedented convenience for the early detection of NCDs, breaking through the previous limitations of people's understanding of health assessment. The SHSQ-25 can therefore be applied to a wider cross-cultural population to promote cost-effective and time-efficient clinical health screening [9, 24].

3.2 Objective Measurements Enhance the Reliability of SHSQ-25

SHSQ-25 is self-reported and subjective tool for health measure. Given the complexity and diversity of suboptimal health symptoms, objective biological measures were included as additional health biomarkers to support for the subjective assessment of suboptimal health. Biological measures are highly valuable in assessing health conditions and forecasting the development of disease. The following two categories of biomarkers were investigated on the association with suboptimal health status: anthropological metrics and general biological indicators (Table 2). Our multi-empirical studies have found that several anthropological metrics and general biological indicators correlate with suboptimal health status and can be used as adjunctive predictive biomarkers, including diastolic blood pressures, systolic blood pressures, body mass index, smoking index, total cholesterol, triglycerides, low-density lipoprotein

Table 1 Example of the application of SHSQ-25 at different ethnic groups

SHSQ-25	Study design	Study population	Sample size (number of participants)	Reference
Chinese version	Cross-sectional study	Chinese population	2799	Yan et al. (2009) [5]
	Cross-sectional study	Chinese workers	3405	Yan et al. (2012) [11]
	Cross-sectional study	Chinese workers	386	Yan et al. (2015) [18]
	Prospective cohort study	Chinese population	4313	Wang et al. (2016) [26] Wang et al. (2017) [28] Ge et al. (2019) [29]
	Case-control study	Chinese population	588	Alzain et al. (2017) [30]
	Cross-sectional study	Chinese urban workers	868	Yan et al. (2018) [21]
	Cross-sectional study	Chinese college students	4119	Hou et al. (2018) [31]
	Cross-sectional study	Chinese nurses	6107	Zhu et al. (2020) [32]
	Cross-sectional study	Northern Chinese population	3524	Ding et al. (2020) [33]
	Case-control study	Chinese population	2861	Wang et al. (2020) [34]
	Case-control study	Chinese undergraduate students	60	Wang et al. (2021) [10]
	Cross-sectional study	Chinese Taiwanese	66	Kung et al. (2021) [35]
	Case-control study	Chinese population	248	Meng et al. (2022) [36]
	Cross-sectional study	Chinese medical students	2741	Zhang et al. (2022) [37]
	Cross-sectional study	Chinese domestic tourists	360	Guo et al. (2022) [38]
English version	Case-control study	Ghanaian population	505	Adua et al. (2017) [27]
	Prospective cohort study	Ghanaian pregnant women	593	Anto et al. (2019) [39] Anto et al. (2021) [40]
	Case-control study	Ghanaian pregnant women	593	Anto et al. (2020) [41] Anto et al. (2022) [42]
	Case-control study	Ghanaian population	262	Adua et al. (2019) [43]
	Cross-sectional study	Ghanaian population	263	Adua et al. (2021) [24]
Russian version	Cross-sectional study	Russia urban population	459	Kupaev et al. (2016) [22]
Korean version	Cross-sectional study	Korean population	460	Guo et al. (2022) [23]

Table 2 Example of the objective marker of SHS

Objective Marker of SHS			Reference
Anthropological metrics		Smoking index, body mass index, systolic blood pressures, diastolic blood pressures	Wang et al. (2014) [7]
General biological indicators	Biochemical indexes	Total cholesterol, triglycerides, low-density lipoprotein cholesterol, plasma cortisol	Wang et al. (2014) [7]
	Molecular biomarkers	Telomere length	Alzain et al. (2017) [30]
		N-glycans (e.g., IgG N-glycosylation)	Adua et al. (2019) [43]
		Metabolic biomarkers (e.g., sphingosine, pregnanolone, taurolithocholate sulfate, and cervonyl carnitine)	Wang et al. (2020) [34]
		Glucocorticoid receptor mRNA	Yan et al. (2015) [18]
		Intestinal microbiota	Sun et al. (2019) [45]
	Subclinical status	Endothelial dysfunction	Kupaev et al. (2016) [22]
		Oxidative stress and its related complication	Anto et al. (2020) [41]

cholesterol, plasma cortisol, endothelial dysfunction, oxidative stress and its related complications [9, 18, 22, 40, 43]. Since SHS is an intermediate state between health and a diagnosable illness, biological changes in metabolomics, glycomics, proteomics, and telomere length may offer valuable insights into the assessment of SHS for chronic disease stratification. Molecular biological measures including intestinal microbiota, glucocorticoid receptor mRNA, N-glycans (e.g., IgG N-glycosylation), and metabolic biomarkers (e.g., sphingosine, pregnanolone, taurolithocholate sulfate, and cervonyl carnitine) can serve as potential predictive biomarkers of suboptimal health status [34, 36, 44]. Moreover, short relative telomere length has been discovered to be significantly correlated with SHS [30].

4 Paradigm Shift from Reactive to Predictive, Preventive, and Personalized Medicine

Many countries are marching into aging societies rapidly. An estimated 727 million people were 65 or older in 2020, totalling 9.3% of the world's population. This number is expected to more than double to over 1.5 billion people by 2050 [46]. Importantly, aging is characterized by declining physiological functions and greater susceptibility to chronic inflammation and aging-related diseases. The prevalence of these chronic diseases has risen accordingly [47]. Therefore, predictive, preventive, and personalized medicine (PPPM) has been proposed as a response to the public health challenges posed by this demographic shift. PPPM is "the new integrative concept in the health care sector that enables to predict individual predisposition before onset of the disease, to provide targeted preventive measures and create personalized treatment algorithms tailored to the person" [48]. PPPM is the medicine of the future as a proactive approach in the practices of effective population/community-based health survey, early prevention, patient stratification, and customization of optimal treatment protocols, forgoing traditional reactive medical practices [49].

The notion of SHS fits well with the PPPM paradigm. More specifically, as an effective sentinel for NCDs, SHS provides a critical window of opportunity for PPPM [9]. Based on the proven potential associations between SHS and NCDs (e.g., type 2 diabetes, cardiovascular diseases, cognitive impairment), chronic diseases can be predicted and even prevented before the initiation of pathologies [9]. Therefore, in-depth insight into SHS may motivate a shift in the medical paradigm from reactive to preventative, i.e., PPPM, facilitating a two-way translation of basic scientific research and clinical treatment: suboptimal health innovation from bench to bedside [7]. In addition, the future is bound to be a new era of "personalized medicine." Due to the significant differences in individuals' living circumstances, physical characteristics and personalities, PPPM places greater emphasis on individual idiosyncrasies [9]. Future treatment plans will therefore be tailored to each individual patients' information [50]. Timely assessments and effective interventions for suboptimal health are a cost-efficient way for NCDs prevention, control, and personalized management, thereby enhancing people's health and life quality and reducing the societal burden [12]. The combination of the subjective questionnaire (SHSQ-25) and objective biomarkers (e.g., metabolites, glycans, glucocorticoids, telomere length, and microbiota) for SHS allows for rapid, accurate and cost-effective identification of subclinical symptoms, making SHS an effective tool for early detection, tailored prevention, and personalized treatment of NCDs [50].

5 Conclusion and Recommendations

Modern Western Medicine, based on evidence, emphasizes the treatment of disease symptoms, while Traditional Chinese Medicine, experience-based, focuses on the improvement of the overall state of individuals [51]. We hope to build a bridge between modern Western Medicine and Traditional Chinese Medicine through the lens of SHS and combine their strengths for the systematic evaluation, treatment, and prevention of NCDs. From a PPPM perspective, SHS innovation from the bench to the bedside boosts predictive, preventive and personalized healthcare for vulnerable populations with NCDs. We are currently experimenting with interdisciplinary research incorporating social science to propose an alternative perspective on suboptimal health research (e.g., **apply tourism as a health intervention for dementia**—aiming to promote the overall health of society) (Fig. 2) [38].

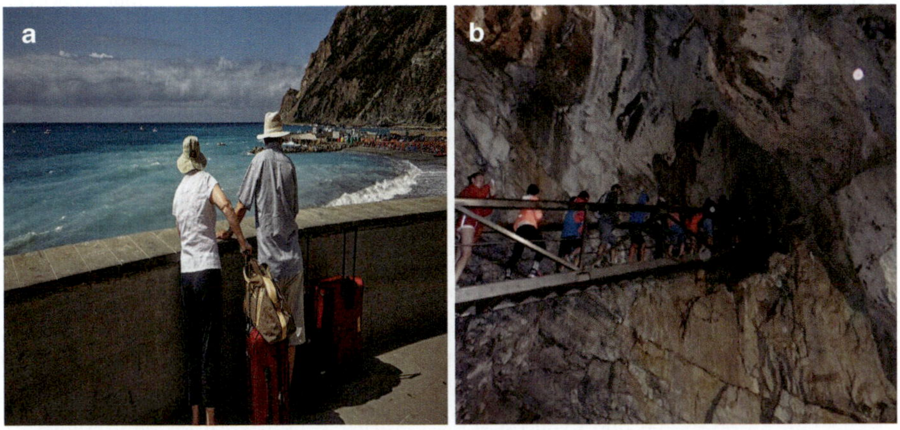

Fig. 2 (**a**, **b**) Composite illustrative image—Holidays and nature exploration can help to improve health and well-being of individuals interested in their health support and relax. (Source: (**a**) https://www.ecu.edu.au/newsroom/articles/research/travel-therapy-could-holidays-help-mental-health-and-wellbeing [52]. (**b**) Authors' internal archive)

Based on positive psychology, travel experiences contribute to individuals' health and well-being through improving the functions of cognitive, affective, conative, and sensorial components [53]. Tourism may, therefore, be a potential non-medical intervention for individuals suffering from SHS or even chronic diseases via prevention and treatment. More specifically, travelers with SHS can enhance their physical and psychological functioning to facilitate the recovery from SHS and prevent from deteriorating to chronic conditions while travelers with chronic diseases can use travel as a therapeutic alternative to alleviate their symptoms and sufferings [54] (Fig. 2). This interdisciplinary work serves as an important provocation bridging medical science and social science, filling key knowledge gaps in medical and tourism literature. In the future, our team will further promote this "hand-in-hand" collaboration between Western and Chinese Medicine and between medical science and social science to improve the health and well-being of people globally.

Appendix 1: SHSQ-25

Here we provide the reader with the references for the particular versions of SHSQ-25 questionnaire in four languages.

English Version

Yan YX, Liu YQ, Li M, Hu PF, Guo AM, Yang XH et al (2009) Development and evaluation of a questionnaire for measuring suboptimal health status in urban Chinese. J Epidemiol 19(6):333–341. https://doi.org/10.2188/jea.je20080086

Chinese Version

Yan YX, Dong J, Liu YQ, Yang XH, Li M, Shia G et al (2012) Association of suboptimal health status and cardiovascular risk factors in urban Chinese workers. J Urban Health 89(2):329–338. https://doi.org/10.1007/s11524-011-9636-8

Russian Version

Kupaev V, Borisov O, Marutina E, Yan YX, Wang W (2016) Integration of suboptimal health status and endothelial dysfunction as a new aspect for risk evaluation of cardiovascular disease. EPMA J 7(1):19. https://doi.org/10.1186/s13167-016-0068-0.

Korean Version

Guo Z, Zheng YL, Wen J, Garcia M, Balmer L, Wang W (2022) Translation and cross-cultural validation of a precision health tool, the Suboptimal Health Status Questionnaire-25 (SHSQ-25), in Korean. J Glob Health 12:04077. https://doi.org/10.7189/jogh.12.04077.

References

1. Wang W (2020) Cardiovascular health in China: low level vs high diversity. Lancet Reg Health West Pac 3:100038. https://doi.org/10.1016/j.lanwpc.2020.100038
2. WHO (2021) Non communicable diseases. https://www.who.int/news-room/fact-sheets/detail/noncommunicable-diseases. Accessed 30 Sep 2022
3. Duarte AA, Mohsin S, Golubnitschaja O (2018) Diabetes care in figures: current pitfalls and future scenario. EPMA J 9(2):125–131. https://doi.org/10.1007/s13167-018-0133-y
4. Polivka J Jr, Polivka J, Pesta M, Rohan V, Celedova L, Mahajani S, Topolcan O, Golubnitschaja O (2019) Risks associated with the stroke predisposition at young age: facts and hypotheses in light of individualized predictive and preventive approach. EPMA J 10(1):81–99. https://doi.org/10.1007/s13167-019-00162-5
5. Yan YX, Liu YQ, Li M, Hu PF, Guo AM, Yang XH, Qiu JJ, Yang SS, Shen J, Zhang LP, Wang W (2009) Development and evaluation of a questionnaire for measuring suboptimal health status in urban Chinese. J Epidemiol 19(6):333–341. https://doi.org/10.2188/jea.je20080086
6. Stein DJ (2013) What is a mental disorder? A perspective from cognitive-affective science. Can J Psychiatry 58(12):656–662. https://doi.org/10.1177/070674371305801202
7. Wang W, Russell A, Yan Y (2014) Traditional Chinese medicine and new concepts of predictive, preventive and personalized medicine in diagnosis and treatment of suboptimal health. EPMA J 5(1):4. https://doi.org/10.1186/1878-5085-5-4
8. WHO (2020) WHO remains firmly committed to the principles set out in the preamble to the Constitution. https://www.who.int/about/governance/constitution. Accessed 30 Sep 2022
9. Wang W, Yan Y, Guo Z, Hou H, Garcia M, Tan X, Anto EO, Mahara G, Zheng Y, Li B, Kang T, Zhong Z, Wang Y, Guo X, Golubnitschaja O (2021) All around suboptimal health—a joint position paper of the suboptimal health study consortium and European Association for predic-

tive, preventive and personalised medicine. EPMA J 12(4):403–433. https://doi.org/10.1007/s13167-021-00253-2
10. Wang H, Tian Q, Zhang J, Liu H, Zhang J, Cao W, Zhang X, Li X, Wu L, Song M, Kong Y, Wang W, Wang Y (2021) Blood transcriptome profiling as potential biomarkers of suboptimal health status: potential utility of novel biomarkers for predictive, preventive, and personalized medicine strategy. EPMA J 12(2):103–115. https://doi.org/10.1007/s13167-021-00238-1
11. Yan YX, Dong J, Liu YQ, Yang XH, Li M, Shia G, Wang W (2012) Association of suboptimal health status and cardiovascular risk factors in urban Chinese workers. J Urban Health 89(2):329–338. https://doi.org/10.1007/s11524-011-9636-8
12. Wang W (2012) Suboptimal health: a potential preventive instrument for non-communicable disease control and management. J Transl Med 10(2):1
13. Mayosi BM, Flisher AJ, Lalloo UG, Sitas F, Tollman SM, Bradshaw D (2009) The burden of non-communicable diseases in South Africa. Lancet 374(9693):934–947. https://doi.org/10.1016/s0140-6736(09)61087-4
14. Chan KY, Wang W, Wu JJ, Liu L, Theodoratou E, Car J, Middleton L, Russ TC, Deary IJ, Campbell H, Wang W, Rudan I (2013) Epidemiology of Alzheimer's disease and other forms of dementia in China, 1990-2010: a systematic review and analysis. Lancet 381(9882):2016–2023. https://doi.org/10.1016/s0140-6736(13)60221-4
15. Schmidt MI, Duncan BB, Azevedo e Silva G, Menezes AM, Monteiro CA, Barreto SM, Chor D, Menezes PR (2011) Chronic non-communicable diseases in Brazil: burden and current challenges. Lancet 377(9781):1949–1961. https://doi.org/10.1016/s0140-6736(11)60135-9
16. Yu X, Wang W (2021) A rapidly aging world in the 21st century: hopes from Glycomics and unraveling the biomarkers of aging with the sugar code. OMICS 25(4):242–248. https://doi.org/10.1089/omi.2021.0016
17. Wang W, Yan Y (2012) Suboptimal health: a new health dimension for translational medicine. Clin Transl Med 1(1):28. https://doi.org/10.1186/2001-1326-1-28
18. Yan YX, Dong J, Liu YQ, Zhang J, Song MS, He Y, Wang W (2015) Association of suboptimal health status with psychosocial stress, plasma cortisol and mRNA expression of glucocorticoid receptor α/β in lymphocyte. Stress 18(1):29–34. https://doi.org/10.3109/10253890.2014.999233
19. Moynihan R, Doust J, Henry D (2012) Preventing overdiagnosis: how to stop harming the healthy. BMJ 344:e3502. https://doi.org/10.1136/bmj.e3502
20. Aaron SD, Boulet LP, Reddel HK, Gershon AS (2018) Underdiagnosis and overdiagnosis of asthma. Am J Respir Crit Care Med 198(8):1012–1020. https://doi.org/10.1164/rccm.201804-0682CI
21. Yan YX, Wu LJ, Xiao HB, Wang S, Dong J, Wang W (2018) Latent class analysis to evaluate performance of plasma cortisol, plasma catecholamines, and SHSQ-25 for early recognition of suboptimal health status. EPMA J 9(3):299–305. https://doi.org/10.1007/s13167-018-0144-8
22. Kupaev V, Borisov O, Marutina E, Yan YX, Wang W (2016) Integration of suboptimal health status and endothelial dysfunction as a new aspect for risk evaluation of cardiovascular disease. EPMA J 7(1):19. https://doi.org/10.1186/s13167-016-0068-0
23. Guo Z, Meng R, Zheng Y, Li X, Zhou Z, Yu L, Tang Q, Zhao Y, Garcia M, Yan Y, Song M, Balmer L, Wen J, Hou H, Tan X, Wang W (2022) Translation and cross-cultural validation of a precision health tool, the suboptimal health status Questionnaire-25, in Korean. J Glob Health 12:04077. https://doi.org/10.7189/jogh.12.04077
24. Adua E, Afrifa-Yamoah E, Frimpong K, Adama E, Karthigesu SP, Anto EO, Aboagye E, Yan Y, Wang Y, Tan X, Wang W (2021) Construct validity of the suboptimal health status Questionnaire-25 in a Ghanaian population. Health Qual Life Outcomes 19(1):180. https://doi.org/10.1186/s12955-021-01810-z
25. Wang W, Tan X (2019) Suboptimal health status and cardiovascular deficits. In: Golubnitschaja O (ed) Flammer syndrome. Advances in predictive, preventive and personalised medicine. Springer, Cham, p 11. https://doi.org/10.1007/978-3-030-13550-8_17

26. Wang Y, Ge S, Yan Y, Wang A, Zhao Z, Yu X, Qiu J, Alzain MA, Wang H, Fang H, Gao Q, Song M, Zhang J, Zhou Y, Wang W (2016) China suboptimal health cohort study: rationale, design and baseline characteristics. J Transl Med 14(1):291. https://doi.org/10.1186/s12967-016-1046-y
27. Adua E, Roberts P, Wang W (2017) Incorporation of suboptimal health status as a potential risk assessment for type II diabetes mellitus: a case-control study in a Ghanaian population. EPMA J 8(4):345–355. https://doi.org/10.1007/s13167-017-0119-1
28. Wang Y, Liu X, Qiu J, Wang H, Liu D, Zhao Z, Song M, Song Q, Wang X, Zhou Y, Wang W (2017) Association between ideal cardiovascular health metrics and suboptimal health status in Chinese population. Sci Rep 7(1):14975. https://doi.org/10.1038/s41598-017-15101-5
29. Ge S, Xu X, Zhang J, Hou H, Wang H, Liu D, Zhang X, Song M, Li D, Zhou Y, Wang Y, Wang W (2019) Suboptimal health status as an independent risk factor for type 2 diabetes mellitus in a community-based cohort: the China suboptimal health cohort study. EPMA J 10(1):65–72. https://doi.org/10.1007/s13167-019-0159-9
30. Alzain MA, Asweto CO, Zhang J, Fang H, Zhao Z, Guo X, Song M, Zhou Y, Chang N, Wang Y, Wang W (2017) Telomere length and accelerated biological aging in the China suboptimal health cohort: a case-control study. OMICS 21(6):333–339. https://doi.org/10.1089/omi.2017.0050
31. Hou H, Feng X, Li Y, Meng Z, Guo D, Wang F, Guo Z, Zheng Y, Peng Z, Zhang W, Li D, Ding G, Wang W (2018) Suboptimal health status and psychological symptoms among Chinese college students: a perspective of predictive, preventive and personalised health. EPMA J 9(4):367–377. https://doi.org/10.1007/s13167-018-0148-4
32. Zhu J, Ying W, Zhang L, Peng G, Chen W, Anto EO, Wang X, Lu N, Gao S, Wu G, Yan J, Ye J, Wu S, Yu C, Yue M, Huang X, Xu N, Ying P, Chen Y, Tan X, Wang W (2020) Psychological symptoms in Chinese nurses may be associated with predisposition to chronic disease: a cross-sectional study of suboptimal health status. EPMA J 11(4):551–563. https://doi.org/10.1007/s13167-020-00225-y
33. Ding G, Zhao X, Wang Y, Song D, Chen D, Deng Y, Xing W, Dong H, Zhou Y, Li D, Hou H (2020) Evaluation of the relationship between cognitive impairment and suboptimal health status in a northern Chinese population: a cross-sectional study. J Glob Health 10(1):010804. https://doi.org/10.7189/jogh.10.010804
34. Wang H, Tian Q, Zhang J, Liu H, Zhang X, Cao W, Zhang J, Anto EO, Li X, Wang X, Liu D, Zheng Y, Guo Z, Wu L, Song M, Wang Y, Wang W (2020) Population-based case-control study revealed metabolomic biomarkers of suboptimal health status in Chinese population-potential utility for innovative approach by predictive, preventive, and personalized medicine. EPMA J 11(2):147–160. https://doi.org/10.1007/s13167-020-00200-7
35. Kung YY, Kuo TBJ, Lai CT, Shen YC, Su YC, Yang CCH (2021) Disclosure of suboptimal health status through traditional Chinese medicine-based body constitution and pulse patterns. Complement Ther Med 56:102607. https://doi.org/10.1016/j.ctim.2020.102607
36. Meng X, Wang B, Xu X, Song M, Hou H, Wang W, Wang Y (2022) Glycomic biomarkers are instrumental for suboptimal health status management in the context of predictive, preventive, and personalized medicine. EPMA J 13(2):195–207. https://doi.org/10.1007/s13167-022-00278-1
37. Zhang M, Zhou Z, Tao X, Huang L, Zhu E, Yu L, Liu H (2022) Prevalence of subhealth status and its effects on mental health and smartphone addiction: a cross-sectional study among Chinese medical students. Rev Assoc Med Bras (1992) 68(2):222–226. https://doi.org/10.1590/1806-9282.20210977
38. Guo Z, Wen J, Zheng D, Yulu Z, Hou H, Wang W (2022) Proposing an avenue for suboptimal health research through the lens of tourism. J Glob Health 12:03058. https://doi.org/10.7189/jogh.12.03058
39. Anto EO, Roberts P, Coall D, Turpin CA, Adua E, Wang Y, Wang W (2019) Integration of suboptimal health status evaluation as a criterion for prediction of preeclampsia is strongly rec-

ommended for healthcare management in pregnancy: a prospective cohort study in a Ghanaian population. EPMA J 10(3):211–226. https://doi.org/10.1007/s13167-019-00183-0
40. Anto EO, Coall DA, Addai-Mensah O, Wiafe YA, Owiredu W, Obirikorang C, Annani-Akollor ME, Adua E, Tawiah A, Acheampong E, Asamoah EA, Wang X, Opoku S, Boakye DK, Hou H, Wang Y, Wang W (2021) Early gestational profiling of oxidative stress and angiogenic growth mediators as predictive, preventive and personalised (3P) medical approach to identify suboptimal health pregnant mothers likely to develop preeclampsia. EPMA J 12(4):517–534. https://doi.org/10.1007/s13167-021-00258-x
41. Anto EO, Roberts P, Coall DA, Adua E, Turpin CA, Tawiah A, Wang Y, Wang W (2020) Suboptimal health pregnant women are associated with increased oxidative stress and unbalanced pro- and antiangiogenic growth mediators: a cross-sectional study in a Ghanaian population. Free Radic Res 54(1):27–42. https://doi.org/10.1080/10715762.2019.1685668
42. Anto EO, Coall DA, Asiamah EA, Afriyie OO, Addai-Mensah O, Wiafe YA, Owiredu W, Obirikorang C, Annani-Akollor ME, Titiloye NA, Adua E, Acheampong E, Adu EA, Opoku S, Anto AO, Tawiah A, Wang Y, Wang W (2022) Placental lesions and differential expression of pro-and anti-angiogenic growth mediators and oxidative DNA damage marker in placentae of Ghanaian suboptimal and optimal health status pregnant women who later developed preeclampsia. PloS One 17(3):e0265717. https://doi.org/10.1371/journal.pone.0265717
43. Adua E, Memarian E, Russell A, Trbojević-Akmačić I, Gudelj I, Jurić J, Roberts P, Lauc G, Wang W (2019) Utilization of N-glycosylation profiles as risk stratification biomarkers for suboptimal health status and metabolic syndrome in a Ghanaian population. Biomark Med 13(15):1273–1287. https://doi.org/10.2217/bmm-2019-0005
44. Wang W (2022) Glycomedicine: the current state of the art. Engineering 26(7). https://doi.org/10.1016/j.eng.2022.03.009
45. Sun Q, Xu X, Zhang J, Sun M, Tian Q, Li Q, Cao W, Zhang X, Wang H, Liu J, Zhang J, Meng X, Wu L, Song M, Liu H, Wang W, Wang Y (2020) Association of suboptimal health status with intestinal microbiota in Chinese youths. J Cell Mol Med 24(2):1837–1847. https://doi.org/10.1111/jcmm.14880
46. UN (2020) World population ageing 2020 highlights. https://www.un.org/development/desa/pd/sites/www.un.org.development.desa.pd/files/undesa_pd-2020_world_population_ageing_highlights.pdf. Accessed 30 Sep 2022
47. Jaul E, Barron J (2017) Age-related diseases and clinical and public health implications for the 85 years old and over population. Front Public Health 5:335. https://doi.org/10.3389/fpubh.2017.00335
48. Golubnitschaja O, Kinkorova J, Costigliola V (2014) Predictive, preventive and personalised medicine as the hardcore of 'Horizon 2020': EPMA position paper. EPMA J 5(1):6. https://doi.org/10.1186/1878-5085-5-6
49. Nabbout R, Kuchenbuch M (2020) Impact of predictive, preventive and precision medicine strategies in epilepsy. Nat Rev Neurol 16(12):674–688. https://doi.org/10.1038/s41582-020-0409-4
50. Wang W, Özdemir V (2019) Glycomics and personalized glycomedicine. OMICS 23(12):599–600. https://doi.org/10.1089/omi.2019.0177
51. Zhang M, Moalin M, Haenen G (2019) Connecting west and east. Int J Mol Sci 20(9):2333. https://doi.org/10.3390/ijms20092333
52. ECU Newsroom (2023) 'Travel therapy': could holidays help mental health and wellbeing?. https://www.ecu.edu.au/newsroom/articles/research/travel-therapy-could-holidays-help-mental-health-and-wellbeing
53. Wen J, Zheng D, Hou H, Phau I, Wang W (2022) Tourism as a dementia treatment based on positive psychology. Tour Manag 92:104556. https://doi.org/10.1016/j.tourman.2022.104556
54. Wen J, Zheng D, Hu F (2022) The emerging concept of travel therapy in health science: will it be applied to tourists visiting sub-frigid climate zones? Frigid Zone Med 2:200. https://doi.org/10.2478/fzm-2022-00042

What Is the Routine Mitochondrial Health Check-Up Good For? A Holistic Approach in the Framework of 3P Medicine

Olga Golubnitschaja

Abbreviations

3PM	Predictive, preventive and personalised medicine
AD	Atopic dermatitis
AF	Atrial fibrillation
ATP	Adenosine triphosphate
BHI	Bioenergetics health index
BRB	Blood–retinal barrier
CFS	Chronic fatigue syndrome
cGAS/STING	Cyclic GMP-AMP Synthase/Stimulator of Interferon Genes
COVID	Corona virus disease
CTD	Connective tissue dysregulation
DAKD	Diabetes associated kidney disease
DM	Diabetes mellitus
DR	Diabetic retinopathy
ECM	Extracellular matrix
ESRD	End stage renal disease
FSP	Flammer syndrome phenotype
HIF1-alpha	Hypoxia inducible factor 1 alpha subunit
IL-18	Interleukin 18

O. Golubnitschaja (✉)
3P Medicine Research Unit, University Hospital, Rheinische Friedrich-Wilhelms Universität Bonn, Bonn, Germany

European Association for Predictive, Preventive and Personalised Medicine, Brussels, Belgium
e-mail: olga.golubnitschaja@ukbonn.de

H. Podbielska, M. Kapalla (eds.), *Predictive, Preventive, and Personalised Medicine: From Bench to Bedside*, Advances in Predictive, Preventive and Personalised Medicine 17, https://doi.org/10.1007/978-3-031-34884-6_3

IL-1β	Interleukin 1β
IS	Ischemic stroke
MAVS	Mitochondria-associated adaptor molecule
MHI	Mitochondrial health index
MHQC	Mitochondrial health quality control
MIA	Maternal immune activation
MRI	Magnetic resonance imaging
mtDNA	Mitochondrial Deoxyribonucleic acid
mtDNA-CN	Mitochondrial deoxyribonucleic acid- copy number
NLRP3	Nucleotide-binding domain, Leucine-Rich–containing family, Pyrin domain-containing-3 protein
NRF2	Nuclear factor erythroid 2–related factor 2
OSAS	Obstructive sleep apnoea syndrome
PDR	Proliferative diabetic retinopathy
PPPM	Predictive, preventive and personalised medicine
RMEC	Retinal microvascular endothelial cells
ROS	Reactive oxygen species
SARS-CoV-2	Severe acute respiratory syndrome coronavirus 2
TLR9	Toll-like receptor 9
ZBP1	Z-DNA binding protein 1

1 By Regulating Whole-Body Physiological Functions, Mitochondria Are at the "Forefront" of Holistic PPPM Approach

As the "powerhouse" of eukaryotic cells, mitochondria regulate whole-body physiological functions. The super-ordinated position mitochondria have secured for themselves via two pillars, namely as the main energy producer and genotoxic stress sentinel in the human body. Depending on the tissue type, with 2000 to 8000 per cell mitochondria are the most abundant subcellular organelle. For example, in heart, up to 70% of mass is created by mitochondria as the dominant organelle and powerful tissue remodelling modulator. Mitochondrial DNA (mtDNA) is lean on repair mechanisms and, therefore, very damage prone—the features which favour mtDNA for carrying out the role of a potent genotoxic stress sentinel in affected cells, tissues and organs. The proposed mechanisms consider mtDNA as the systemic second messenger of the cellular stress and a direct activator of the nuclear DNA repair machinery towards genotoxic conditions traced that, however, under progressing pathophysiological conditions, such as malignant transformation, may result in chemoresistance of cancer tissue [1]. Contextually, inhibiting mitochondrial metabolism is a new strategy in cancer therapeutic treatment [2].

Mitochondria evolve to sense any kind of stressors (environmental, metabolic, neuro/endocrine) and stress mediators (e.g., glucocorticoids and sex hormones, etc.). Responding to stress conditions, mitochondria undergo dynamic morphological and functional changes and generate signals of adaptation. Being situated in close proximity to the nucleus, mitochondria are capable to regulate human genome and cellular fate (health and death) via epigenetic mechanisms [3].

Mitochondrial disorders are described amongst the most frequent inborn defects in metabolism causing mainly dysfunction of the oxidative phosphorylation system composed of the electron transport chain and ATP-synthase [4]. The genetic defects underlie about a half of all registered mitochondrial diseases.

Mitochondrial health and bioenergetics health are tightly linked together (Fig. 1). Their indexation has been proposed for quantifying mitochondrial functionality and energetic efficacy [5].

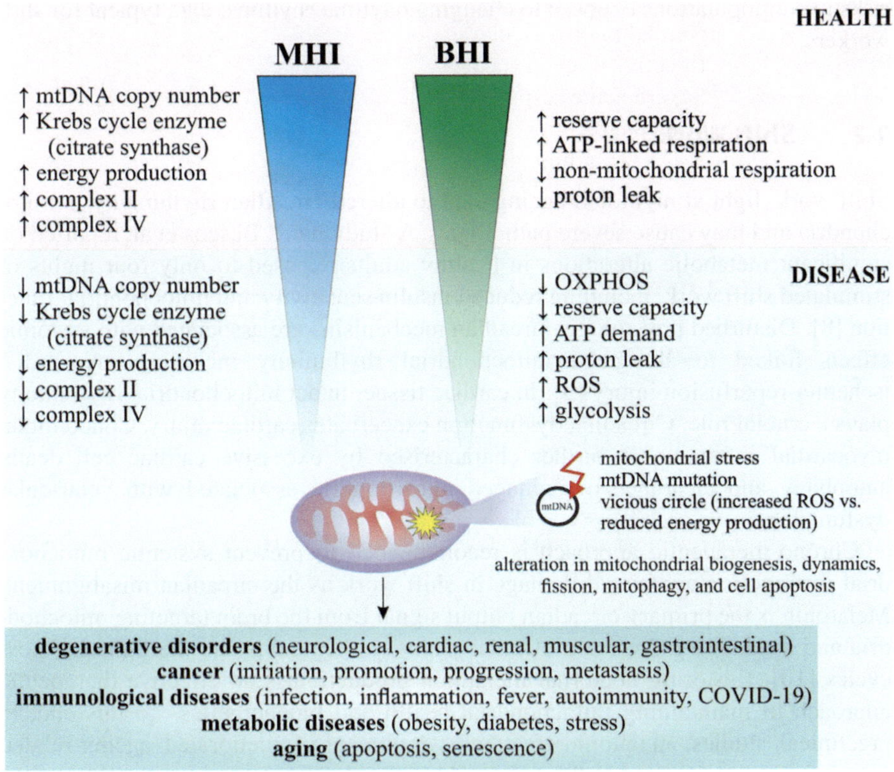

Fig. 1 MHI and BHI in health and disease. *mtDNA* mitochondrial DNA, *MHI* mitochondrial health index, *BHI* bioenergetic health index, *OXPHOS* oxidative phosphorylation, *ATP* adenosine triphosphate [5]

1.1 Mitochondrial Dynamics and Circadian Rhythmicity

Mitochondria are responsive to environmental stimuli such as high and low temperature, genotoxic environment, tobacco smoking, etc. To adapt to the ever-changing environment, mitochondria are highly dynamic in their shape and functionality. Loss of this flexibility known as "imbalanced mitochondrial dynamics" is associated with severe systemic disorders and represent as attractive therapeutic target in broad spectrum of human pathologies [6].

Accumulating research data demonstrate that mitochondrial morphology, generation of mitochondrial mass as well as mitochondrial respiration and ROS (reactive oxygen species) production—all directly depend on a circadian clock aligned to the light-darkness cycles [7]. Preclinical studies suggested that molecular clock disturbances lead to changed mitochondrial respiration. This knowledge is essential for better understanding abrogated mitochondrial rhythmicity and associated health risks in subpopulations exposed to changing daytime rhythms, e.g., typical for shift workers.

1.2 Shift Work

Shift work, light at night and ageing lead to altered circadian rhythmicity in mitochondria and may cause severe pathologies. A study by R. Bescos et al. reported on significant metabolic alterations in healthy adults exposed to only four nights of stimulated shift work, including reduced insulin sensitivity and mitochondrial function [8]. Disturbed physiologic circadian mechanisms are associated with systemic effects linked to abrogated mitochondrial rhythmicity including myocardial ischemia-reperfusion injury [9]. In cardiac tissue, intact mitochondrial rhythmicity plays a crucial role. Circadian dysfunction exacerbates cardiac injury. Concomitant myocardial infarction is further characterised by excessive cardiac cell death, autophagy and clearance of damaged mitochondria associated with ventricular dysfunction.

Chrono-therapeutic approach is recommended to prevent systemic mitochondrial dysfunction-associated damage in shift work as the circadian misalignment. Melatonin is the primary circadian output signal from the brain targeting mitochondria and modulating diverse molecular pathways depending on the light-darkness cycles [10]. Restoring nocturnal melatonin production is an effective therapeutic approach in maintaining mitochondrial health and bioenergetics. To this end, in preclinical studies, melatonin treatment significantly ameliorated ageing-related impairments in mitochondrial function [11].

1.3 Chronic Stress, Fatigue and Mitochondrial Burnout

As described above, mitochondria are adaptive to environmental stressors. However, chronic stress overload may cause imbalanced mitochondrial dynamics leading to mitochondrial burnout with systemic effects and downstream pathologies. For example, toxicological studies demonstrated clear associations between chronic exposure to pesticides, severe mitochondrial injury and chronic diseases including cancers, diabetes mellitus, Parkinson's and Alzheimer's diseases, amyotrophic lateral sclerosis as well as reproductive dysfunction and inborn defects [12]. Experiments with the site-specific irradiation exposure revealed genotoxic insult to nuclear and mitochondrial DNA with downstream regulation events stabilising genome to costs of mitochondrial autophagy. Mitochondrial autophagy eliminates damaged mtDNA to prevent endonuclease G-mediated genome instability [13].

Four pillars are considered to functionally link stress reactions with mitochondria [14], namely

- Energy resources provided by functional mitochondria are decisive for an adequate stress response at molecular, cellular, organ and systemic levels.
- Adequate hormonal regulation is governed by healthy mitochondria.
- Mitochondrial, neuroendocrine and metabolic stress regulation is physiologically performed in a reciprocal manner.
- Behavioural patterns in psychologic distress response strongly depend on the mitochondrial health.

Under chronic psychologic distress conditions, metabolic and neuroendocrine stress mediators cause imbalanced mitochondrial dynamics and burnout followed by sustainable functional recalibration and allostatic load of mitochondria affecting brain tissue and cognitive functions, endocrine and immune systems synergistically involved into development of psychosomatic deficits and inadequate reactions towards non-compensated stress overload. Corresponding molecular and cellular mechanisms (epigenetic control of signalling and metabolic pathways) play the key role in the mitochondrial burnout promoted systemic dysfunction and cascading associated pathologies. Contextually, individual psychosocial experiences and resulting emotion response directly reflects the level of mitochondrial health which is an attractive target in behavioural medicine and well-being PPPM approach in the entire population.

Mitochondrial burnout is further linked to the mitochondrial mass variability, intra-mitochondrial calcium homeostasis, mitochondrial membrane potential, the level of oxidation and apoptosis/mitophagy under a non-compensated stress overload [15].

As the key stress-modulator, mitochondria influence all aspects of the stress response including systemic cortisol and catecholamine levels [14] differentiating between adequate (healthy controls) and abnormal (chronic fatigue, amongst others) stress response.

Metabolic shifts detected in the chronic fatigue syndrome (CFS) are extremely complex including irregularities in the energetic profiles, amino acids/nucleotides/nitrogens/hormones patterns and oxidative stress response associated metabolites—all directly related to compromised mitochondrial functionality [16]. In turn, over 60% of patients with mitochondrial disease report excessive symptomatic fatigue and over 30%—severe, functionally limiting fatigue symptoms [17]. CFS is frequently diagnosed in relation to clinically established comorbidities which are many of associated with CFS that additionally complicate CFS treatment. Biological underpinning of CFS presentation revealed functional involvement of compromised mitochondrial health and immune system, shifted circadian rhythm / melatonin production and gut microbiome profiles, involvement of autonomic nervous and endogenous opioidergic systems, amongst others [18]. All the interacting systems involved suggest that an understanding of the CFS complicity may significantly contribute to the patient stratification and cost-effective PPPM implementation in management of fibromyalgia, depression, migraine and dementia, amongst others.

To achieve and study the CFS, a repeated forced swimming test has been applied to healthy mice. After 25 days of the forced swimming exercise, the level of fatigue has been investigated utilising mitochondria fraction in gastrocnemius muscle: the level of pyruvate dehydrogenase was significantly decreased in mitochondria of the forced swimming mice (CFS model) [19]. The authors proposed potentially beneficial effects by utilising sodium dichloroacetate for the treatment to prevent fatigue-like behaviour in CFS.

Studies dedicated to the adaptive mechanisms demonstrated that a well-controlled balance between fission and fusion is critical for maintaining mitochondrial health and functionality, when mitochondrial are exposed to excessive environmental and metabolic stressors. On the one hand, specifically the fusion is an adaptive mechanism for stress mitigation by mixing complementary contents of partially damaged mitochondria. On the other hand, fission is essential to create new mitochondria increasing the mitochondrial mass but also contributing to the mitochondrial health quality control by removal of severely damaged mitochondria and facilitating apoptosis [20], e.g., under non-compensated stress overload. Extracellular release of fragmented mtDNA is a reliable biomarker for the non-compensated stress overload and predisposition to downstream pathologies related to the compromised mitochondrial health. Chronic accumulation of damage-associated molecular patterns including mtDNA fragments have been demonstrated as inducing downstream inflammatory response via pattern-recognition receptors (such as NLRP3 inflammasome, TLR9, cGAS/STING and ZBP1) leading to chronic inflammation observed, for example in autoimmune disorders such as type 1 diabetes mellitus, Sjögren's syndrome and rheumatoid arthritis, amongst others [21].

2 Microvascular Deficits and Silent Lacunar Brain Lesions in Flammer Syndrome: A Case Presentation for Implementing PPPM Strategies

Individuals with the Flammer syndrome phenotype (FSP) are known to suffer from primary vasospasm, increased endothelin-1 level and pronounced sensitivity to psychological distress and cold stress provocation [22]. Several disorders have been associated with FSP such as connective tissue deficits, migraine, tinnitus, normal-tension glaucoma and highly aggressive cancer subtypes [23, 24], amongst others—all, in turn, are tightly linked with mitochondrial impairments [5, 25, 26]. The best acknowledged FSP attributes associated with mitochondrial injury are shifted circadian rhythms, increased blood endothelin-1 levels and disturbed microcirculation resulting in subtle ischemia-reperfusion events [27, 28].

Recently, a detailed presentation of FSP was performed in the context of ischemic stroke vulnerability in the population and the call for multi-professional expertise for implementing advanced PPPM strategies [29]. The topic-dedicated case report demonstrated the spectrum of signs and symptoms of the Flammer syndrome including high stress-sensitivity and strong vasospastic reactions under stress conditions accompanied with a significantly increased endothelin-1 level (3.2 pg/mL) in blood serum, low body mass index, low blood pressure, migraine with aura, retinal ischemic lesions diagnosed early in life, connective tissue impairments and corresponding pregnancy complications. Mitochondrial test demonstrated strongly compromised health quality according to the expertise of 3PMedicon [29]. Recommended brain-MRI revealed micro-angiopathy, lacunar microinfarction zones and white matter hyper-intensities and micro-haemorrhages—see Fig. 2 [30]. Since brain lacunar microinfarction is an independent and best acknowledged predictor of ischemic stroke predisposition, the authors conclude the essentiality of PPPM

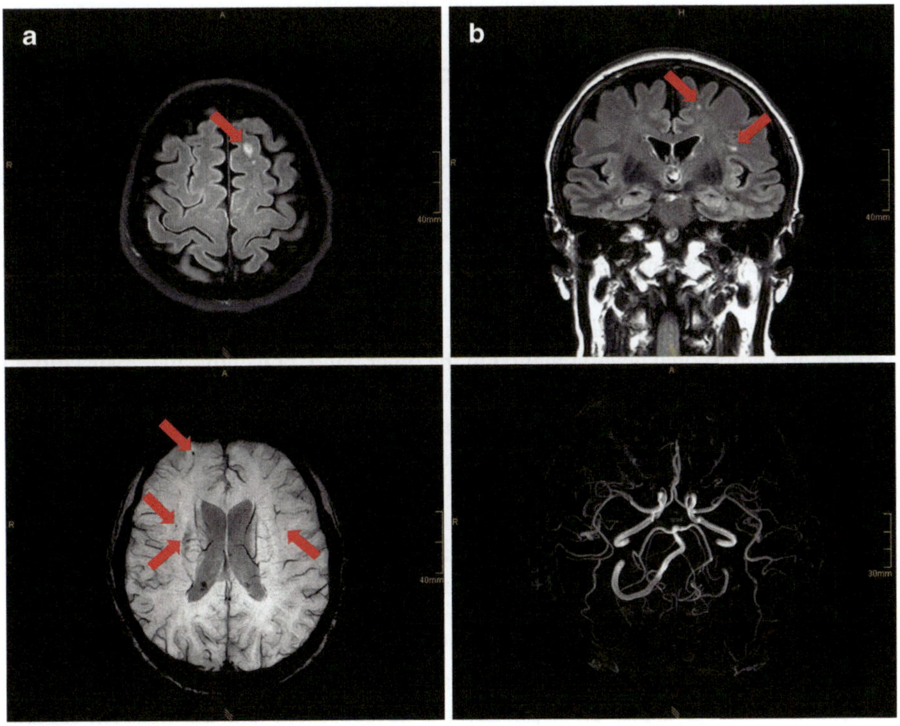

Fig. 2 FSP case report [30]: Brain-MRI demonstrated signs of micro-angiopathy; several lacunar microinfarction zones (**a**, **b**), white matter hyper-intensities and micro-haemorrhages

implementation to the FSP considered a suboptimal health condition. Obviously mitochondrial health quality control is highly appropriate for diagnostics and targeted prevention of downstream pathologies in FSP-individuals.

3 Compromised Mitochondrial Health in Critical Illnesses: Prominent Examples

3.1 Mitochondrial Dysfunction in the Ageing-Related Metabolic Disorders

Organismal ageing is associated with progressive metabolic changes, reduced cellular functions and systemic deterioration of multiple tissues synergistically causing vulnerability to the ageing-related disorders. Mitochondrial burnout plays the key role in accelerated ageing and associated pathologies, such as diabetes mellitus type 2, cancers, neurodegenerative and cardiovascular diseases. Accumulated research data suggest that accelerated ageing and related diseases are caused by insufficient energy supply associated with mitochondrial dysfunction that could be restored by a variety of interventions such as mitochondrial-targeted therapy also linked to the longevity-pathways [31].

3.2 Female and Male Reproductive Health

Infertility is frequently liked to an accelerated ageing. To this end, mitochondria create a high portion of the cytoplasm in oocytes which are the largest cells in mammalians. Furthermore, the number of mitochondria per cell is considered the highest in oocytes that is essential to effectively support oocytes' maturation, fertilisation and initial embryonic development [32]. The total number of mitochondria as well as the mitochondria functionality—both are decreasing in oocytes with progressing age. Consequently, mitochondrial dysfunction in oocytes negatively impacts their quality, fertility and embryonal development. On the other hand, preventive therapies tailored to the mitochondrial health have been proposed as promoting oocyte rejuvenation.

The mtDNA quantity inversely correlates to sperm quality being implicated in energy production, redox equilibrium and calcium regulation and apoptotic pathways—all essential for flagellar motility, capacitation, acrosome reaction and gametic fusion. Therefore, mitochondrial health is central for the spermatozoa metabolism and quality presenting an attractive target for the male fertility [33].

Specifically mitochondria-targeted antioxidants significantly improve semen quality and their overall reproductive performance utilised for artificial insemination [34].

Finally, mitochondria are the key regulator in the synthesis of sex hormones such as oestrogen that is decisive for phenotypic development and downstream regulation of mental and behavioural patterns [35]. Therefore, mitochondrial health is crucial for all aspects of reproductive function in humans.

3.3 Pathologic Pregnancy

Accumulated research data demonstrate the association between the maternal immune activation (MIA) during pregnancy and offspring neuropsychiatric disorder risks, where mitochondria play the role of the mediator. Furthermore, mitochondrial dysfunction is evident in preclinical MIA models and human neurodevelopmental disorders [36]. This is the new concept of the pathophysiology of mental health disorders which originate from the exposure to MIA and mitochondrial dysfunction during pregnancy that makes mitochondrial health to an attractive target for the pre-pregnancy check-up and adapted therapeutic approach [24].

3.4 Connective Tissue Dysregulation

Mitochondrial dysfunction has been demonstrated as the key player in the connective tissue dysregulation (CTD) [37]. Noteworthy, incidence of CTD tends to increase specifically in young populations and is attributed to changing environmental conditions such as an environmental stress that mitochondria are extremely sensitive to. Furthermore, there is a broad spectrum of pathologies linked to CTD and developing early in life including severe complications in pregnancy, eye disorders, aortic aneurism, pulmonary fibrosis and musculoskeletal disorders, amongst others [24, 38]. Intact energy metabolism and extracellular matrix functionality—together orchestrate and maintain tissue organisation. In turn, mitochondrial dysfunction, imbalanced hypoxic-ischemic events, extracellular matrix (ECM) remodelling and chronic low-grade inflammation are implicated in the disease progression. To this end, ECM remodelling is performed by metalloproteinases under mitochondrial redox control mechanism [39]. Shifted redox control by disordered mitochondria lead to abnormal / extensive ECM remodelling which has been implicated to the cancer progression and metastatic disease, ischemia/reperfusion injury, atherosclerosis, arthritis and neuro/degeneration.

3.5 Atrial Fibrillation (AF)

Worldwide AF is the most prevalent and progressive type of cardiac arrhythmias and an independent risk factor of the downstream development of heart failure and ischemic stroke. Despite steadily improving treatment modalities, still they are only moderately effective in the AF severity progression. Mitochondrial health is compromised in AF, due to highly increased demand towards the energy supply associated with the accelerated atrial activation (both electrical and mechanical) of the heart rate characteristic for AF. Mitochondrial damage and dysfunction are pre evidence the dominant contributor to the retarding cardiomyocyte function and cell population in AF. Contextually, targeted mitochondrial therapies are considered a promising approach for diagnostics and therapeutic interventions to advance overall AF management [40].

3.6 Ischemic Stroke

The pivotal role of mitochondria in ischemic stroke (IS) prediction, prevention and treatment has been recently demonstrated based on the abundant research data available [5]. Worldwide, stroke is the leading cause of physical and intellectual disability in adults, and a cost-effective and timely therapy approach are considered problematic. Mitochondria are a major target in hypoxic/ischemic injury, and the mitochondrial health quality control (MHQC) was proposed an attractive target for the ischemic stroke risk assessment, neuroprotective therapies and improved individual outcomes [5, 41–44]. Furthermore, (MHQC) is of great clinical utility for predicting and preventing cerebral small vessel disease causing one in five stroke cases and considered a leading cause of cognitive impairment and dementia [45]. Finally, compromised mitochondrial health was detected in the peri-infarct zone of young adults and associated with poor recovery prognosis [46].

3.7 Skin Disorders

At the organismal level, the skin has the main protector against foreign bodies and toxic invasions maintaining physiologic body homeostasis despite noxious environments. In the skin, there is a reciprocal relationship between the physiologic functionality of mitochondria and melatonin metabolism. To this end, mitochondria act as a central hub of melatonin metabolism which, in turn, is indispensable for physiological skin functions and for an effective protection of the cutaneous homeostasis against environmental invasiveness and toxicity. In the skin, melatonin-mitochondria axis attenuates adverse systemic effects such as those associated with the UV-light exposure, pro-inflammatory and carcinogenic processes [47]. Furthermore, specifically functional melatonin metabolism effectively operates against mitochondrial injury and dysfunction modulating mitochondrion redox control and bioenergetic homeostasis and demonstrating significant anti-apoptotic effects, therewith allowing for an adequate cellular adaptive response to skin injury and effective repair.

Contextually, there is a clear reciprocity between the mitochondrial and skin health: common as well as rare skin pathologies demonstrate mitochondrial involvement; in turn, there is a dermal manifestation of primary mitochondrial diseases. This reciprocity led to developing therapeutics targeted in the skin health utilising an ATP production boost and free radical scavenging highly attractive for both clinical and aesthetic purposes. Bioactive compounds effective for improving mitochondrial function have proved effective against aged and diseased skin [48].

3.7.1 Atopic Dermatitis (AD, Also *Atopic Eczema/Neurodermitis*)

AD is the most common inflammatory skin disease characterised by cutaneous inflammation and associated deficient epidermal barrier. Recently performed differential proteomics investigated epidermis of healthy versus AD skin lesions revealed an impaired activation of the NRF2-antioxidant pathway and reduced mitochondrial proteins in the diseased epidermis [49].

Moreover, an increased oxidative stress was demonstrated as being specific for AD-lesions. Treatment with MitoQ largely corrected the AD profile suggesting mitochondria as a specific target for mitigation AD-lesions [50]. Finally, dietary vitamin D supplementation has been proposed to be effective for AD treatment [51]. To this end, vitamin D-related metabolites support mitochondrial function [52], and the vitamin D—mitochondria cross-talk seems to be essential for maintaining skin health.

3.8 Impaired Wound Healing

During wound healing, stage-specific changes in mitochondrial metabolism coordinate the physiologic healing process: for the subpopulation of early-stage pro-inflammatory wound macrophages, an excessive mitochondrial ROS production and HIF-1alpha stabilisation are highly specific, whereas the late-stage wound macrophages are characterised by IL-4Ralpha-mediated mitochondrial respiration and mitohormesis [53]. Furthermore, factors which negatively influence mitochondrial health also may impair healing such as excessive environmental, psychologic and metabolic stress, oxygenation defects, ageing, alcohol overuse, smoking and nutritional deficits, amongst others. Therefore, treatments targeted to the mitochondrial health are of particular interest for maintaining physiological healing [54].

Finally, keloid scars are caused by tissue injury leading to impaired healing and predisposition to cancerous lesions. Research data demonstrated compromised mitochondrial health as being highly relevant for developing keloid scars [55] that is highly indicative for complex treatments involving mitochondria as the specific target.

3.9 Cancers

Under excessive stress, mitochondrial respiratory chain dysfunction induces NOX-associated overproduction of cellular ROS. The escalated ROS generation is utilised by cancer cells as a messenger to stimulate cell proliferation under oxidative stress conditions further promoting pro-carcinogenic genetic instability. As discussed above, mtDNA is more susceptible to the ROS-associated damage and mutagenesis than the nuclear genome, since mtDNA lacks histone protection, possesses highly limited DNA repair capacity, and is in close proximity to the electron transport chain. Consequently, the level of mtDNA mutations is 10–20 times higher than this of chromosomal DNA that plays an important role in the cancer initiation at the site of damaged mitochondria [56].

Accumulated evidence suggests that mitochondrial DNA copy number (mtDNA-CN) is considered an important indicator of mitochondrial dysfunction and an easily quantifiable parameter useful for the health risk assessment towards chronic diseases associated with mitochondrial impairment such as diabetes mellitus and cancer [57]. Indeed, an excessive mitochondrial fission promotes the pro-tumorigenic phenotype [58]. However, meta-analytical studies demonstrate that mtDNA-CN may be increased in some malignancies but decreased in others [59] that argues against simplistic measurements and interpretation of mtDNA-CN alone.

3.10 Sleep Disorders

In mitochondrial disorders, sleep complaints are prevalent and amongst them specifically the sleep-disordered breathing (e.g., obstructive sleep apnoea syndrome OSAS associated with decreased microcirculation, impaired aerobic metabolism and muscle dysfunction and contribute to upper airway obstruction during sleep) was reported as being the most typical sleep disorder [60]. To this end, an excessive damage to the mtDNA was demonstrated for patients diagnosed with OSAS [61].

Mitochondria display circadian oscillation and are involved in the sleep-wake cycle [62]. Physiological sleep patterns and good quality of sleep is essential for systemic effects such as repair mechanisms and has a defensive role against oxidative damage. Contextually being linked to the oxidative stress, insomnia is associated with compromised mitochondrial health, depression and anxiety disorders as well as a severe damage to immune and cardiovascular systems [63]. Furthermore, molecular biological analysis of the fatal familial insomnia terminal stages confirmed severe impairments in the mitochondrial function and protein synthesis machinery associated with the extensive neuron loss detected in mediodorsal thalamus [64].

Also excessive daytime sleepiness investigated in persons diagnosed with the posttraumatic stress disorders (such as military personnel) demonstrated shifted expression patterns of genes involved in mitochondrial bioenergetics [65].

3.11 Psychiatric Disorders

Autism, Schizophrenia, bipolar and major depressive disorders share common epi/genetic risk factors as well as symptoms of metabolic alterations and mitochondrial dysfunction [66]. Being impaired to a various degree, mitochondrial function and downstream redox balance and brain energetics are implicated in pathophysiology of psychiatric disorders. Moreover, mitochondrial dysfunction was proposed to be circuit-specific for the developmental stage of corresponding pathology that makes mitochondria to the primary target for the patient stratification and cost-effective personalised treatment of psychiatric disorders. Specifically for the major depressive disorder this would be an excellent solution, since nearly 50% of these patients under treatment never reach remission [67]. The incidence of depression continues to increase worldwide and conditions associated with the COVID-19 pandemic have significantly accelerated these trends. The underlying pathomechanisms demonstrate synergistic effects of social stress on mitochondrial injury and inflammation together facilitating the stress-related depression [67]: non-compensated stress overload damage mitochondria which in turn release cell-free mtDNA and trigger neuroinflammatory processes in brain [68]. At the cellular level, mitochondrial dysfunction is reflected in an impaired neuroplasticity and neurotransmission in brain [69]. Contextually, therapeutic interventions focused on modulating mitophagy are under development to treat depression effectively.

3.12 Endocrine Disorders

Mitochondria are critical organelles for endocrine health: the steroid hormone biosynthesis is performed in mitochondria which provide energy for hormone production and trafficking. Endocrine dysfunction is frequently observed in patients diagnosed with mitochondrial diseases and clearly reflected in significantly decreased intracellular production as well as diminished extracellular secretion of hormones. The most frequently described endocrine dysregulation in patients with inborn mitochondrial dysfunction is Diabetes mellitus. Other types of endocrine manifestations include growth hormone deficiency, hypogonadism, adrenal dysfunction, hypoparathyroidism and thyroid disease. Mitochondria-associated endocrine dysfunction generally occurs at the multisystem level that makes mitochondria to the unique target for developing innovative therapeutic approaches for maintaining endorine health [70].

3.13 Kidney Disease

The kidney function essentially demonstrates high level of dynamicity and therefore demands an extraordinary large amount of energy for performing the entire spectrum of activities including maintaining the body's metabolism, plasma haemodynamics, electrolytes and water homeostasis, nutrients reabsorption and hormone secretion. After the heart, kidney demonstrates the second highest mitochondrial count and oxygen consumption [71]. Contextually, the mitochondrial health status is pivotal for maintaining all kidney functions adequate, and mitochondria-targeted therapeutics attract a lot of attention for maintaining mitochondria homeostasis, in order to prevent downstream kidney injury and disease progression. One of the best examples is the diabetes associated kidney disease (DAKD) reported as the leading cause of end stage renal disease (ESRD) in the USA. Per evidence, massive alterations in mitochondrial bioenergetics of the kidney cells cause the disease progression from DAKD to ESRD [72]. The central contributing factors are alterations in the mitochondrial dynamics and energetics, non-compensated oxidative stress overload, shifted redox status and metabolic profiles—all innovative targets to delay health-to-disease transition in the kidney.

3.14 Liver Disorders

Due to the central organismal detoxification function of the liver, mitochondria is the key organelle in regulating hepatic redox status and all associated functions. Consequently, mitochondrial dysfunction underlies pathogenesis of acute and chronic liver disorders such as alcoholic and non-alcoholic fatty liver disease, ischemia-reperfusion and drug-induced liver injury, hepatitis and liver cancers [73]. Mitophagy of damaged mitochondria is the critical regulator in the liver patho/physiology. Disordered mitochondrial fusion and fission result in a progressive reduction of functional mitochondria leading to the excessive necrosis and apoptosis, organ failure and metabolic dysfunction of the liver—all clearly demonstrated for the ischemia-reperfusion injury as a main complication of hepatectomy, liver transplantation, trauma and hypovolemic shock [74]. Corresponding protective measures consider mitochondrial health maintaining therapeutic strategies as promising for prevention and cost-effective treatment of liver pathologies.

3.15 Eye Disorders

3.15.1 Retinal Microvascular Endothelial Cells Dysfunction

As discussed above, environmental and metabolic stress stimuli cause mitochondrial damage releasing mtDNA into the cytosol and cell-free mtDNA fragments. Released mtDNA then drives the activation of non-infectious (sterile) inflammation implemented downstream, for example, in the retinal microvascular endothelial cells (RMECs) dysfunction playing the central role in the inner endothelial blood–retinal barrier (BRB) and BRB breakdown. Per evidence, both RMEC dysfunction and BRB breakdown frequently occurs in posterior-segment eye diseases, causing loss of vision [75].

3.15.2 Myopia

Connective tissue deficits/disease is associated with mitochondrial impairments (upstream) and on the other hand with a broad spectrum of associated pathological conditions (downstream) such as myopia and glaucoma [24]. Although, the mechano-biology underlying connective tissue remodelling differs between both diseases, the asymmetric remodelling of the optic nerve head in a myopic eye significantly increases risks of glaucoma development and mechanical insult of retinal ganglion cell axons [76].

3.15.3 Glaucoma

Mitochondrial dysfunction is associated with normal- and high-tension glaucoma—both are multifactorial diseases with characteristic optic nerve degeneration leading to blindness. Dysfunctional mitochondria trigger sterile inflammation via NLRP3 inflammasome activation, liberation of IL-1β and IL-18 and interferon signalling. Mitochondrial associated ER membrane contacts and the mitochondria-associated adaptor molecule MAVS can activate NLRP3 inflammasome signalling. In parallel, the mitochondrial ATP production is significantly reduced that synergistically results in downward spiral accelerating degeneration process. These pathomechanisms occur in retinal ganglion cells, microglia cells and astrocytes [77]. In several glaucoma models demonstrated upstream decrease in the mitochondrial mass and in the mitochondria-encoded electron transport chain transcripts prior to the hypoxic retinal ganglion cells loss (downstream) [78].

Finally, it has been demonstrated that glaucoma prediction is possible in vulnerable subpopulations such as individuals with the Flammer syndrome phenotype: disease-specific biomarker-panels are detectable in the body fluids including significant alterations in mitochondrial protein setup, stress response, ischemia-reperfusion signalling, blood–brain barrier breakdown and tissue remodelling associated pathways, amongst others [79–83].

3.15.4 Diabetic Retinopathy

Proliferative diabetic retinopathy (DR) is the leading cause of blindness in the working-age population. DR screening is currently ineffective, since the disease remains undetected until irreversible damage occurs. DM associated small vessel disease and neuro-retinal changes synergistically result in conversion of DR into PDR. Characteristic pathomechanisms include progressive mitochondrial and retinal cell damage, chronic sterile inflammation, neovascularisation and reduced visual field. Mitochondrial health control is strongly recommended for advanced DR management. To this end, particularly multiomic tear fluid analysis is considered as instrumental for predicting DR clinical manifestation and disease progression [84].

3.15.5 Early Cataract

Mitochondrial dysfunction is implicated to the cataract development—corresponding pathomechanisms involved shifted redox control [85].

To prevent early cataract manifestation, phenotype-specific screening has been suggested; compromised mitochondrial health is involved in the proposed phenotype [86].

3.16 Neurodegeneration

Accumulating research data have identified several overlapping pathomechanisms involved in a broad spectrum of neurodegenerative disorders such as cognitive decline, Alzheimer's and Parkinson's diseases, diabetic retinopathy and neuropathy as well as glaucoma, amongst others. Per evidence, these pathomechanisms include non-compensated oxidative stress, mitochondrial dysfunction, neuroinflammation and significant metabolic alteration [87, 88].

3.17 Musculoskeletal Degenerative Disorders

Musculoskeletal system disorders have been reported as associated with a degeneration of supporting tissues due to pro-inflammatory micro-environments. Affected chondrocytes, osteoblasts and synoviocytes exhibit extensive mitochondrial injury and cell death, cartilage degeneration, bone erosion and musculoskeletal degeneration. An artificial transfer of exogenous functional mitochondria has been proposed as highly innovative and effective therapy approach to restore mitochondrial functionality by replacing malfunctioning mitochondria with their healthy and functional counterparts. This innovative approach is expected to reverse the failed metabolic status of musculoskeletal tissues by restoring mitochondrial bioenergetics [89].

3.18 Respiratory Diseases

Since mitochondria do sense and respond to the upstream processes pivotal for respiratory diseases such as environmental insults, exposure to toxic pollutants, infections and tobacco smoke, they are well-known modulators of patho/physiological processes influencing airway structure, functions, airway remodelling and hyper-responsiveness [90]. To this end, allergic asthma is tightly associated with mitochondrial dysfunction, reduced ATP production, imbalanced oxidative stress and abnormal calcium homeostasis. Particularly in the lung—an oxygen-rich organ, defective mitochondria play the key role in the pro-inflammatory mechanisms of lung fibrosis and excessive airways cells' apoptosis [91]. Due to the redox-dependent modulation of the cell signalling, antioxidant treatment were suggest to mitigate asthma-associated hyper-responsiveness of airways. However, general antioxidant compounds have proven clinically ineffective against asthma [92]. In contrast, specifically mitochondria-targeted medication (smooth muscle remodelling) is considered highly promising treatment for asthma prevention and mitigation of its severe forms [93].

3.19 Long COVID

Chronic fatigue syndrome (CFS) is highly relevant for a big portion of patients infected with SARS-CoV-2 who suffer from CFS symptoms for a couple of months that is called a "long COVID". Accumulated research data indicate mitochondrial involvement into pathophysiology of both CFS and "long COVID" suggesting high clinical utility of mitochondrial health check-up and therapeutic approaches focused on the mitochondrial health [94].

4 Conclusions and Outlook in the Framework of 3P Medicine

Mitochondria, as the "powerhouse" of eukaryotic cells, play the key role in the cell fate (proliferation, differentiation, growth and death) as well as systemic events and effects including stress response towards environmental changes, redox balance, the innate and acquired immunity as well as severity of the acute and chronic disorders.

This key role makes mitochondria to an attractive target in treating a variety of disorders ranging from metabolic alterations, ischemia-reperfusion events, chronic inflammatory and respiratory diseases, mood disorders, to neurodegeneration and malignancies. For example, metabolic alterations associated with the mitochondrial dysfunction are considered causal for the insulin resistance and type 2 diabetes mellitus. Metformin, which is the widely prescribed DMT2-medication, also retards aging in model organisms and reduces the incidence of aging-related diseases such as neurodegenerative disease and cancer in humans [95]. It is widely accepted that the mitochondrion is a primary target of metformin responsible for its anti-glycaemic effect. Furthermore, specifically due to its primary effects on the complex I of mitochondrial electron transport chain, metformin inhibits cancer cell growth that is particularly relevant for DMT2 patients strongly predisposed to particularly aggressive cancers with poor outcomes [96].

Well controlled mitochondrial dynamics (mitochondrial mass in corresponding tissue, fission, fusion, biogenesis and mitophagy) is pivotal for their functionality, and can be pharmacologically manipulated. In clinical trials, creatine, coenzyme Q10 and antioxidants targeted specifically to mitochondria demonstrate remarkable effects on restoring mitochondrial bioenergetics, for example, in treating neurodegenerative processes [97]. In case of mitochondrial deficient conditions leading to depleted energy production and ROS excess, proposed compensatory mechanisms of targeted treatments prompt mitochondria to enhance ATP production by overexpressed antioxidants and respiratory complex subunits, for example using bezafibrate (resulting in activation of the PPAR-PGC-1 alpha axis), resveratrol and metformin (AMPK activation), as well as using Sirt1 agonists (quercetin and isoflavone-derived compounds) [97]. Further pharmacological strategies utilise dietary antioxidant supplements targeted to mitochondria (L-carnitine, coenzyme Q10, MitoQ10) and triggering Nrf2/antioxidant response by oleanolic acid derivatives (triterpenoids).

Holistic treatment strategies considering mitochondria as the cellular genotoxic stress "sentinel", are focused on restoring and maintaining mitochondrial homeostasis utilising systemic effects by supervised physical activity, keto-diet application, mitigation measures focused on reduced exposure to stress and vitamin therapy, amongst others. Towards the latter, vitamin D—mitochondria axis is considered an attractive target for restoring mitochondrial-associated homeostasis stabilising downstream physiologic processes. To this end, vitamin D deficiency is a worldwide pandemic resulting in multifaceted pathological processes and development of severe disorders including cardiovascular deficits, malignant transformation and neuro/degeneration via non-compensated oxidative stress, pro-inflammatory signalling and mitochondrial damage. Vitamin D values below 25 ng/mL have been associated with abnormal vascular smooth muscle contraction and disturbance in calcium homeostasis and mitochondrial metabolism [98]. Vitamin D deficiency is frequently accompanied with symptoms of skeletal muscle myopathy such as muscle weakness and fatigue. Contextually, vitamin D- mitochondrial axis is pivotal for maintaining mitochondrial health and functionality within skeletal muscle and mitigating fatigue [52]. Furthermore, there is an evident association between microbiome abnormalities and mitochondrial stress [99].

Finally, there is an evident reciprocity between mitochondrial and organismal health status: compromised mitochondrial health is reflected in systemic damage as well as organismal health-to-disease transition is reflected in an altered mitochondrial signalling. Contextually, mitochondrion acts as a natural biosensor integrated into human cells, and the routine non-invasive mitochondrial health quality control test is a powerful tool for the holistic predictive diagnostic approach in PPPM-framework highly recommended at the level of primary and secondary care for

- the whole-body health quality check-up,
- pre-pregnancy check-up,
- health-to-disease transition check-up,
- accompanying diagnostics in sport medicine and supervised physical activities,
- accompanying diagnostics in physiotherapeutic and well-being services,
- therapy efficacy monitoring for personalised treatments (e.g., chronic fatigue; burnout syndrome and sleep disorders; eye, skin, kidney, liver and respiratory diseases, endocrine and cardiovascular impairments, musculoskeletal- and neuro-degenerative disorders, depression, etc.).

Table 1 presents prominent conditions which mitochondrial health quality test is essential for to predict disease development and progression, to apply targeted prevention and treatments tailored to the person as well as to monitor treatment efficacy.

Table 1 A brief list of conditions under which mitochondrial health is known to be compromised and, therefore, its monitoring may be of a great practical benefit in application of 3P medicine in future healthcare

Conditions	Prominent examples and clarifying notes
Environmental and professional occupation risks with adverse effects on mitochondrial health status	
Exposure to ionising radiation/aggressive particles	Professional occupation; environmental (geo-specific natural radiation and artificial) contamination; long and frequent flights
Toxic environment	Heavy metals; toxic chemicals; extensive air pollution, amongst others
Electromagnetic smog	Natural (geo-specific) and artificial (e.g., mobiles) sources of electromagnetic irradiation
Shift work	Changing physiologic circadian rhythms
Non-physiologic time-frame of the job performance	Different from an individual circadian rhythm
Socio-economic and lifestyle associated risks	
Malnutrition	Suboptimal/deficient dietary patterns
Suboptimal life style	Stress overload, sedentary lifestyle, deficits in physiologic needs
Extensive body activities	Physical distress

Table 1 (continued)

Conditions	Prominent examples and clarifying notes
Genetic risks	
Family predisposition to chronic/severe disorders	Inborn genetic information leading to metabolic shifts and increased risks of rare and major disorders such as diabetes mellitus type 1, autoimmune disorders, stroke, cancers and neuro/degenerative pathologies, amongst others
Highly relevant medical conditions	
Suboptimal health conditions	Health-to-disease transition linked to decreasing mitochondrial health quality
Vascular status associated conditions	Increased endothelin-1 level, vascular stiffness, primary and secondary vasospasm, low and high blood pressure, ischemia-reperfusion, Flammer syndrome, etc.—all potentially linked to mitochondrial damage
Migraine and headache	
Tinnitus	
Hormonal stress	
Psychologic distress, autism spectrum condition	Mitochondrial burnout
Burnout syndrome	
Chronic fatigue	
Abnormal sleep patterns	
Inadequate stress response and behavioural patterns	
Psycho-trauma and post-traumatic stress disorder	
Musculoskeletal deficits and impairments	Mitochondrial impairments to be diagnosed and treated
Frequent acute infections	
Chronic inflammation and associated conditions	
Prolonged and impaired wound healing	
Microbiome shifts and pathogenic bio-flora	Mitochondrial stress is highly indicative for systemic effects caused by bio-toxins; relevant sources of information: body fluids, skin, oral and vaginal cavities, digestive and urogenital tracts, airways, wounds, etc.
Digestion-associated deficits	Multifaceted involvement of mitochondria to be considered for diagnostics and treatments tailored to the person
Allergies	
Asthma	
Local deficits of unclear aetiology	Eyes, skin, hair, nails, connective tissue etc.
Accelerated ageing	Higher biologic age against chronologic one—decreased mitochondrial functionality
Major disorders in the population	Mitochondrial component is essential to be considered for the holistic approach
Rehabilitation	
Medications	

Table 1 (continued)

Conditions	Prominent examples and clarifying notes
Acute viral and bacterial infections	Anti-biotics, immunisation and pain-killers—all are known to cause mitochondrial damage and dysfunction
Vaccinations	
Frequent acute and chronic pain	
Complex treatment of multifactorial syndromes and diseases	Mitochondrial component has to be considered in secondary prevention and monitoring of the therapy efficacy
Routine health condition check-up recommended for targeted prevention	
Regular health status check-up	Protection against health-to-disease transition
Pre-pregnancy check-up	Preventable pregnancy complications
Sport medicine	Protection against negative side-effects
Physical exercise couching	Improved individual outcomes
High performance athletes couching	Reaching top-achievements and preventing life-threatening conditions

References

1. Wu Z, Sainz AG, Shadel GS (2021) Mitochondrial DNA: cellular genotoxic stress sentinel. Trends Biochem Sci 46(10):812–821. https://doi.org/10.1016/j.tibs.2021.05.004
2. Vasan K, Werner M, Chandel NS (2020) Mitochondrial metabolism as a target for cancer therapy. Cell Metab 32(3):341–352. https://doi.org/10.1016/j.cmet.2020.06.019
3. Picard M, McEwen BS (2018) Psychological stress and mitochondria: a conceptual framework. Psychosom Med 80(2):126–140. https://doi.org/10.1097/PSY.0000000000000544
4. Fernandez-Vizarra E, Zeviani M (2021) Mitochondrial disorders of the OXPHOS system. FEBS Lett 595(8):1062–1106. https://doi.org/10.1002/1873-3468.13995
5. Koklesova L, Mazurakova A, Samec M, Kudela E, Biringer K, Kubatka P, Golubnitschaja O (2022) Mitochondrial health quality control: measurements and interpretation in the framework of predictive. EPMA J 13(2):177–193. https://doi.org/10.1007/s13167-022-00281-6
6. Whitley BN, Engelhart EA, Hoppins S (2019) Mitochondrial dynamics and their potential as a therapeutic target. Mitochondrion 49:269–283. https://doi.org/10.1016/j.mito.2019.06.002
7. de Goede P, Wefers J, Brombacher EC, Schrauwen P, Kalsbeek A (2018) Circadian rhythms in mitochondrial respiration. J Mol Endocrinol 60(3):R115–R130. https://doi.org/10.1530/JME-17-0196
8. Bescos R, Boden MJ, Jackson ML, Trewin AJ, Marin EC, Levinger I, Garnham A, Hiam DS, Falcao-Tebas F, Conte F, Owens JA, Kennaway DJ, McConell GK (2018) Four days of simulated shift work reduces insulin sensitivity in humans. Acta Physiol (Oxf) 223(2):e13039. https://doi.org/10.1111/apha.13039
9. Rabinovich-Nikitin I, Kirshenbaum LA (2022) Circadian regulated control of myocardial ischemia-reperfusion injury. Trends Cardiovasc Med. https://doi.org/10.1016/j.tcm.2022.09.003
10. Munmun F, Witt-Enderby PA (2021) Melatonin effects on bone: implications for use as a therapy for managing bone loss. J Pineal Res 71(1):e12749. https://doi.org/10.1111/jpi.12749
11. Ahluwalia A, Patel K, Hoa N, Brzozowska I, Jones MK, Tarnawski AS (2021) Melatonin ameliorates aging-related impaired angiogenesis in gastric endothelial cells via local actions on mitochondria and VEGF-survivin signaling. Am J Physiol Gastrointest Liver Physiol 321(6):G682–G689. https://doi.org/10.1152/ajpgi.00101.2021

12. Mostafalou S, Abdollahi M (2013) Pesticides and human chronic diseases: evidences, mechanisms, and perspectives. Toxicol Appl Pharmacol 268(2):157–177. https://doi.org/10.1016/j.taap.2013.01.025
13. Chao T, Shih HT, Hsu SC, Chen PJ, Fan YS, Jeng YM, Shen ZQ, Tsai TF, Chang ZF (2021) Autophagy restricts mitochondrial DNA damage-induced release of ENDOG (endonuclease G) to regulate genome stability. Autophagy 17(11):3444–3460. https://doi.org/10.1080/15548627.2021.1874209
14. Picard M, McEwen BS, Epel ES, Sandi C (2018) An energetic view of stress: focus on mitochondria. Front Neuroendocrinol 49:72–85. https://doi.org/10.1016/j.yfrne.2018.01.001
15. Méthot SJ, Proulx S, Brunette I, Rochette PJ (2020) Chronology of cellular events related to mitochondrial burnout leading to cell death in Fuchs endothelial corneal dystrophy. Sci Rep 10(1):5811. https://doi.org/10.1038/s41598-020-62602-x
16. Armstrong CW, McGregor NR, Butt HL, Gooley PR (2014) Metabolism in chronic fatigue syndrome. Adv Clin Chem 66:121–172. https://doi.org/10.1016/b978-0-12-801401-1.00005-0
17. Gorman GS, Elson JL, Newman J, Payne B, McFarland R, Newton JL, Turnbull DM (2015) Perceived fatigue in highly prevalent and debilitating in patients with mitochondrial disease. Neuromuscul Disord 25(7):563–566. https://doi.org/10.1016/j.nmd.2015.03.001
18. Anderson G, Maes M (2020) Mitochondria and immunity in chronic fatigue syndrome. Prog Neuropsychopharmacol Biol Psychiatry 103:109976. https://doi.org/10.1016/j.pnpbp.2020.109976
19. Ohba T, Domoto S, Tanaka M, Nakamura S, Shimazawa M, Hara H (2019) Myalgic encephalomyelitis/chronic fatigue syndrome induced by repeated forced swimming in mice. Biol Pharm Bull 42(7):1140–1145. https://doi.org/10.1248/bpb.b19-00009
20. Youle RJ, van der Bliek AM (2012) Mitochondrial fission, fusion, and stress. Science 337(6098):1062–1065. https://doi.org/10.1126/science.1219855
21. Barrera MJ, Aguilera S, Castro I, Carvajal P, Jara D, Molina C, González S, González MJ (2021) Dysfunctional mitochondria as critical players in the inflammation of autoimmune diseases: potential role in Sjögren's syndrome. Autoimmun Rev 20(8):102867. https://doi.org/10.1016/j.autrev.2021.102867
22. Konieczka K, Ritch R, Traverso CE, Kim DM, Kook MS, Gallino A, Golubnitschaja O, Erb C, Reitsamer HA, Kida T, Kurysheva N, Yao K (2014) Flammer syndrome. EPMA J 5(1):11. https://doi.org/10.1186/1878-5085-5-11
23. Golubnitschaja O (ed) (2019) Flammer syndrome—from phenotype to associated pathologies, prediction, prevention and personalisation V.11. ISBN 978-3-030-13549-2 ISBN 978-3-030-13550-8 (eBook). https://doi.org/10.1007/978-3-030-13550-8
24. Evsevieva M, Sergeeva O, Mazurakova A, Koklesova L, Prokhorenko-Kolomoytseva I, Shchetinin E, Birkenbihl C, Costigliola V, Kubatka P, Golubnitschaja O (2022) Pre-pregnancy check-up of maternal vascular status and associated phenotype is crucial for the health of mother and offspring. EPMA J 13(3):351. https://doi.org/10.1007/s13167-022-00294-1
25. Liskova A, Samec M, Koklesova L, Kudela E, Kubatka P, Golubnitschaja O (2021) Mitochondriopathies as a clue to systemic disorders - analytical tools and mitigating measures in context of predictive, preventive, and personalized (3P) medicine. IJMS 22(4):2007. https://doi.org/10.3390/ijms22042007
26. Koklesova L, Samec M, Liskova A, Zhai K, Büsselberg D, Giordano FA, Kubatka P, Golunitschaja O (2021) Mitochondrial impairments in aetiopathology of multifactorial diseases: common origin but individual outcomes in context of 3P medicine. EPMA J 12(1):27–40. https://doi.org/10.1007/s13167-021-00237-2
27. Torres Crigna A, Link B, Samec M, Giordano FA, Kubatka P, Golubnitschaja O (2021) Endothelin-1 axes in the framework of predictive, preventive and personalised (3P) medicine. EPMA J 12(3):1–41. https://doi.org/10.1007/s13167-021-00248-z
28. Golubnitschaja O, Liskova A, Koklesova L, Samec M, Biringer K, Büsselberg D, Podbielska H, Kunin AA, Evsevyeva ME, Shapira N, Paul F, Erb C, Dietrich DE, Felbel D, Karabatsiakis A, Bubnov R, Polivka J, Polivka J Jr, Birkenbihl C, Fröhlich H, Hofmann-Apitius M, Kubatka P (2021) Caution, "normal" BMI: health risks associated with potentially masked individ-

ual underweight EPMA position paper 2021. EPMA J 12(3):1–22. https://doi.org/10.1007/s13167-021-00251-4
29. 3Pmedicon. https://3pmedicon.de/en/
30. Golubnitschaja O, Potuznik P, Polivka J Jr, Pesta M, Kaverina O, Pieper CC, Kropp M, Thumann G, Erb C, Karabatsiakis A, Stetkarova I, Polivka J, Costigliola V (2022) Ischemic stroke of unclear aetiology: a case-by-case analysis and call for a multi-professional predictive, preventive and personalised approach. EPMA J 13(4):535–545. https://doi.org/10.1007/s13167-022-00307-z
31. Amorim JA, Coppotelli G, Rolo AP, Palmeira CM, Ross JM, Sinclair DA (2022) Mitochondrial and metabolic dysfunction in ageing and age-related diseases. Nat Rev Endocrinol 18(4):243–258. https://doi.org/10.1038/s41574-021-00626-7
32. van der Reest J, Cecchino GN, Haigis MC, Kordowitzki P (2021) Mitochondria: their relevance during oocyte ageing. Ageing Res Rev 70:101378. https://doi.org/10.1016/j.arr.2021.101378
33. Boguenet M, Bouet PE, Spiers A, Reynier P, May-Panloup P (2021) Mitochondria: their role in spermatozoa and in male infertility. Hum Reprod Update 27(4):697–719. https://doi.org/10.1093/humupd/dmab001
34. Masoudi R, Asadzadeh N, Sharafi M (2021) Effects of freezing extender supplementation with mitochondria-targeted antioxidant Mito-TEMPO on frozen-thawed rooster semen quality and reproductive performance. Anim Reprod Sci 225:106671. https://doi.org/10.1016/j.anireprosci.2020.106671
35. Shaw GA (2021) Mitochondria as the target for disease related hormonal dysregulation. Brain Behav Immun Health 18:100350. https://doi.org/10.1016/j.bbih.2021.100350
36. Gyllenhammer LE, Rasmussen JM, Bertele N, Halbing A, Entringer S, Wadhwa PD, Buss C (2022) Maternal inflammation during pregnancy and offspring brain development: the role of mitochondria. Biol Psychiatry Cogn Neurosci Neuroimaging 7(5):498–509. https://doi.org/10.1016/j.bpsc.2021.11.003
37. Schaefer PM, Scherer Alves L, Lvova M, Huang J, Rathi K, Janssen K, Butic A, Yardeni T, Morrow R, Lott M, Murdock D, Song A, Keller K, Garcia BA, Francomano CA, Wallace DC (2022) Combination of common mtDNA variants results in mitochondrial dysfunction and a connective tissue dysregulation. Proc Natl Acad Sci U S A 119(45):e2212417119. https://doi.org/10.1073/pnas.2212417119
38. Effendi WI, Nagano T (2022) Connective tissue growth factor in idiopathic pulmonary fibrosis: breaking the bridge. Int J Mol Sci 23(11):6064. https://doi.org/10.3390/ijms23116064
39. Nelson KK, Melendez JA (2004) Mitochondrial redox control of matrix metalloproteinases. Free Radic Biol Med 37(6):768–784. https://doi.org/10.1016/j.freeradbiomed.2004.06.008
40. Pool L, Wijdeveld LFJM, de Groot NMS, Brundel BJJM (2021) The role of mitochondrial dysfunction in atrial fibrillation: translation to Druggable target and biomarker discovery. Int J Mol Sci 22:8463. https://doi.org/10.3390/ijms22168463
41. Yang J-L, Mukda S, Chen S-D (2018) Diverse roles of mitochondria in ischemic stroke. Redox Biol 16:263–275. https://doi.org/10.1016/j.redox.2018.03.002
42. Ham PB, Raju R (2017) Mitochondrial function in hypoxic ischemic injury and influence of aging. Prog Neurobiol 157:92–116. https://doi.org/10.1016/j.pneurobio.2016.06.006
43. Anzell AR, Maizy R, Przyklenk K, Sanderson TH (2018) Mitochondrial quality control and disease: insights into ischemia-reperfusion injury. Mol Neurobiol 55:2547–2564. https://doi.org/10.1007/s12035-017-0503-9
44. He Z, Ning N, Zhou Q, Khoshnam SE, Farzaneh M (2020) Mitochondria as a therapeutic target for ischemic stroke. Free Radic Biol Med 146:45–58. https://doi.org/10.1016/j.freeradbiomed.2019.11.005
45. Teng Z, Dong Y, Zhang D, An J, Lv P (2017) Cerebral small vessel disease and post-stroke cognitive impairment. Int J Neurosci 127:824–830. https://doi.org/10.1080/00207454.2016.1261291
46. Nahirney PC, Reeson P, Brown CE (2016) Ultrastructural analysis of blood-brain barrier breakdown in the peri-infarct zone in young adult and aged mice. J Cereb Blood Flow Metab 36:413–425. https://doi.org/10.1177/0271678X15608396

47. Slominski AT, Zmijewski MA, Semak I, Kim TK, Janjetovic Z, Slominski RM, Zmijewski JW (2017) Melatonin, mitochondria, and the skin. Cell Mol Life Sci 74(21):3913–3925. https://doi.org/10.1007/s00018-017-2617-7
48. Sreedhar A, Aguilera-Aguirre L, Singh KK (2020) Mitochondria in skin health, aging, and disease. Cell Death Dis 11(6):444. https://doi.org/10.1038/s41419-020-2649-z
49. Koch M, Kockmann T, Rodriguez E, Wehkamp U, Hiebert P, Ben-Yehuda Greenwald M, Stölzl D, Beer HD, Tschachler E, Weidinger S, Werner S, Auf dem Keller U (2023) Quantitative proteomics identifies reduced NRF2 activity and mitochondrial dysfunction in atopic dermatitis. J Invest Dermatol 143(2):220–231.e7. https://doi.org/10.1016/j.jid.2022.08.048
50. Leman G, Pavel P, Hermann M, Crumrine D, Elias PM, Minzaghi D, Goudounèche D, Roshardt Prieto NM, Cavinato M, Wanner A, Blunder S, Gruber R, Jansen-Dürr P, Dubrac S (2022) Mitochondrial activity is upregulated in nonlesional atopic dermatitis and amenable to therapeutic intervention. J Invest Dermatol 142(10):2623–2634.e12. https://doi.org/10.1016/j.jid.2022.01.035
51. Kim MJ, Kim SN, Lee YW, Choe YB, Ahn KJ (2016) Vitamin D status and efficacy of vitamin D supplementation in atopic dermatitis: a systematic review and meta-analysis. Nutrients 8(12):789. https://doi.org/10.3390/nu8120789
52. Ashcroft SP, Fletcher G, Philp AM, Jenkinson C, Das S, Hansbro PM, Atherton PJ, Philp A (2021) Diet-induced vitamin D deficiency reduces skeletal muscle mitochondrial respiration. J Endocrinol 249(2):113–124. https://doi.org/10.1530/JOE-20-0233
53. Willenborg S, Sanin DE, Jais A, Ding X, Ulas T, Nüchel J, Popović M, MacVicar T, Langer T, Schultze JL, Gerbaulet A, Roers A, Pearce EJ, Brüning JC, Trifunovic A, Eming SA (2021) Mitochondrial metabolism coordinates stage-specific repair processes in macrophages during wound healing. Cell Metab 33(12):2398–2414.e9. https://doi.org/10.1016/j.cmet.2021.10.004
54. Sanchez MC, Lancel S, Boulanger E, Neviere R (2018) Targeting oxidative stress and mitochondrial dysfunction in the treatment of impaired wound healing: a systematic review. Antioxidants (Basel) 7(8):98. https://doi.org/10.3390/antiox7080098
55. Javad F, Day PJ (2012) Protein profiling of keloidal scar tissue. Arch Dermatol Res 304(7):533–540. https://doi.org/10.1007/s00403-012-1224-6
56. Luo Y, Ma J, Lu W (2020) The significance of mitochondrial dysfunction in cancer. Int J Mol Sci 21(16):5598. https://doi.org/10.3390/ijms21165598
57. Memon AA, Vats S, Sundquist J, Li Y, Sundquist K (2022) Mitochondrial DNA copy number: linking diabetes and cancer. Antioxid Redox Signal 37(16–18):1168–1190. https://doi.org/10.1089/ars.2022.0100
58. Srinivasan S, Guha M, Kashina A, Avadhani NG (2017) Mitochondrial dysfunction and mitochondrial dynamics-the cancer connection. Biochim Biophys Acta Bioenerg 1858(8):602–614. https://doi.org/10.1016/j.bbabio.2017.01.004
59. Filograna R, Mennuni M, Alsina D, Larsson NG (2021) Mitochondrial DNA copy number in human disease: the more the better? FEBS Lett 595(8):976–1002. https://doi.org/10.1002/1873-3468.14021
60. Brunetti V, Della Marca G, Servidei S, Primiano G (2021) Sleep disorders in mitochondrial diseases. Curr Neurol Neurosci Rep 21(7):30. https://doi.org/10.1007/s11910-021-01121-2
61. Lacedonia D, Carpagnano GE, Crisetti E, Cotugno G, Palladino GP, Patricelli G, Sabato R, Foschino Barbaro MP (2015) Mitochondrial DNA alteration in obstructive sleep apnea. Respir Res 16(1):47. https://doi.org/10.1186/s12931-015-0205-7
62. Beaupre LMM, Brown GM, Braganza NA, Kennedy JL, Gonçalves VF (2022) Mitochondria's role in sleep: novel insights from sleep deprivation and restriction studies. World J Biol Psychiatry 23(1):1–13. https://doi.org/10.1080/15622975.2021.1907723
63. Heyat MBB, Akhtar F, Sultana A, Tumrani S, Teelhawod BN, Abbasi R, Kamal MA, Muaad AY, Lai D, Wu K (2022) Role of oxidative stress and inflammation in insomnia sleep disorder and cardiovascular diseases: herbal antioxidants and anti-inflammatory coupled with insomnia detection using machine learning. Curr Pharm Des 28:3618. https://doi.org/10.2174/1381612829666221201161636

64. Frau-Méndez MA, Fernández-Vega I, Ansoleaga B, Tech RB, Tech MC, Del Rio JA, Zerr I, Llorens F, Zarranz JJ, Ferrer I (2017) Fatal familial insomnia: mitochondrial and protein synthesis machinery decline in the mediodorsal thalamus. Brain Pathol 27(1):95–106. https://doi.org/10.1111/bpa.12408
65. Pattinson CL, Guedes VA, Edwards K, Mithani S, Yun S, Taylor P, Dunbar K, Kim HS, Chen Lai C, Roy MJ, Gill JM (2020) Excessive daytime sleepiness is associated with altered gene expression in military personnel ad veterans with posttraumatic stress disorder: an RNA sequencing study. Sleep 43(9):zsaa036. https://doi.org/10.1093/sleep/zsaa036
66. Kim Y, Vadodaria KC, Lenkei Z, Kato T, Gage FH, Marchetto MC, Santos R (2019) Mitochondria, metabolism, and redox mechanisms in psychiatric disorders. Antioxid Redox Signal 31(4):275–317. https://doi.org/10.1089/ars.2018.7606
67. Hollis F, Pope BS, Gorman-Sandler E, Wood SK (2022) Neuroinflammation and mitochondrial dysfunction Link social stress to depression. Curr Top Behav Neurosci 54:59–93. https://doi.org/10.1007/7854_2021_300
68. Tripathi A, Scaini G, Barichello T, Quevedo J, Pillai A (2021) Mitophagy in depression: pathophysiology and treatment targets. Mitochondrion 61:1–10. https://doi.org/10.1016/j.mito.2021.08.016
69. Bansal Y, Kuhad A (2016) Mitochondrial dysfunction in depression. Curr Neuropharmacol 4(6):610–618. https://doi.org/10.2174/1570159x14666160229114755
70. Chow J, Rahman J, Achermann JC, Dattani MT, Rahman S (2017) Mitochondrial disease and endocrine dysfunction. Nat Rev Endocrinol 13(2):92–104. https://doi.org/10.1038/nrendo.2016.151
71. Duann P, Lin PH (2017) Mitochondria damage and kidney disease. Adv Exp Med Biol 982:529–551. https://doi.org/10.1007/978-3-319-55330-6_27
72. Ahmad AA, Draves SO, Rosca M (2021) Mitochondria in diabetic kidney disease. Cell 10(11):2945. https://doi.org/10.3390/cells10112945
73. Ma X, McKeen T, Zhang J, Ding WX (2020) Role and mechanisms of mitophagy in liver diseases. Cell 9(4):837. https://doi.org/10.3390/cells9040837
74. Zhang H, Yan Q, Wang X, Chen X, Chen Y, Du J, Chen L (2021) The role of mitochondria in liver ischemia-reperfusion injury: from aspects of mitochondrial oxidative stress, mitochondrial fission, mitochondrial membrane permeable transport pore formation, mitophagy, and mitochondria-related protective measures. Oxid Med Cell Longev 2021:6670579. https://doi.org/10.1155/2021/6670579
75. Guo Y, Gu R, Gan D, Hu F, Li G, Xu G (2020) Mitochondrial DNA drives noncanonical inflammation activation via cGAS-STING signaling pathway in retinal microvascular endothelial cells. Cell Commun Signal 18(1):172. https://doi.org/10.1186/s12964-020-00637-3
76. Grytz R, Yang H, Hua Y, Samuels BC, Sigal IA (2020) Connective tissue remodeling in myopia and its potential role in increasing risk of glaucoma. Curr Opin Biomed Eng 15:40–50. https://doi.org/10.1016/j.cobme.2020.01.001
77. Jassim AH, Inman DM, Mitchell CH (2021) Crosstalk between dysfunctional mitochondria and inflammation in glaucomatous neurodegeneration. Front Pharmacol 12:699623. https://doi.org/10.3389/fphar.2021.699623
78. Jassim AH, Fan Y, Pappenhagen N, Nsiah NY, Inman DM (2021) Oxidative stress and hypoxia modify mitochondrial homeostasis during glaucoma. Antioxid Redox Signal 35(16):1341–1357. https://doi.org/10.1089/ars.2020.8180
79. Golubnitschaja O, Flammer J (2007) What are the biomarkers for glaucoma? Surv Ophthalmol 52(Suppl 2):S155–S161. https://doi.org/10.1016/j.survophthal.2007.08.011
80. Golubnitschaja O, Yeghiazaryan K, Flammer J (2010) Key molecular pathways affected by glaucoma pathology: is predictive diagnosis possible? EPMA J 1(2):237–244. https://doi.org/10.1007/s13167-010-0031-4
81. Yeghiazaryan K, Flammer J, Orgül S, Wunderlich K, Golubnitschaja O (2009) Vasospastic individuals demonstrate significant similarity to glaucoma patients as revealed by gene expression profiling in circulating leukocytes. Mol Vis 15:2339–2348

82. Golubnitschaja O (2018) The keyrole of multiomics in the predictive, preventive and personalised medical approach towards glaucoma management. Klin Monbl Augenheilkd 235(2):146–150. https://doi.org/10.1055/s-0044-101164
83. Zhan X, Li J, Guo Y, Golubnitschaja O (2021) Mass spectrometry analysis of human tear fluid biomarkers specific for ocular and systemic diseases in the context of 3P medicine. EPMA J 12(4):449–475. https://doi.org/10.1007/s13167-021-00265-y
84. Kropp M, Golubnitschaja O, Mazurakova A, Koklesova L, Sargheini N, Vo T-TKS, de Clerck E, Polivka J, Potuznik P, Polivka J, Stetkarova I, Kubatka P, Thumann G (2023) Diabetic retinopathy as the leading cause of blindness and early predictor of cascading complications—risks and mitigation. EPMA J 14(1):21. https://doi.org/10.1007/s13167-023-00314-8
85. Wu H, Yu Y, David L, Ho Y-S, Lou MF (2014) Glutaredoxin 2 (Grx2) gene deletion induces early onset of age-dependent cataracts in mice. J Biol Chem 289(52):36125–36139. https://doi.org/10.1074/jbc.M114.620047
86. Horga A, Bugiardini E, Manole A, Bremner F, Jaunmuktane Z, Dankwa L, Rebelo AP, Woodward CE, Hargreaves IP, Cortese A, Pittman AM, Brandner S, Polke JM, Pitceathly RDS, Züchner S, Hanna MG, Scherer SS, Houlden H, Reilly MM (2019) Autosomal dominant optic atrophy and cataract "plus" phenotype including axonal neuropathy. Neurol Genet 5(2):e322. https://doi.org/10.1212/NXG.0000000000000322
87. Pugazhenthi S, Qin L, Reddy PH (2017) Common neurodegenerative pathways in obesity, diabetes, and Alzheimer's disease. Biochim Biophys Acta Mol Basis Dis 1863(5):1037–1045. https://doi.org/10.1016/j.bbadis.2016.04.017
88. Song T, Song X, Zhu C, Patrick R, Skurla M, Santangelo I, Green M, Harper D, Ren B, Forester BP, Öngür D, Du F (2021) Mitochondrial dysfunction, oxidative stress, neuroinflammation, and metabolic alterations in the progression of Alzheimer's disease: a meta-analysis of in vivo magnetic resonance spectroscopy studies. Ageing Res Rev 72:101503. https://doi.org/10.1016/j.arr.2021.101503
89. Bourebaba L, Kornicka-Garbowska K, Galuppo L, Marycz K (2022) Artificial mitochondrial transfer (AMT) for the management of age-related musculoskeletal degenerative disorders: an emerging avenue for bone and cartilage metabolism regulation. Stem Cell Rev Rep 18(6):2195–2201. https://doi.org/10.1007/s12015-022-10357-5
90. Prakash YS, Pabelick CM, Sieck GC (2017) Mitochondrial dysfunction in airway disease. Chest 152(3):618–626. https://doi.org/10.1016/j.chest.2017.03.020
91. Qian L, Mehrabi Nasab E, Athari SM, Athari SS (2022) Mitochondria signaling pathways in allergic asthma. J Invest Med 70(4):863–882. https://doi.org/10.1136/jim-2021-002098
92. Michaeloudes C, Abubakar-Waziri H, Lakhdar R, Raby K, Dixey P, Adcock IM, Mumby S, Bhavsar PK, Chung KF (2022) Molecular mechanisms of oxidative stress in asthma. Mol Aspects Med 85:101026. https://doi.org/10.1016/j.mam.2021.101026
93. Esteves P, Celle A, Berger P, Trian T (2020) Bronchial smooth muscle mitochondria: a new target for asthma therapy? Rev Mal Respir 37(3):201–204. https://doi.org/10.1016/j.rmr.2020.02.004
94. Wood E, Hall KH, Tate W (2021) Role of mitochondria, oxidative stress and the response to antioxidants in myalgic encephalomyelitis/chronic fatigue syndrome: a possible approach to SARS-CoV-2 'long-haulers'? Chronic Dis Transl Med 7(1):14–26. https://doi.org/10.1016/j.cdtm.2020.11.002
95. Soukas AA, Hao H, Wu L (2019) Metformin as anti-aging therapy: is it for everyone? Trends Endocrinol Metab 30(10):745–755. https://doi.org/10.1016/j.tem.2019.07.015
96. Cebioglu M, Schild HH, Golubnitschaja O (2010) Cancer predisposition in diabetics: risk factors considered for predictive diagnostics and targeted preventive measures. EPMA J 1(1):130–137. https://doi.org/10.1007/s13167-010-0015-4
97. Teresa VT (2014) Mitochondrial biogenesis: pharmacological approaches. Curr Pharm Des 20(35):5507–5509. https://doi.org/10.2174/138161282035140911142118
98. Sanz R, Mazzei L, Santino N, Ingrasia M, Manucha W (2020) Vitamin D-mitochondria cross-talk could modulate the signaling pathway involved in hypertension development: a transla-

tional integrative overview. Clin Investig Arterioscler 32(4):144–155. https://doi.org/10.1016/j.arteri.2020.02.002
99. Boyko N, Golubnitschaja O (eds) (2023) Microbiome in 3P medicine strategies—the first exploitation guide. ISSN 2211-3495 ISSN 2211-3509 (electronic) Advances in Predictive, Preventive and Personalised Medicine ISBN 978-3-031-19563-1 ISBN 978-3-031-19564-8 (eBook). https://doi.org/10.1007/978-3-031-19564-8

Prehabilitation as an Integral Procedure in Predictive, Preventive, and Personalized Medicine and Modern and Effective Healthcare

Barbara Mrázová, Marko Kapalla, Dávid Liška, Igor Martuliak, Martina Flašková, Ján Mráz, and Ľubomír Marko

Abbreviations

5A's	Ask, Advise, Assess, Assist, Arrange
6MWT	6-min walk test
AAR	Abbreviated variation of the 5A's—Ask, Assist, Refer
BJA	British journal of anesthesia
BMI	Body Mass Index
CI	Confidence interval
DrEaMing	Drinking eating and mobilizing
DRM	Disease-related malnutrition
ERAS	Enhanced recovery after surgery
ESPEN	European Society for Clinical Nutrition and Metabolism

Barbara Mrázová and Marko Kapalla contributed equally.

B. Mrázová (✉) · M. Kapalla · I. Martuliak · M. Flašková · J. Mráz · Ľ. Marko
F.D. Roosevelt University General Hospital of Banská Bystrica, Banská Bystrica, Slovakia

D. Liška
Department of Physical Education and Sports, Faculty of Arts, Matej Bel University, Banská Bystrica, Slovak Republic

H. Podbielska, M. Kapalla (eds.), *Predictive, Preventive, and Personalised Medicine: From Bench to Bedside*, Advances in Predictive, Preventive and Personalised Medicine 17, https://doi.org/10.1007/978-3-031-34884-6_4

FFMI	Fat-free mass index
FITT	F—frequency, I—intensity, T—time, T—type
HR	Hazard ratio
IGF	Insulin-like growth factor
PPPM/3 PM	Predictive, preventive and personalized medicine
SD	Standard deviation
SF-36	36-item short form health survey
SHS	Suboptimal health state
TCAM	Traditional complementary and alternative medicine
TUG	Timed up-and-go

1 Introduction

1.1 History of Prehabilitation

One of the first use of the term "prehabilitation" can be traced back to the beginning of 1940s of the twentieth century [1]. Originally it was understood as the procedure dedicated to solve health-related problems prior to the recruitment or prior to the unwanted manifestation during a military operation. In parallel, the pre-placement examinations of the employees in the industry were introduced by W.A. Sawyer in 1942 [2].

Later on, in 1952, in the German journal, the term "preoperative" is used in relation to the preoperative breathing exercise in thoracic surgery [3].

In the beginning of the 1980s the meaning of the "prehabilitation" changed and it is now defined as "the process of expanding patient's functional and psychological capacity to reduce potential deleterious effects of a significant stressor, which is the surgical procedure itself" [4]. The Cambridge dictionary defines "prehabilitation" in medical context as "activities done by someone before they have a medical operation in order to improve their physical strength and help them to recover more quickly after the operation" [5]. According to the BJA Education journal, prehabilitation is "the practice of enhancing a patient's functional capacity before surgery, with the aim of improving postoperative outcomes" [6]. The Collins dictionary defines "prehabilitation" as "the preparation of patients prior to major surgical procedures to enhance general health and well-being with the outcome of decreasing morbidity and mortality" [7].

Prehabilitation has also been defined as "a process on the cancer continuum of care that occurs between the time of cancer diagnosis and the beginning of acute treatment and includes physical and psychological assessments that establish a baseline functional level, identify impairments, and provide interventions that promote physical and psychological health to reduce the incidence and/or severity of future impairments" [8].

Nowadays, in principle, every definition of "prehabilitation" is in primary connection with surgery. When we take a closer look at this topic, we come to the conclusion that "prehabilitation" is an important part of the majority of medical protocols dedicated to the best preparation of the patient for the particular medical procedure. As an example we may take cancer treatment—chemotherapy, radiotherapy and hormonal treatment, can, undoubtedly, have a negative impact on health or the functionality of the organs [9]. Poor physical condition and poor, or inappropriate, dietary habits have been identified as important reasons for low adherence to neo-adjuvant treatment resulting in an inability to respond to it, while it is known that the more late adjuvant treatment starts as result of poor physical condition, the higher is the mortality [10].

Clearly, knowing the growing field of PPPM/3 PM, prehabilitation can, and should, use all accumulated and published scientific knowledge, technologies and tools, including research into the suboptimal health status [11] of a specific patient who is to go through scheduled therapeutic/surgical procedure, result of which depends on the patient's specific health status. In our opinion, this condition should be assessed using available medical technologies in order to predict potential problems and to prevent them with adequate preventive measures, whether it is personalized nutritional support based on a biochemical analysis of the patient's blood and other biological samples, specific physical exercises to increase fitness, psychological support, disease-related patient education about scheduled disease or procedure, chronic pain prediction, assessment of mitochondrial health and function, as discussed in another chapter of this book, as well as identification of negative environmental factors that need to be suppressed and health-supporting environmental factors that need to be enhanced in all relevant fields like obstetrics, oncology, organ transplantation, surgery, dental care, neurodegenerative diseases, genetic diseases, pandemic management and other areas of healthcare (Fig. 1).

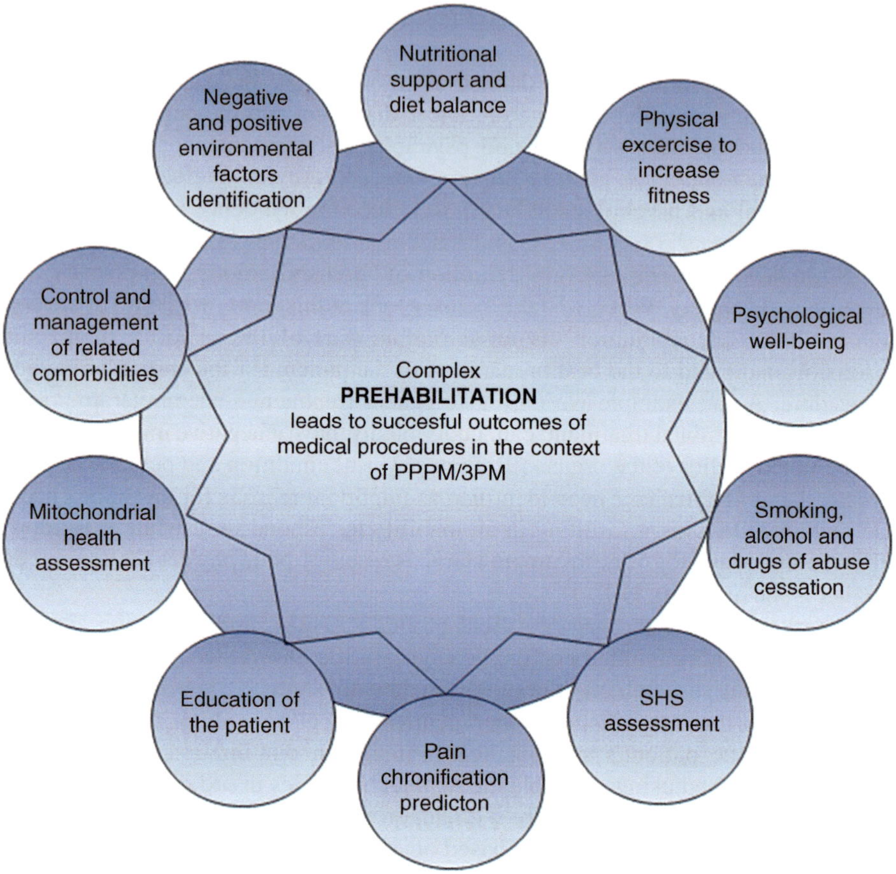

Fig. 1 Complex prehabilitation in the context of PPPM/3 PM should be multimodal and include also other health-supporting activities apart of the standard ones which are nutrition, physical activity, psychological well-being, smoking cessation, and control of related comorbidities. Here we suggest enhancing the process of prehabilitation with inclusion of particular questionnaires focused on identification of suboptimal health state (SHS), pain chronification prediction, mitochondrial health assessment, cessation of smoking, alcohol consumption and drugs of abuse, particular health-problem-related education of the patient, control and management of related comorbidities, and identification of environmental factors having negative influence on health and worsening disease state, or on the contrary, having positive influence on health which may increase the chances for better outcome of the desired medical procedure and speed up the consequent recovery. Providing, of course, that the particular medical procedure is not provided under an emergency situation when there is no time for complex prehabilitation as outlined in this figure

2 Prehabilitation

2.1 Multimodal Approach of Prehabilitation

Prehabilitation requires a well-designed approach from several disciplines, the so-called multi-modal prehabilitation, requiring a fundamental change of the current medical care paradigm [12].

Although this is a long-term vision, we suggest initially focusing on patients at high risk of postoperative morbidity and mortality, such as elderly surgical patients who are weak (frail) and unprepared for the significant burden of a particular procedure [13, 14]. In the later stages of the implementation of prehabilitation processes, as already suggested by several researchers [15], the hospital should offer prehabilitation for a much wider spectrum of patients and, as we believe, also for other than surgical patients who need specific medical procedures.

The basis of any multimodal prehabilitation approach (exercise and adequate physical activity, nutrition improvement and adjustment, psychological support and well-being, patient education, etc.) is a personalized intervention with the possibility of prediction, which prevents negative clinical outcomes.

From the point of view of rapid recovery after a given surgical or other medical procedure, and from the point of view of regaining physical strength, prehabilitation has the potential to increase the chances of returning home earlier and to engage in the usual activities that were performed before the undertaken procedure. Last but not least, it is also expected that supported and accelerated recovery will have an impact on the economy, effectiveness and utilization of beds available in hospitals, as well as on the use of limited financial resources in the health care system in any country worldwide [12].

The following are the basic elements of prehabilitation:

- Physical training through exercise.
- Nutritional support and supplementation.
- Mental support, patient education, and patient empowerment.
- Cessation of smoking and behavioral changes.
- Control of related comorbidities.

2.1.1 The Reason for Multimodal Approach in Prehabilitation

Exercise without nutrition will not increase muscle mass. Nutrition is better utilized in combination with training. For training a good mental state is mandatory and on the other hand the effort of training will be rewarding for your mental state. Moreover, ultimate goal is to generate persistent behavioral changes through all elements [16].

In one randomized trial, 77 patients undergoing colorectal resection for cancer received a home-based intervention consisting of moderate aerobic and resistance exercises, as well as nutritional counseling with protein supplementation and relaxation exercises, beginning either 4 weeks before surgery (prehabilitation group), or immediately after hospital discharge (control group). Both groups continued the regimen for 8 postoperative weeks. The primary functional capacity outcome was the 6-min walk test. Better 8 week 6-min walk test scores were noted in the prehabilitation group (+23.7 with standard deviation (SD) 54.8 m versus −21.8 with SD 80.7 m, with a mean difference of 45.4 m (95% CI 13.9–77.0)). Also, a higher proportion of patients in the prehabilitation group recovered to an exercise capacity greater than their baseline at 8 postoperative weeks (84 vs. 62%) [17].

Similar interventions and improvements were noted in another randomized trial of prehabilitation before colorectal cancer surgery with additional supervised exercise sessions during the first three postoperative days [18]. In a meta-analysis that included these two randomized trials together with one prospective cohort study [19], multimodal plus nutritional prehabilitation was associated with improved disease-free survival 5 years after colorectal cancer surgery (hazard ratio (HR) 0.45, 95% CI 0.21–0.93; 202 total patients) [15, 20].

One international multicenter, randomized controlled trial with two study groups (714 patients) in progress, with inclusion of four prehabilitation interventions (in-hospital high-intensity endurance and strength training, high-protein nutrition supplementation, smoking cessation, and psychological support) [21] have as primary outcomes postoperative complications (assessed with the Comprehensive Complication Index [22]) at the 30 days of follow-up and functional capacity (assessed with the 6 min walk test) measured 4 weeks after surgery and compared to baseline and additionally directly after prehabilitation and 8 weeks after surgery. Notably, 86% of patients in the prehabilitation group recovered baseline functional capacity within four postoperative weeks compared with 40% in the control group [15, 21]. The authors concluded that prehabilitation programs are feasible, effective, and safe [15].

Research on prehabilitation has focused primarily on patients undergoing elective cardiac surgery [15, 23], and major gastrointestinal or hepatobiliary cancer surgery [15, 20, 21]. In some centers, patients undergoing other types of major surgery are candidates for prehabilitation, such as those undergoing joint replacement surgery [15, 24–26] or major vascular surgery [15, 27]. Some authors, however, propose offering prehabilitation for all surgical patients [15].

In the context of the implementing PPPM principles within hospital health care processes [28], we suggest that prehabilitation be included in standard therapeutic procedures in every hospital that wants to improve the level of care provided and thus apply PPPM in routine practice, which will certainly benefit patients. We are aware that the practical implementation of this vision will not be easy but we are also sure that the well-organized cooperation of all interested parties, including those at the international level, who want to change the current disease-oriented philosophy to future healthcare, oriented to prediction, prevention and a personalized approach can accelerate beneficial changes.

2.2 Exercise and Physical Activity (Rehabilitation) as Element of Prehabilitation

In the last decade, there has been a growing awareness that the success of treatment itself depends not only on technical surgical skills, radiation therapy, and targeted therapy, but also on the patient's overall physical and mental condition [29]. At present, the purpose of treatment for patients is to shorten hospital stays, to release patients who are relatively self-sufficient, in good physical condition, to home care, and then to work to improve the patient's functional status [30]. In medical terminology, this continuous care process in the cancer patient, which is provided since cancer diagnosis, and also includes nutritional support, support of physical and mental health to reduce the incidence and severity of future complications, can be called prehabilitation [31].

Personalized treatment of any disease, especially cancer, is indeed a major challenge. Exercise without nutrition will not increase muscle mass, and, on the other hand, nutrition is better utilized in combination with adequate training. A good mental state is mandatory for training, and in return the effort of training will be rewarding for patient's mental state [16]. Therefore, rehabilitation is an essential part of prehabilition but cannot be confused with prehabilitation itself. Rehabilitation is a potentially effective strategy to improve the functional status and quality of life of patients [32]. Exercise interventions are known to alleviate or prevent the deleterious effects of cancer and treatment [33]. Rehabilitation provides also an opportunity to improve the health care of cancer patients [33]. The evidence for exercise in the care of cancer patients is largely positive.

Rehabilitation includes a complex process that improves the course of the disease, reduces the functional impairment, accelerates the reconvalescence of the patient and faster return to the family and working environment [34]. Patient rehabilitation is focused on restoring functional state and integration of the patient into society [35]. The complexity of the prehabilitation and rehabilitation processes is given by the fact that the patient is understood as a person who may have both physical and mental difficulties. In more serious cases, these impairments are associated with damage to work potential and disability. Due to the increasing number of surviving colorectal cancer patients, there is a growing need for an effective program before, during, and after treatment [36]. Rehabilitation is one of the basic components of treatment to improve the health of a patient [37]. Basic rehabilitation therapies include exercise [38]. The purpose of prehabilitation is to achieve maximum benefit in terms of improving the functional and mental state of the patient [39]. Physical activity plays an important role for the cardiovascular system and muscle function and mass maintenance, which are critical factors for the postoperative recovery of a patient [40].

Physical performance of patients is a multidimensional concept that involves body function related to movement. Exercise, together with other components of prehabilitation plays an important protective and therapeutic role in patients with colorectal cancer [33]. Although the link between exercise and the prevention of colorectal cancer appears clear, the molecular mechanism underlying the protective effect of exercise is not yet clear [41]. The link between the protective and therapeutic benefits of exercise and cancer can be explained by several mechanisms. These mechanisms include an explanation for metabolic dysregulation, which includes the effect of exercise on insulin resistance, glucose metabolism, and insulin-like growth factor (IGF) [42]. Physical activity reduces insulin resistance and insulin levels affecting the IGF pathway and indirectly reduces the risk of colorectal cancer, recurrence, and mortality [43]. Another significant effect of exercise is the effect on adiposity, which includes, in particular, the effect on leptin and adinopectin [44]. Another possible explanation is the effect on oxidative stress, inflammation, and impaired immune function. Another important effect is the effect of exercise on myokines and interleukins [45].

Current recommendations for physical activity and exercise in prehabilitation include 150 min of moderate or 75 min of vigorous physical activity per week. Exercise prescription should follow the FITT principles:

F—frequency (how often).
I—intensity (how hard).
T—time (how long).
T—type (what kind of exercise).

The recommendations for exercise are based on the guideline of 150 min per week, aerobic training should occur at least every second day for 30–45 min, in duration at a moderate level of intensity (50–75% of age predicted maximum heart rate). The exercise itself may be of different type—aerobic component, resistance, flexibility, balance exercises. It must be tailored to suit the needs and physiological status of each patient and designed and supervised by qualified personnel.

Even for the patient who is unable or does not want to embark on training program, health benefits can still be acquired by increasing activities of daily living—light walk, stair climbing, gardening, housework, dancing, swimming, hiking, biking [12].

2.2.1 Patient Examination and Setting Up Training in Terms of Prehabilitation

The effectiveness of rehabilitation depends on a comprehensive and interdisciplinary approach [46]. Current procedures emphasize rehabilitation as an important part of surgical treatment [47]. There is growing evidence for the benefits of rehabilitation in various cancers [48–51]. The rehabilitation model currently focuses on optimizing treatment for cancer patients. Rehabilitation is a complex model and its mutual integration into the health system represents a potential benefit for patients. Most patients have reduced function. Functional examination plays an important role in rehabilitation, where it is possible to use several functional examinations.

2.2.2 6-Minute Walk Test

The 6-min walk test is a submaximal exercise test used to assess aerobic capacity and endurance in various pathological conditions [52]. The distance traveled in 6 min is used as a result to compare changes in functional capacity in patients. This test can be used in patients of all ages. The test was originally designed to help evaluate a patient with cardiopulmonary problems. It was gradually introduced into other diagnoses [53]. It also plays an important role in the examination of colorectal cancer with respect to the functional fitness of patients [54]. The 6-min walk test gives information on the patient's functional capacity and provides important information on all systems during physical activity, including the pulmonary and cardiovascular systems. To perform the test, it is necessary to measure the range in which patients will perform the test.

2.2.3 Chair Stand Test

The chair stand test is a test for testing the strength and endurance of the legs in older adults [55]. It is part of a senior functional test battery. The chair stand test evaluates the functional strength of the lower limbs, balance, and the risk of falling in older adults. The evaluation of the test is based on the amount of time. During the test, the patient sits in a standing and sitting chair five times. A stopwatch and a standard height chair with a straight back are important to perform the test. If the test is performed correctly, the patient sits with a straight back and is supported. The patient is also instructed to rest his hands on his chest and then sit down and rise five times as quickly as possible. The shorter the time to complete the test, the better the indicator of the test result.

2.2.4 Timed Up-and-Go Test (TUG)

This test is mainly used in the elderly population. TUG focuses on the functional ability of patients and the assessment of fall risk [56]. In patients with colorectal cancer, it can represent a benefit in determining the physical impairment caused by colorectal cancer [56]. A stool and stopwatch are required to perform the test. The patient sits in a chair to perform the test correctly. His feet are placed in place marked by a line. After the start signal, the patient gets up from the chair and walks a distance of 3 m. The clinician records the time the patient walked the specified distance and returned to the stool.

2.2.5 SF36 Quality of Life Questionnaire

The quality of life questionnaire was created on the basis of the requirement of adequate evaluation of therapies in medicine. The SF36 questionnaire is a standardized form to evaluate patient quality of life [57]. SF36 contains 36 questions, the results of which are scored. SF36 addresses a set of general, coherent, and easy-to-apply questions about patients' quality of life.

Two types of exercise are most often used in the rehabilitation of patients. It is resistance exercise and aerobic exercise.

2.2.6 Resistance Training

Resistance exercise using resistance to stimulate muscle contraction. It is important to maintain a slow controlled movement during strength training. During strength training, it is possible to increase the load due to the patient's health. Strength training consisting of concentric and eccentric muscle contraction is a safe, simple, and effective intervention to induce muscle hypertrophy, increase muscle strength, and improve the patient's functional condition before and after surgery/medical procedure.

2.2.7 Aerobic Exercise

This type of physical activity is one of the most common. During aerobic training, the patient exercises at a moderate load intensity. Aerobic exercise is known to induce an increase in skeletal muscle mitochondria. Muscle mitochondrial cells are able to adapt to aerobic training. Aerobic exercise begins with warming up in the form of 10 min of light activity and dynamic stretching. As a form of aerobic exercise it is possible to use walking, Nordic walking, swimming, cycling. Exercises focused on the aerobic component in patients are applied twice a week.

2.2.8 Respiratory Exercises

Respiratory rehabilitation is a therapy for patients with symptoms related to impaired lung function. It has been started in patients with chronic obstructive pulmonary disease. It is a standard treatment for patients with lung cancer. Respiratory rehabilitation is aimed at improving the physical and mental condition of the patient. The primary purpose of respiratory rehabilitation is to improve the patient's physical function, functional condition, and quality of life.

2.2.9 Goals of Physical Activity as Element of Prehabilitation

- To identify patients with poor physical conditioning (6MWT, cardiopulmonary exercise testing).
- To prescribe a targeted and individualized exercise program (cardiovascular, resistance, flexibility, balance training).
- To encourage daily physical activity that totals at least 30 min per day.
- To reduce sitting or sedentary time.
- To change long term behavior to include a more active lifestyle [12].

2.3 Nutritional Optimization, Nutritional Balance as Elements of Prehabilitation

The rate of development of postoperative malnutrition for a given individual depends upon their preexisting nutritional status before the surgery, the nature and complexity of the surgical procedure, the degree of postoperative hypermetabolism, and their ability to consume an optimal number of calories [58]. Starvation during metabolic stress from any type of injury differs from fasting under physiological conditions [59].

The stress of surgery or trauma creates a catabolic state, increasing protein and energy utilization. Macronutrients (fat, protein, and glycogen) from the labile reserves of fat tissue and skeletal muscle are redistributed to more metabolically active tissues such as the liver and visceral organs. This response can lead to the onset of protein calorie malnutrition (defined as a negative balance of 100 g of nitrogen and 10,000 kcal) within a few days [58, 60–62].

Definitions of malnutrition often include an "unbalanced nutritional state" that leads to "alterations in body composition" and "diminished function" [63]. An unbalanced nutritional state refers to both over- and undernutrition [64].

With an increasing percentage of obese people in the Western world is malnutrition often not realized and Disease-related Malnutrition (DRM) frequently not recognized and therefore untreated [65].

According to ESPEN (European Society for Clinical Nutrition and Metabolism) diagnostic criteria for malnutrition according to two options [65].

- option 1: BMI <18.5 kg/m^2,
- option 2: combined: weight loss >10% or > 5% over 3 months and reduced BMI or a low fat-free mass index (FFMI).

Reduced BMI is <20 or < 22 kg/m^2 in patients younger and older than 70 years, respectively. Low FFMI is <15 and < 17 kg/m^2 in females and males, respectively.

From the prehabilitation point of view it is important to note that nearly 50% of patients admitted to hospital are malnourished or at risk of malnutrition [66]. The American Society for Enhanced Recovery and Perioperative Quality estimates that two out of three patients undergoing gastrointestinal surgery are malnourished, which renders them three times more likely to suffer perioperative complications and five times more likely to die [67].

Malnutrition is associated with a poorer response to cancer treatment [68], increased susceptibility to infection, poor wound healing, increased frequency of decubitus ulcers, overgrowth of bacteria in the gastrointestinal tract, abnormal nutrient losses through the stool [58, 69–71] and hypoalbuminemia is associated with post-surgical mortality, increased morbidity and length of stay [68].

Perioperative nutritional supplementation has been shown in a recent meta-analysis of 56 trials including 6370 patients to decrease postoperative infectious and non-infectious complications, and also length of stay in patients undergoing gastrointestinal cancer surgery [72, 73].

2.3.1 Synergy Between Feeding and Exercise

Speaking of nutrition, we have to emphasize the fact that lean tissue accretion will not occur without a positive protein balance, with protein synthesis exceeding protein breakdown. Stable isotope studies suggest net muscle protein balance postexercise remains negative until amino acids are available [74–76]. It is the synergistic effect of feeding- and exercise-induced stimulation of muscle protein synthesis that positively impacts protein balance, to a greater extent than either feeding or exercise could alone. Repeated bouts of resistance exercise and protein feeding stimulate lean tissue gains which is essential for a better and quicker recovery after surgery and a healthier life [74, 75]. It is important to keep in mind that for training a good mental state is mandatory.

2.3.2 Goals of Nutritional Optimization as Element of Prehabilitation

- To identify patients who are malnourished.
- To better understand how the patient is eating and to identify where deficiencies are occurring.
- To provide feedback as to how the patient can optimize their nutrition.
- To provide appropriate nutritional supplementation [12].
- Minimize starvation.
- Prevent pre and postoperative malnutrition.
- Support anabolism for recovery [65].
- Although additional nutritional considerations will be required for surgical subspecialities and to provide personalized patient care, these basic nutrition principles hold true for all cases [74].
- In addition, given the rising proportion of cancer patients who are obese at diagnosis, the prehabilitative window and rehabilitative window are potentially an opportunity to embed new lifestyle behaviors [68].

2.4 Psychological Well-Being as Element of Prehabilitation

Preoperative anxiety, depression and low self-efficacy are consistently associated with worse physiological surgical outcomes and postoperative quality of life. This has led to the emergence of psychological prehabilitation and the trimodal approach to prehabilitation, incorporating psychological intervention as well as exercise and nutritional optimization [77].

2.4.1 The Reasons for Psychological Well-Being as a Part of Prehabilitation

Increasingly, evidence suggests that psychological factors have an impact on both physiological and psychological surgical outcomes in the short as well as long term [77].

A systematic research identified 16 eligible studies summarized the association between psychological factors and physiological outcomes affecting the site of surgery, namely wound healing and postoperative complications in the first month after surgery. However, there was significant heterogeneity across the studies, overall, trait and state anxiety, state anger, active coping, subclinical depression, and intramarital hostility appeared to complicate recovery, while dispositional optimism, religiousness, anger control, low pain expectations, and external locus of control seemed to promote healing. Psychological interventions (guided relaxation, couple support visit, and psychiatric interview) also appeared to favor recovery. Psychological factors unrelated to surgical outcomes included loneliness, perceived social support, anger expression, and trait anger [78].

Another review with inclusion of 29 studies evaluated the effect of mood, attitudinal factors, personality and coping mechanisms on complications, pain and analgesic use, functional recovery, length of hospital stay and ratings of physical recovery [79].

Psychological factors can also affect both acute and chronic postoperative pain [77]. Anxiety is one of the four factors that predict acute postoperative pain as was identified in qualitative systematic review including 48 trials and 23,037 patients [80] and there is a high level of evidence for the predictive value of pre-surgical depression, psychological vulnerability and chronic stress on the risk of chronic pain after surgery [81].

2.4.2 The Ways to Achieving Mental Well-Being in Terms of Prehabilitation

A recent Cochrane review of 105 studies from all surgical specialties synthesized the evidence of psychological preparation and postoperative outcomes of pain, return to normal activities (behavioral recovery), length of hospital stay and negative effect in adults undergoing elective surgery. They evaluated a broad range of psychological interventions including: procedural information (information about what, when and how processes will happen); sensory information (what the experience will feel like and what other sensations they may have, for example, taste, smell); behavioral instruction (telling patients what they need to do); cognitive intervention (techniques that aim to change how people think); relaxation techniques; hypnosis; and emotion-focused interventions (techniques that aim to help people to manage their feeling) [77, 82]. Such interventions should be proposed as preoperative education programs [77].

2.4.3 Goals of Psychological Well-Being as Element of Prehabilitation

- To identify patients who require psychological interventions.
  To provide anxiety reducing techniques for all patients, based on preference [12].

2.5 Pain Management in Prehabilitation

As we discuss in another chapter of this book dedicated to pain chronification prediction and to the reasons for including its assessment into the processes of prehabilitation in context of PPPM/3 PM, psychological factors affect pain perception in a fundamental way. Pain is a complex, multidimensional perception with a diversity of its quality, intensity, duration, location, as well as perception of its discomfort, while the intensity and degree of discomfort of pain are not directly dependent on the cause and extent of tissue damage. In particular, situational and emotional psychological factors present in the experience of pain can fundamentally change the intensity and quality of pain perception. As the pain suddenly reaches the brain, the thalamus redirects its feelings to other cortical and subcortical parts of the Pain matrix, which are also associated with emotions, attention, and memory. This explains why emotions have such an effect on how we feel [83].

Every chronic pain develops from acute pain. The onset of acute pain is associated with tissue damage through various mechanisms (e.g., mechanical damage, burns, infection, inflammation, genetic disorders, etc.) and thus the integrity of the biological structures and functions of the individual. Therefore, fear (= the first affective phase of pain) and anxiety of its persistence are naturally associated with its occurrence. For the patient's adaptation to pain and further development of the painful state, his/her current attitude is essential to actual acute pain. Thus, it is essentially a question of whether he/she accepts it as a positive and necessary signal, or succumbs to the fear of pain and, by excessive obsession and catastrophe, neurotizes its further development and thus creates the conditions for neural sensitization and pain chronification. This creates a gradually deepening suffering, which is a complex of negative affective and cognitive processes. The affective component of suffering is characterized by anxiety, anger, and depression (= second affective phase of pain), the cognitive component of suffering includes views on pain and its impact on the sufferer, most often devaluing his whole life and perception of the environment [84].

In addition to the evidence describing the importance of psychological factors on physiological outcomes after surgery, emerging data suggest psychological state before cancer surgery may have an impact on longer term quality of life and well-being [77]. Higher pre-surgical depression and lower self-efficacy to manage illness were significantly associated with poorer trajectories of recovery [85]. Within the field of oncology, an emphasis on reductions in stress and anxiety are emerging increasingly [77].

Therefore we suggest that pain chronification prediction should be included in the process of prehabilitation as a part of practical implementation of PPPM/3 PM in the routine processes of future healthcare, as we discuss in more details in the dedicated chapter of this book (see also Fig. 1).

2.6 Smoking and Other Cessations as Element of Prehabilitation

Patients should be strongly encouraged to cease smoking as part of any prehabilitation program [86]. The perioperative period is considered to be a "teachable moment" when the need for surgery might serve as a driver for permanent behavioral changes including smoking cessation [86–88]. Cigarette smoking is a risk factor for several perioperative pulmonary, cardiovascular, and wound healing complications. Limited evidence suggests that risks are also associated with "vaping" (i.e., use of electronic cigarettes [e-cigarettes]) as a method for consumption of nicotine (or other substances such as cannabis) [89]. Smoking increases the risk of postoperative morbidity and mortality. Smoking cessation before surgery reduces the risk of complications [86].

2.6.1 The Way to Cease Smoking in Terms of Prehabilitation

One of the possible way is "The 5A's" (**Ask** about tobacco use, **Advise** quitting, **Assess** readiness to quit, **Assist** smokers ready to quit, **Arrange** follow-up) or abbreviated variation "AAR" (**Ask** about tobacco use, **Assist**—Offer advice to quit and assistance to make a plan, including prescribing cessation medication, **Refer** to behavioral support resources to continue treatment after the visit) [90–92].

At this point we have to essentially emphasize that, logically, it is not only the cessation of smoking that is important, although it is the most pronounced one within the standard elements of prehabilitation, but also cessation of body intoxication from other resources such as, for example, alcohol, drugs of abuse, environment, food, beverages, is important from the perspective of more complex prehabilitation under the changed paradigm of healthcare brought by PPPM/3 PM.

2.7 Importance of Prehabilitation Before Major Surgery in Context of PPPM

Successful surgery does not depend exclusively on the procedure alone but, rather, on how quickly and efficiently the patient can return to his normal life. With increasing awareness of ERAS (Enhanced Recovery After Surgery) protocols, prehabilitation as an integral part of preoperative period takes on larger dimensions.

Improving preoperative functional capacity together with following best-evidence practice medicine, may be a tool to safely and effectively raise the number of patients suitable for curative-intent surgical procedures [12].

It follows from the above mentioned that a successful operation depends on a combination of technical surgical skills and, on the other hand, also on metabolic interventional therapy "tailored" to the patient's metabolic status. This includes providing appropriate nutritional, physical and psychological support. Suitable perioperative management may be vital for long-term outcome in oncology patients [93, 94]. Half of the patients still manifest a degree of incapacity 3 months after major elective abdominal surgery [95]. Major surgery reduces 40% of physiological reserve. Four weeks after discharge patients report pain, physical fatigue, reduced appetite, trouble sleeping, reduced ability to concentrate [96]. Functional capacity may not be fully recovered up to 6–9 weeks [97] and so for the elderly patients, at 8 weeks, at most one third and at 6 months after surgery only 50% recover to preoperative levels [95, 98].

Due to the increasing age of patients undergoing major abdominal surgery there is a subsequent increase in postoperative complications, prolonged hospital stays, mortality rates and also health care costs. "Frail" elderly patients frequently develop delirium as a sever complication. The primary study outcome of one single-center controlled before-and-after study, in progress, is to reduce the incidence of delirium in elderly patients regarding of major abdominal surgery applying principles of multicomponent prehabilitation pathway [99].

There is emerging evidence suggesting that many of the negative effects of major surgery can be reduced through the attenuation of surgical stress, not only due to intraoperative (minimally invasive surgery [99], fluid management [100], etc.), or postoperative (e.g., "fast track" early nutrition, mobilization [101]) interventions but also with the effort to focus on the preoperative period and accelerate convalescence [21].

Despite this evidence, surgical prehabilitation is not yet a component of routine clinical practice. Prehabilitation as a multicomponent approach requires an interdisciplinary cooperation, as it offers a shift from the current healthcare paradigm, just as PPPM/3 PM represents a paradigm change, and these two changes are well in agreement. Preoperative period proposes the best opportunity for preventive targeted (personalized) interventions in order to improve more effective healthcare and postoperative recovery [12].

Preoperative prehabilitation involve four main pillars and goals—nutritional optimization (recognition of malnourished patients, identification deficiencies in patient's eating, provision of holistic nutritional management including nutritional supplementation, etc.), exercise and physical activity (individualized exercise program, combining aerobic, and intensity training) and psychological well-being (anxiety and stress reducing techniques, interventions to improve cognitive function) [12]. As a part of prehabilition patients should be profusely support to cease smoking [85]. Additionally to these elements of multimodal approach, we suggest that prehabilitation, from the perspective of PPPM/3 PM, should also include other elements as already highlighted in Fig. 1.

2.8 Peri-Operative, Intraoperative Prehabilitation and PPPM/3 PM

The optional surgery pathways provide the caregiver an opportunity for significant changes in the attitude the care is arranged—instead of taking provider convenience into fundamental consideration the patient needs are primarily considered. Redesigning peri-operative pathways helps to improve the provided care for the patient and increase the quality of services, patient's satisfaction, public health as well as healthcare value, defined as outcome per unit of currency [102]. Episodic peri-operative care in some systems accounts for over half of hospital costs [103].

Multidisciplinary medical care of patient from the intention of undergoing surgery until full recovery is defined as peri-operative medicine [104, 105]. Peri-operative medicine is a new and rapidly evolving clinical science that is well in agreement with the attitude of PPPM, and respond to the needs of a population of patients with more complex medical management. Peri-operative medicine means the ability to prepare patients beyond the traditional anesthetic and surgical care of a single patient (personalization) in the early, preventive peri-operative period [106]. Elective peri-operative care helps to rationalize and redesign more advantageous patients care. Providing patients care with the possibility of predicting the risk of adverse outcome, the so-called risk-adapted approach, improve the value of healthcare delivery [102].

The goal is patient-centered care of their own, their wishes, expectations, opinions, on the other hand management around surgical procedure resulting in their best interest, adequate preparation for the surgery and enhanced recovery after surgery [102].

Avoiding "wrong-patient surgery," serving patient's best interests with improved patient-physician experience, together with effective management of comorbidities with the intention of mitigating the risk of major surgery, cooperation with pain clinics, that and lot more at the same time offer the preoperative period [107].

During the preoperative period, patients may be more susceptible to behavior change interventions. Smoking cessation, alcohol cessation, nutritional optimization and physical activity and exercise. Such changes in behavior at a time when patients may feel very limited control of their immediate destiny may have significant psychological benefit and may be long-lasting which also highlights possible population health benefits.

Regarding intra-operative care the published data support the idea that numerous factors provided for the patients do not follow provable evidence and/or a comprehensive medical basis which results in the situation when particular factors are not essentially those which one might expect in everyday life. Even if we may consider alternatives for these factors resulting from the patient and surgery-specific characteristics (e.g., age, risk factors, duration of surgery, amount of blood loss), the most significant effect would have anesthesia and providers of surgery. (e.g., fluid therapy) [108]. On the basis of related studies and examinations we support the opinion that intra-operative care must essentially be standardized to provide particular standard level of quality and patterns of care for wide spectrum of patients, as well as it must be personalized/individualized in order to include patient-specific characteristics which might be unique and important for good result [102].

2.9 Management of Comorbidities as Important Element of Prehabilitation

The growing prevalence of comorbid conditions [103], and harmful lifestyle characteristics (e.g., inactivity, unbalanced diet, stress, intoxication from environment and other resources, cigarette smoking, alcohol abuse, etc.) coupled with an understanding that some surgery may be unnecessary or even harmful [109] are driving a re-appraisal of peri-operative processes. Patients who are candidates for surgery are often not ready for it [102].

Risk of problems after surgery, or a medical procedure in general, is the product of particular probability(ies) consequently leading to undesirable outcome(s). The probability of a particular peri-operative episode is determined by both, patient characteristics and healthcare characteristics (taking into consideration all aspects of peri-operative care and surgery itself). Together, these risk determinants can be preventively reduced by implementation of particular changes in peri-operative procedures. We distinguish between permanent risk factors and modifiable risk factors which may be adjusted or changed ahead of the scheduled time of the surgery or a medical procedure. There are, of course, several factors such as age, sex or genetic predispositions which can't be changed. Other factors, on the other hand, have the potential for modification or for being influenced; for example, emphysema, myocardial injury, anemia, reversible airway disease can be partly resolved. Among risk factors that can be substantially modified, if the patient is properly motivated and well instructed, there are factors such as consumption of alcohol and tobacco, drugs, low physical activity, unbalanced diet, psychological stress—all related to life style and behavior [102] and are well in agreement with the attitude of PPPM/3 PM.

2.10 Postoperative Procedures, DrEaMing, in Relation to Prehabilitation and PPPM/3 PM

Patients with an uncomplicated recovery should be discharged and return to normal life as quickly as possible. Higher-risk patients or patients developing postoperative complications should be provided with the appropriate level of care without delay and on a predictive, preventive, and personalized basis where possible.

Providing care based on effectiveness of use, not traditionally used procedures, more patient-oriented postoperative care, the flexible use of health professional resources to maximize effectiveness and minimizing risks through more effective communication and systematized actions like checklists, risk-adapted management of postoperative period, all this can increase and underpin efficiency of postoperative care.

Patients who achieve Drinking Eating and Mobilizing (DrEaMing) [110] rarely develop postoperative complications, so concept of DrEaMing is solid marker of recovery and benchmark of the effectiveness of peri-operative care [110].

2.11 Conclusion and Recommendations

In conclusion, the idea of prehabilitation and its practical application is enriching the vision of PPPM/3 PM in a very natural and logical way. Although the prehabilitation is being primarily connected to the surgical procedures, it should be, in our opinion, applied to much wider spectrum of personalized medical procedures that would include: surgery, stomatosurgery, plastic surgery, childbirth, application of physiotherapy, pharmacotherapy, radiotherapy, chemotherapy, traditional, complementary and alternative medicine (TCAM), invasive diagnostic procedures, and other.

We suggest that basic elements of prehabilitation should include also other factors and tools as visualized in the complex prehabilitation in Fig. 1. The communities of experts in surgery, oncology, prehabilitation, peri-operative care and postoperative care may benefit from the tools developed under PPPM/3MP and vice versa, the attitudes in the prehabilitation fit very well within PPPM/3 PM and represent a very good example of practical implementation of PPPM from bench to bedside. The conscious cooperation between the experts in all related fields will essentially bring benefits to all patients and gradually prepare the ground for effective future healthcare.

References

1. Rowntree LG (1942) The health of registrants and the president's plan of rehabilitation. Proc Am Philos Soc 85(4):343–348
2. Sawyer WA (1942) Prehabilitation and rehabilitation in industry. J Am Med Assoc 119:419
3. Schneidrzik WE (1952-1953) Significance of preoperative breathing exercise for thoracic surgery, langenbecks. Arch Klin Chir Ver Dtsch Z Chir 273:540–541
4. Carli F, Zavorsky GS (2005) Optimizing functional exercise capacity in the elderly surgical population. Curr Opin Clin Nutr Metab Care 8(1):23–32
5. https://dictionary.cambridge.org/dictionary/english/prehabilitation. Accessed 17 Jul 2022
6. Banguo P, Amoako D (2017) Prehabilitation. BJA Educ 17(12):401–405. https://doi.org/10.1093/bjaed/mkx032
7. https://www.collinsdictionary.com/submission/21810/prehabilitation. Accessed 17 Jul 2022
8. Silver JK, Baima J (2013) Cancer prehabilitation: an opportunity to decrease treatment-related morbidity, increase cancer treatment options, and improve physical and psychological health outcomes. Am J Phys Med Rehabil 92(8):715–727. https://doi.org/10.1097/PHM.0b013e31829b4afe; PMID: 23756434
9. Jones LW, Eves ND, Haykowsky M, Freedland SJ, Mackey JR (2009) Exercise intolerance in cancer and the role of exercise therapy to reverse dysfunction. Lancet Oncol 10(6):598–605. https://doi.org/10.1016/S1470-2045(09)70031-2; PMID: 19482248
10. Gao P, Huang XZ, Song YX, Sun JX, Chen XW, Sun Y, Jiang YM, Wang ZN (2018) Impact of timing of adjuvant chemotherapy on survival in stage III colon cancer: a population-based study. BMC Cancer 18(1):234. https://doi.org/10.1186/s12885-018-4138-7

11. Yan YX, Liu YQ, Li M, Hu PF, Guo AM, Yang XH, Qiu JJ, Yang SS, Shen J, Zhang LP, Wang W (2009) Development and evaluation of a questionnaire for measuring suboptimal health status in urban. Chin J Epidemiol 19(6):333–341. https://doi.org/10.2188/jea.je20080086
12. Scheede-Bergdahl C, Minnella EM, Carli F (2019) Multi-modal prehabilitation: addressing the why, when, what, how, who and where next? Anaesthesia 74(Suppl 1):20–26. https://doi.org/10.1111/anae.14505
13. Gurlit S, Gogol M (2019) Prehabilitation is better than cure. Curr Opin Anaesthesiol 32(1):108–115. https://doi.org/10.1097/ACO.0000000000000678
14. Chan SP, Ip KY, Irwin MG (2019) Peri-operative optimisation of elderly and frail patients: a narrative review. Anaesthesia 74(Suppl 1):80–89. https://doi.org/10.1111/anae.14512
15. Joyce MF, Azocar RJ (2020) Prehabilitation for anesthesia and surgery. In: Post TW (ed) UpToDate. UpToDate, Waltham, MA; https://www.uptodate.com/contents/prehabilitation-for-anesthesia-and-surgery?search=prehabilitation&source=search_result&selectedTitle=1~19&usage_type=default&display_rank=1#H3780502168. Accessed 29 Jul 2022
16. International Prehabilitation Society 2018–2020. Activities—International Prehabilitation Society; https://prehabsociety.com/activities/. Accessed 8 Jan 2022
17. Gillis C, Li C, Lee L, Awasthi R, Augustin B, Gamsa A, Liberman AS, Stein B, Charlebois P, Feldman LS, Carli F (2014) Prehabilitation versus rehabilitation: a randomized control trial in patients undergoing colorectal resection for cancer. Anesthesiology 121(5):937–947. https://doi.org/10.1097/ALN.0000000000000393
18. Bousquet-Dion G, Awasthi R, Loiselle SÈ, Minnella EM, Agnihotram RV, Bergdahl A, Carli F, Scheede-Bergdahl C (2018) Evaluation of supervised multimodal prehabilitation programme in cancer patients undergoing colorectal resection: a randomized control trial. Acta Oncol 57(6):849–859. https://doi.org/10.1080/0284186X.2017.1423180
19. Li C, Carli F, Lee L, Charlebois P, Stein B, Liberman AS, Kaneva P, Augustin B, Wongyingsinn M, Gamsa A, Kim DJ, Vassiliou MC, Feldman LS (2013) Impact of a trimodal prehabilitation program on functional recovery after colorectal cancer surgery: a pilot study. Surg Endosc 27(4):1072–1082. https://doi.org/10.1007/s00464-012-2560-5
20. Trépanier M, Minnella EM, Paradis T, Awasthi R, Kaneva P, Schwartzman K, Carli F, Fried GM, Feldman LS, Lee L (2019) Improved disease-free survival after prehabilitation for colorectal cancer surgery. Ann Surg 270(3):493–501. https://doi.org/10.1097/SLA.0000000000003465
21. van Rooijen S, Carli F, Dalton S, Thomas G, Bojesen R, Le Guen M, Barizien N, Awasthi R, Minnella E, Beijer S, Martínez-Palli G, van Lieshout R, Gögenur I, Feo C, Johansen C, Scheede-Bergdahl C, Roumen R, Schep G, Slooter G (2019) Multimodal prehabilitation in colorectal cancer patients to improve functional capacity and reduce postoperative complications: the first international randomized controlled trial for multimodal prehabilitation. BMC Cancer 19(1):98. https://doi.org/10.1186/s12885-018-5232-6
22. Slankamenac K, Nederlof N, Pessaux P, de Jonge J, Wijnhoven BP, Breitenstein S, Oberkofler CE, Graf R, Puhan MA, Clavien PA (2014) The comprehensive complication index: a novel and more sensitive endpoint for assessing outcome and reducing sample size in randomized controlled trials. Ann Surg 260(5):757–762. https://doi.org/10.1097/SLA.0000000000000948; discussion 762–3
23. McCann M, Stamp N, Ngui A, Litton E (2019) Cardiac prehabilitation. J Cardiothorac Vasc Anesth 33(8):2255–2265. https://doi.org/10.1053/j.jvca.2019.01.023
24. Chen H, Li S, Ruan T, Liu L, Fang L (2018) Is it necessary to perform prehabilitation exercise for patients undergoing total knee arthroplasty: meta-analysis of randomized controlled trials. Phys Sportsmed 46(1):36–43. https://doi.org/10.1080/00913847.2018.1403274; Erratum in: Phys Sportsmed 2018 Sep;46(3):399–403
25. Jahic D, Omerovic D, Tanovic AT, Dzankovic F, Campara MT (2018) The effect of prehabilitation on postoperative outcome in patients following primary total knee arthroplasty. Med Arch 72(6):439–443. https://doi.org/10.5455/medarh.2018.72.439-443

26. Clode NJ, Perry MA, Wulff L (2018) Does physiotherapy prehabilitation improve presurgical outcomes and influence patient expectations prior to knee and hip joint arthroplasty? Int J Orthop Trauma Nurs 30:14–19. https://doi.org/10.1016/j.ijotn.2018.05.004
27. Benson R, McGregor G, Shehata M, Imray C (2019) Optimising fitness for major vascular surgery. BMJ 366:l5002. https://doi.org/10.1136/bmj.l5002
28. Lapuníková M, Sklenková I, Bečková Z, Ďurajová V, Kubáň J, Kapalla M. Vision of the essential extension of health-related services provided in the hospital as an initial step towards future healthcare and practical realization of predictive, preventive and personalized medicine. In Golubnitschaja O, Topolcan O, Kucera R. et al. (eds) 10th Anniversary of the European association for predictive, preventive and personalised (3P) medicine—EPMA world congress supplement 2020. EPMA J. 2020; 11, 1–133. https://doi.org/10.1007/s13167-020-00206-1
29. Líška D, Stráska B, Pupiš M (2020) Physical therapy as an adjuvant treatment for the prevention and treatment of cancer. Klin Onkol 33(2):101–106; Scopus, 33
30. Kim DW, Kang SB, Lee SY, Oh HK, In MH (2013) Early rehabilitation programs after laparoscopic colorectal surgery: evidence and criticism. World J Gastroenterol 19(46):8543–8551. https://doi.org/10.3748/wjg.v19.i46.8543
31. Líška D, Rutkowski RS (2021) Breast rehabilitation. Rehabilitácia pri rakovine prsníka. Klinicka Onkol 34(1):14–19. https://doi.org/10.48095/ccko202114
32. Djurasić L, Pavlović A, Zarić N, Palibrk I, Basarić D, Djordjević VR (2012) The effects of early rehabilitation in patients with surgically treated colorectal cancer. Acta Chir Iugosl 59(3):89–91. https://doi.org/10.2298/aci1203089d
33. Singh B, Hayes SC, Spence RR, Steele ML, Millet GY, Gergele L (2020) Exercise and colorectal cancer: a systematic review and meta-analysis of exercise safety, feasibility and effectiveness. Int J Behav Nutr Phys Act 17(1):122. https://doi.org/10.1186/s12966-020-01021-7
34. Wade DT (2020) What is rehabilitation? An empirical investigation leading to an evidence-based description. Clin Rehabil 34(5):571–583. https://doi.org/10.1177/0269215520905112
35. Wong CL, Lee HHC, Chang SC (2016) Colorectal cancer rehabilitation review. J Cancer Res Pract 3(2):31–33. https://doi.org/10.1016/j.jcrpr.2015.07.001
36. Akimoto N, Ugai T, Zhong R, Hamada T, Fujiyoshi K, Giannakis M, Wu K, Cao Y, Ng K, Ogino S (2021) Rising incidence of early-onset colorectal cancer—a call to action. Nat Rev Clin Oncol 18(4):230–243. https://doi.org/10.1038/s41571-020-00445-1
37. Durrand J, Singh SJ, Danjoux G (2019) Prehabilitation. Clin Med 19(6):458–464. https://doi.org/10.7861/clinmed.2019-0257
38. Blanchard S, Glasgow P (2019) A theoretical model for exercise progressions as part of a complex rehabilitation programme design. Br J Sports Med 53(3):139–140. https://doi.org/10.1136/bjsports-2017-097486
39. Dekker J, de Groot V, Ter Steeg AM, Vloothuis J, Holla J, Collette E, Satink T, Post L, Doodeman S, Littooij E (2020) Setting meaningful goals in rehabilitation: rationale and practical tool. Clin Rehabil 34(1):3–12. https://doi.org/10.1177/0269215519876299
40. Koo CY, Tai BC, Chan DKH, Tan LL, Tan KK, Lee CH (2021) Chemotherapy and adverse cardiovascular events in colorectal cancer patients undergoing surgical resection. World J Surg Oncol 19(1):21. https://doi.org/10.1186/s12957-021-02125-5
41. Hojman P, Gehl J, Christensen JF, Pedersen BK (2018) Molecular mechanisms linking exercise to cancer prevention and treatment. Cell Metab 27(1):10–21. https://doi.org/10.1016/j.cmet.2017.09.015
42. Kang DW, Lee J, Suh SH, Ligibel J, Courneya KS, Jeon JY (2017) Effects of exercise on insulin, IGF axis, adipocytokines, and inflammatory markers in breast cancer survivors: a systematic review and meta-analysis. Cancer Epidemiol Biomarkers Prev 26(3):355–365. https://doi.org/10.1158/1055-9965.EPI-16-0602
43. Komninou D, Ayonote A, Richie JP, Rigas B (2003) Insulin resistance and its contribution to colon carcinogenesis. Exp Biol Med (Maywood) 228(4):396–405. https://doi.org/10.1177/153537020322800410

44. Sturgeon K, Digiovanni L, Good J, Salvatore D, Fenderson D, Domchek S, Stopfer J, Galantino ML, Bryan C, Hwang WT, Schmitz K (2016) Exercise-induced dose-response alterations in adiponectin and leptin levels are dependent on body fat changes in women at risk for breast cancer. Cancer Epidemiol Biomarkers Prev 25(8):1195–1200. https://doi.org/10.1158/1055-9965.EPI-15-1087
45. Son JS, Chae SA, Testroet ED, Du M, Jun HP (2018) Exercise-induced myokines: a brief review of controversial issues of this decade. Expert Rev Endocrinol Metab 13(1):51–58. https://doi.org/10.1080/17446651.2018.1416290
46. Builova TV, Marchenkova LA (2020) Multidisciplinary approach to the rehabilitation of patients with osteoporosis. Vopr Kurortol Fizioter Lech Fiz Kult 97(2):58–67. https://doi.org/10.17116/kurort20209702158
47. Debes C, Aissou M, Beaussier M (2014) Prehabilitation. Preparing patients for surgery to improve functional recovery and reduce postoperative morbidity. Ann Fr Anesth Reanim 33(1):33–40. https://doi.org/10.1016/j.annfar.2013.12.012
48. Barassi G, Bellomo RG, Di Iulio A, Lococo A, Porreca A, Di Felice PA, Saggini R (2018) Preoperative rehabilitation in lung cancer patients: yoga approach. Adv Exp Med Biol 1096:19–29. https://doi.org/10.1007/5584_2018_186
49. Bradley A, Marshall A, Stonehewer L, Reaper L, Parker K, Bevan-Smith E, Jordan C, Gillies J, Agostini P, Bishay E, Kalkat M, Steyn R, Rajesh P, Dunn J, Naidu B (2013) Pulmonary rehabilitation programme for patients undergoing curative lung cancer surgery. Eur J Cardiothorac Surg 44(4):e266–e271. https://doi.org/10.1093/ejcts/ezt381ň
50. Fox L, Wiseman T, Cahill D, Beyer K, Peat N, Rammant E, Van Hemelrijck M (2019) Barriers and facilitators to physical activity in men with prostate cancer: a qualitative and quantitative systematic review. Psychooncology 28(12):2270–2285. https://doi.org/10.1002/pon.5240
51. Dennett AM, Elkins MR (2020) Cancer rehabilitation. J Physiother 66(2):70–72. https://doi.org/10.1016/j.jphys.2020.03.004
52. Giannitsi S, Bougiakli M, Bechlioulis A, Kotsia A, Michalis LK, Naka KK (2019) 6-minute walking test: a useful tool in the management of heart failure patients. Ther Adv Cardiovasc Dis 13:1753944719870084. https://doi.org/10.1177/1753944719870084
53. Schmidt K, Vogt L, Thiel C, Jäger E, Banzer W (2013) Validity of the six-minute walk test in cancer patients. Int J Sports Med 34(7):631–636. https://doi.org/10.1055/s-0032-1323746
54. Pecorelli N, Fiore JF, Gillis C, Awasthi R, Mappin-Kasirer B, Niculiseanu P, Fried GM, Carli F, Feldman LS (2016) The six-minute walk test as a measure of postoperative recovery after colorectal resection: further examination of its measurement properties. Surg Endosc 30(6):2199–2206. https://doi.org/10.1007/s00464-015-4478-1
55. Mehmet H, Yang AWH, Robinson SR (2020) What is the optimal chair stand test protocol for older adults? A systematic review. Disabil Rehabil 42(20):2828–2835. https://doi.org/10.1080/09638288.2019.1575922
56. Kear BM, Guck TP, McGaha AL (2017) Timed up and go (TUG) test. J Prim Care Community Health 8(1):9–13. https://doi.org/10.1177/2150131916659282
57. Lins L, Carvalho FM (2016) SF-36 total score as a single measure of health-related quality of life: scoping review. SAGE Open Med 4:2050312116671725. https://doi.org/10.1177/2050312116671725
58. Romanowski KS, Askari R (2021) Overview of perioperative nutrition support. In: Seres D, Cochran A (eds) UpToDate. UpToDate Inc., Waltham, MA; https://www.uptodate.com/contents/overview-of-perioperative-nutrition-support. Accessed 11 Jul 2022
59. Soeters P, Bozzetti F, Cynober L, Elia M, Shenkin A, Sobotka L (2016) Meta-analysis is not enough: the critical role of pathophysiology in determining optimal care in clinical nutrition. Clin Nutr 35(3):748–757. https://doi.org/10.1016/j.clnu.2015.08.008
60. Gillis C, Carli F (2015) Promoting perioperative metabolic and nutritional care. Anesthesiology 123(6):1455–1472. https://doi.org/10.1097/ALN.0000000000000795
61. Alazawi W, Pirmadid N, Lahiri R, Bhattacharya S (2016) Inflammatory and immune responses to surgery and their clinical impact. Ann Surg 64:73–80

62. Aahlin EK, Tranø G, Johns N, Horn A, Søreide JA, Fearon KC, Revhaug A, Lassen K (2015) Risk factors, complications and survival after upper abdominal surgery: a prospective cohort study. BMC Surg 15:83. https://doi.org/10.1186/s12893-015-0069-2
63. Laur CV, McNicholl T, Valaitis R, Keller HH (2017) Malnutrition or frailty? Overlap and evidence gaps in the diagnosis and treatment of frailty and malnutrition. Appl Physiol Nutr Metab 42(5):449–458. https://doi.org/10.1139/apnm-2016-0652
64. White JV, Guenter P, Jensen G, Malone A, Schofield M, Academy Malnutrition Work Group; A.S.P.E.N. Malnutrition Task Force; A.S.P.E.N. Board of Directors (2012) Consensus statement: academy of nutrition and dietetics and American Society for Parenteral and Enteral Nutrition: characteristics recommended for the identification and documentation of adult malnutrition (undernutrition). J Parenter Enter Nutr 36(3):275–283. https://doi.org/10.1177/0148607112440285
65. Weimann A, Braga M, Carli F, Higashiguchi T, Hübner M, Klek S, Laviano A, Ljungqvist O, Lobo DN, Martindale R, Waitzberg DL, Bischoff SC, Singer P (2017) ESPEN guideline: clinical nutrition in surgery. Clin Nutr 36(3):623–650. https://doi.org/10.1016/j.clnu.2017.02.013
66. Jeejeebhoy KN, Keller H, Gramlich L, Allard JP, Laporte M, Duerksen DR, Payette H, Bernier P, Vesnaver E, Davidson B, Teterina A, Lou W (2015) Nutritional assessment: comparison of clinical assessment and objective variables for the prediction of length of hospital stay and readmission. Am J Clin Nutr 101(5):956–965. https://doi.org/10.3945/ajcn.114.098665; Epub 2015 Mar 4. PMID: 25739926
67. Wischmeyer PE, Carli F, Evans DC, Guilbert S, Kozar R, Pryor A, Thiele RH, Everett S, Grocott M, Gan TJ, Shaw AD, JKM T, Miller TE, Hedrick TL, MD ME, Mythen MG, Bergamaschi R, Gupta R, Holubar SD, Senagore AJ, Abola RE, Bennett-Guerrero E, Kent ML, Feldman LS, Fiore JF Jr, Perioperative Quality Initiative (POQI) 2 Workgroup (2018) American society for enhanced recovery and perioperative quality initiative joint consensus statement on nutrition screening and therapy within a surgical enhanced recovery pathway. Anesth Analg 126(6):1883–1895. https://doi.org/10.1213/ANE.0000000000002743
68. Hu WH, Cajas-Monson LC, Eisenstein S, Parry L, Cosman B, Ramamoorthy S (2015) Preoperative malnutrition assessments as predictors of postoperative mortality and morbidity in colorectal cancer: an analysis of ACS-NSQIP. Nutr J 14:91. https://doi.org/10.1186/s12937-015-0081-5
69. Elwyn DH, Bryan-Brown CW, Shoemaker WC (1975) Nutritional aspects of body water dislocations in postoperative and depleted patients. Ann Surg 182(1):76–85. https://doi.org/10.1097/00000658-197507000-00015
70. Kinney JM, Weissman C (1986) Forms of malnutrition in stressed and unstressed patients. Clin Chest Med 7(1):19–28
71. Santos JI (1994) Nutrition, infection, and immunocompetence. Infect Dis Clin N Am 8(1):243–267
72. Zhang B, Najarali Z, Ruo L, Alhusaini A, Solis N, Valencia M, Sanchez MIP, Serrano PE (2019) Effect of perioperative nutritional supplementation on postoperative complications-systematic review and meta-analysis. J Gastrointest Surg 23(8):1682–1693. https://doi.org/10.1007/s11605-019-04173-5
73. Weimann A, Braga M, Carli F, Higashiguchi T, Hübner M, Klek S, Laviano A, Ljungqvist O, Lobo DN, Martindale RG, Waitzberg D, Bischoff SC, Singer P (2021) ESPEN practical guideline: clinical nutrition in surgery. Clin Nutr 40(7):4745–4761. https://doi.org/10.1016/j.clnu.2021.03.031
74. Gillis C, Wischmeyer PE (2019) Pre-operative nutrition and the elective surgical patient: why, how and what? Anaesthesia 74(Suppl 1):27–35. https://doi.org/10.1111/anae.14506; PMID: 30604414
75. Phillips SM (2004) Protein requirements and supplementation in strength sports. Nutrition 20(7–8):689–695. https://doi.org/10.1016/j.nut.2004.04.009
76. Biolo G, Tipton KD, Klein S, Wolfe RR (1997) An abundant supply of amino acids enhances the metabolic effect of exercise on muscle protein. Am J Phys 273(1 Pt 1):E122–E129. https://doi.org/10.1152/ajpendo.1997.273.1.E122

77. Levett DZH, Grimmett C (2019) Psychological factors, prehabilitation and surgical outcomes: evidence and future directions. Anaesthesia 74(Suppl 1):36–42. https://doi.org/10.1111/anae.14507; PMID: 30604423
78. Mavros MN, Athanasiou S, Gkegkes ID, Polyzos KA, Peppas G, Falagas ME (2011) Do psychological variables affect early surgical recovery? PLoS One 6(5):e20306. https://doi.org/10.1371/journal.pone.0020306
79. Rosenberger PH, Jokl P, Ickovics J (2006) Psychosocial factors and surgical outcomes: an evidence-based literature review. J Am Acad Orthop Surg 14(7):397–405. https://doi.org/10.5435/00124635-200607000-00002
80. Ip HY, Abrishami A, Peng PW, Wong J, Chung F (2009) Predictors of postoperative pain and analgesic consumption: a qualitative systematic review. Anesthesiology 111(3):657–677. https://doi.org/10.1097/ALN.0b013e3181aae87a
81. Hinrichs-Rocker A, Schulz K, Järvinen I, Lefering R, Simanski C, Neugebauer EA (2009) Psychosocial predictors and correlates for chronic post-surgical pain (CPSP)—a systematic review. Eur J Pain 13(7):719–730. https://doi.org/10.1016/j.ejpain.2008.07.015
82. Powell R, Scott NW, Manyande A, Bruce J, Vögele C, Byrne-Davis LM, Unsworth M, Osmer C, Johnston M (2016) Psychological preparation and postoperative outcomes for adults undergoing surgery under general anaesthesia. Cochrane Database Syst Rev 2016(5):CD008646. https://doi.org/10.1002/14651858.CD008646.pub2
83. Martuliak I (2020) Pathophysiology of pain for clinical practice—2nd supplemented edition. Martimed s r.o, Banská Bystrica, p 344; ISBN 978–80–971753-2-0
84. Knotek P (2010) Psychological aspects of chronic pain. In: Treatment of chronic pain. Solen, Olomouc, pp 16–28; ISBN 978–80–87327-45-6
85. Foster C, Haviland J, Winter J, Grimmett C, Chivers Seymour K, Batehup L, Calman L, Corner J, Din A, Fenlon D, May CM, Richardson A, Smith PW, Members of the Study Advisory Committee (2016) Pre-surgery depression and confidence to manage problems predict recovery trajectories of health and wellbeing in the first two years following colorectal cancer: results from the CREW cohort study. PLoS One 11(5):e0155434. https://doi.org/10.1371/journal.pone.0155434
86. Yousefzadeh A, Chung F, Wong DT, Warner DO, Wong J (2016) Smoking cessation: the role of the anesthesiologist. Anesth Analg 122(5):1311–1320. https://doi.org/10.1213/ANE.0000000000001170
87. Older P, Smith R, Courtney P, Hone R (1993) Preoperative evaluation of cardiac failure and ischemia in elderly patients by cardiopulmonary exercise testing. Chest 104(3):701–704. https://doi.org/10.1378/chest.104.3.701
88. Warner DO (2006) Perioperative abstinence from cigarettes: physiologic and clinical consequences. Anesthesiology 104(2):356–367. https://doi.org/10.1097/00000542-200602000-00023
89. Warner DO, Preston P, Subramanyam R (2020) Smoking or vaping: perioperative management. In: Holt NF, Kathuria H (eds) UpToDate. UpToDate Inc, Waltham, MA; https://www.uptodate.com/contents/smoking-or-vaping-perioperative-management. Accessed 17 Jan 2022
90. 2008 PHS Guideline Update Panel, Liaisons, and Staff (2008) Treating tobacco use and dependence: 2008 update U.S. Public Health Service Clinical Practice Guideline executive summary. Respir Care 53(9):1217–1222
91. US Preventive Services Task Force, Krist AH, Davidson KW, Mangione CM, Barry MJ, Cabana M, Caughey AB, Donahue K, Doubeni CA, Epling JW Jr, Kubik M, Ogedegbe G, Pbert L, Silverstein M, Simon MA, Tseng CW, Wong JB (2021) Interventions for tobacco smoking cessation in adults, including pregnant persons: US Preventive Services Task Force recommendation statement. JAMA 325(3):265–279. https://doi.org/10.1001/jama.2020.25019; PMID: 33464343
92. Siu AL, U.S. Preventive Services Task Force (2015) Behavioral and pharmacotherapy interventions for tobacco smoking cessation in adults, including pregnant women: U.S. Preventive Services Task Force recommendation statement. Ann Intern Med 163(8):622–634. https://doi.org/10.7326/M15-2023

93. Horowitz M, Neeman E, Sharon E, Ben-Eliyahu S (2015) Exploiting the critical perioperative period to improve long-term cancer outcomes. Nat Rev Clin Oncol 12:213–226
94. Gustafsson UO, Oppelstrup H, Thorell A, Nygren J, Ljungqvist O (2016) Adherence to the ERAS protocol is associated with 5-year survival after colorectal cancer surgery: a retrospective cohort study. World J Surg 40:1741–1747
95. Lawrence VA, Hazuda HP, Cornell JE, Pederson T, Bradshaw PT, Mulrow CD, Page CP (2004) Functional independence after major abdominal surgery in the elderly. J Am Coll Surg 199(5):762–772. https://doi.org/10.1016/j.jamcollsurg.2004.05.280
96. Jensen MB, Houborg KB, Nørager CB, Henriksen MG, Laurberg S (2011) Postoperative changes in fatigue, physical function and body composition: an analysis of the amalgamated data from five randomized trials on patients undergoing colorectal surgery. Color Dis 13(5):588–593. https://doi.org/10.1111/j.1463-1318.2010.02232.x
97. Salmon P, Hall GM (1997) A theory of postoperative fatigue: an interaction of biological, psychological, and social processes. Pharmacol Biochem Behav 56(4):623–628. https://doi.org/10.1016/s0091-3057(96)00429-7
98. Nicholson A, Lowe MC, Parker J, Lewis SR, Alderson P, Smith AF (2014) Systematic review and meta-analysis of enhanced recovery programmes in surgical patients. Br J Surg 101(3):172–188. https://doi.org/10.1002/bjs.9394
99. Janssen TL, Mosk CA, Wielders D, Seerden TCJ, Steyerberg EW, van Gammeren AJ, de Lange DC, van Alphen R, van der Zee M, de Bruijn RM, de Vries J, Wijsman JH, Ho GH, Gobardhan PD, van der Laan L et al (2019) A multicomponent prehabilitation pathway to reduce the incidence of delirium in elderly patients in need of major abdominal surgery: study protocol for a before-and-after study. BMC Geriatr 19(1):87. https://doi.org/10.1186/s12877-019-1101-7
100. van Rooijen SJ, Huisman D, Stuijvenberg M, Stens J, Roumen RMH, Daams F, Slooter GD (2016) Intraoperative modifiable risk factors of colorectal anastomotic leakage: why surgeons and anesthesiologists should act together. Int J Surg 36(Pt A):183–200. https://doi.org/10.1016/j.ijsu.2016.09.098
101. Kehlet H, Wilmore DW (2008) Evidence-based surgical care and the evolution of fast-track surgery. Ann Surg 248(2):189–198. https://doi.org/10.1097/SLA.0b013e31817f2c1a
102. Grocott MPW, Edwards M, Mythen MG, Aronson S (2019) Peri-operative care pathways: re-engineering care to achieve the 'triple aim'. Anaesthesia 74:90–99. https://doi.org/10.1111/anae.14513
103. Barnett K, Mercer SW, Norbury M, Watt G, Wyke S, Guthrie B (2012) Epidemiology of multimorbidity and implications for health care, research, and medical education: a cross-sectional study. Lancet 380(9836):37–43. https://doi.org/10.1016/S0140-6736(12)60240-2
104. Grocott MP, Pearse RM (2012) Perioperative medicine: the future of anaesthesia? Br J Anaesth 108(5):723–726. https://doi.org/10.1093/bja/aes124
105. The Royal College of Anaesthetists (RCoA) (2015) Perioperative medicine—the pathway to better surgical care. RCoA, London, pp 1–23; https://www.rcoa.ac.uk/sites/default/files/documents/2019-08/Perioperative%20Medicine%20-%20The%20Pathway%20to%20Better%20Care.pdf. Accessed 22 Aug 2022
106. Pasquale MK, Sun SX, Song F, Hartnett HJ, Stemkowski SA (2012) Impact of exacerbations on health care cost and resource utilization in chronic obstructive pulmonary disease patients with chronic bronchitis from a predominantly medicare population. Int J Chron Obstruct Pulmon Dis 7:757–764. https://doi.org/10.2147/COPD.S36997
107. Koepke EJ, Manning EL, Miller TE, Ganesh A, Williams DG, Manning MW (2018) The rising tide of opioid use and abuse: the role of the anesthesiologist. Perioper Med (Lond) 7(1):1–10
108. Lilot M, Ehrenfeld JM, Lee C, Harrington B, Cannesson M, Rinehart J (2015) Variability in practice and factors predictive of total crystalloid administration during abdominal surgery: retrospective two-centre analysis. Br J Anaesth 114(5):767–776. https://doi.org/10.1093/bja/aeu452

109. Glance LG, Osler TM, Neuman MD (2014) Redesigning surgical decision making for high-risk patients. N Engl J Med 370(15):1379–1381. https://doi.org/10.1056/NEJMp1315538
110. Levy N, Mills P, Mythen M (2016) Is the pursuit of DREAMing (drinking, eating and mobilising) the ultimate goal of anaesthesia? Anaesthesia 71(9):1008–1012. https://doi.org/10.1111/anae.13495

Pathophysiology of the Acute Pain Chronification and the Possibilities of Its Prediction and Prevention

Igor Martuliak, Miroslav Ferenčík, Marko Kapalla, and Barbara Mrázová

Abbreviations

3 PM	Predictive, preventive, and personalized medicine
4-HNE	4-hydroxynonenal
CGRP	Calcitonin gene related peptide
CNS	Central nervous system
CVS	Cardiovascular system
DHA	Docosahexaenoic acid
DNA	Deoxyribonucleic acid
EPA	Eicosapentaenoic acid
EPMA	European association for predictive, preventive, and personalized medicine
ERAS	Enhanced recovery after surgery
GIT	Gastrointestinal tract
hs-CRP	High sensitivity C-reactive protein
IASP	International association for the study of pain
IL	Interleukin
LLLT	Low level laser light therapy
MDA	Malondialdehyde
MMP-9	Matrix metalloproteinase 9
MnSOD	Manganese superoxide dismutase
Na^+	Sodium ion

I. Martuliak (✉) · M. Ferenčík · B. Mrázová · M. Kapalla
F.D. Roosevelt University General Hospital of Banská Bystrica, Banská Bystrica, Slovakia
e-mail: imartuliak@nspbb.sk

H. Podbielska, M. Kapalla (eds.), *Predictive, Preventive, and Personalised Medicine: From Bench to Bedside*, Advances in Predictive, Preventive and Personalised Medicine 17, https://doi.org/10.1007/978-3-031-34884-6_5

NGAL	Neutrophil gelatinase-associated lipocalin
NMDA	N-methyl-D-aspartate
NS	Nervous system
NSAIDs	Nonsteroidal anti-inflammatory drugs
PBMT	Photobiomodulation therapy
PPPM	Predictive, preventive, and personalized medicine
PUFA	Polyunsaturated fatty acids
RNA	Ribonucleic acid
RPCQ	Risk of pain chronification questionnaire
SHS	Suboptimal health status
SIRT3	Sirtuin 3
SNRIs	Serotonin norepinephrine reuptake inhibitors
SSRIs	Selective serotonin reuptake inhibitors
TCA	Tricyclic antidepressants
TENS	Transcutaneous electrical nerve stimulation
TNF-α	tumor necrosis factor alpha
TNF-β	tumor necrosis factor beta
TRPV	Transient receptor potential V channel
UGT	Urogenital tract
VAS	Visual analogue scale
VEGF	Vascular endothelial growth factor

1 Educational Background

1.1 Pain

Pain is defined by the International Association for the Study of Pain (IASP) as: "An unpleasant emotional and sensory experience that is associated with, or described as, potential or actual tissue damage. Pain is always subjective".

Pain is a complex sensation, processed by branched, hierarchically arranged neural networks in several cortical and subcortical centers of the brain (the so-called Pain Matrix as a specialized part of the "Neuromatrix") [1–5].

Pain is a subjective perception, each person perceives it individually. It arises during the development of an individual on the basis of repeated experience with pain, with its individual experience and reaction to it. The onset of pain takes place in four basic phases, described in detail by the American neurosurgeon Loeser in 1982. In the so-called **the conceptual model of pain** (Fig. 1) recognizes the phase of nociception (somatic component), pain (sensory component), suffering (affective component), and the phase of subsequent painful behavior (behavioral component) [6].

Acute pain is a symptom, it is a part of many pathological conditions, and diseases. Its role is primarily protective, the pain has a positive, warning meaning for a living organism. Its physiological significance lies in the fact that in the event of an

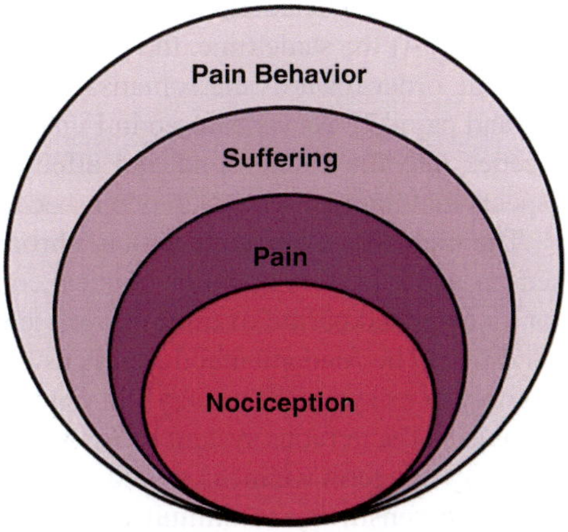

Fig. 1 Biopsychosocial model of chronic pain, Loeser's conceptual model of pain [9]

acute threat, it draws attention to the need to eliminate the cause of the damage to the organism and seek help. It is part of an archetypal attack-escape threat. Acute pain is associated with the activation of a symptomatic nervous autonomic system that responds to a "stress response" to the extent of the intensity of the stimulus and the condition of the nervous system. However, if its intensity is too strong, its metabolic, neurogenic, and immunological changes can seriously damage the patient's health. Acute pain usually lasts as long as the cause of its occurrence, respectively the healing time of the damaged tissue that causes the pain [1]. It usually does not exceed 6 weeks, but it can be considered acute for a maximum of 3–6 months [7].

Chronic pain is more difficult to define, or more precisely several aspects are needed to define it. The most commonly used time point of view defines chronic pain as lasting longer than 3–6 months. In this context, the Doyen of systematic pain treatment prof. John J. Bonica suggested that chronic pain should be defined as "pain that persists for more than one month after the end of a normal healing period, or is associated with a pathological process that causes it to persist or recur for months to years" [8]. Although a certain period of time is required for the onset of chronic pain (i.e., the transition from acute to chronic pain, chronification), the emphasis on time is inaccurate and simplistic in its definition [1]. A similar, often used characteristic of chronic pain, such as "pain lasting longer than the expected healing time" [9], says nothing about its pathophysiological nature.

The distinction between acute and chronic pain is based not only on the time factor, but also on other differences [10]. The fundamental differences defining chronic pain in contrast to acute pain are therefore not only in its symptomatology (especially its duration, its nature, psychological changes, etc.), but especially in the evolving pathophysiological changes. Nervous system accompanied by typical "painful behavior." Chronic pain is a separate disease with complicated aetiology, pathophysiology, and symptoms. Even for the polymorbid patient, it often becomes the most important source of impaired quality of life and suffering. It is the understanding of the manifestations and dynamics of changes in the painful behavior of the patient who can decisively clarify the presence of chronic pain. In some cases, the presence of nociception, a painful afferent from the damaged area, is not even necessary. At the same time, the phases of the conceptual model can develop in the opposite order towards the somatisation of subjective experience of mental suffering and pain [7]. As we can see in Fig. 1, in the case of chronic pain, a nociception recedes into the background and affective, cognitive, evaluative, and behavioral aspects that interact with each other, become more important [11].

The transition from acute pain to chronic, the so-called **Pain chronification** is a serious and relatively common medical condition in which patients suffer from pain for an extended period of time that exceeds the time normally expected to treat the condition. The fundamental differences defining chronic pain versus acute pain are not only in its symptomatology, but especially in the developing pathophysiological changes in the nervous system (NS), which can be described by the term "sensitization." By this term we mean a kind of "sensitization" of the nervous system, i.e., its excessive sensitivity to stimuli and at the same time its excessive reactivity. It expresses an increased response to the supply of information from the environment, which is able to overwhelm, disrupt, and eventually disable the pain inhibitory mechanisms. This process is very dynamic, evolves over time and involves a number of pathological restructuring changes in the nervous system in its metabolism, function, and structure (the so-called **pathological neuroplastic changes**), which can lead to dysfunction and in extreme to failure of transmission and modulation nociceptive systems.

Chronic pain is often referred to as "**pathological**" but also as "**dysfunctional" pain**. It is the understanding of the manifestations and dynamics of changes in the painful behavior of the suffering patient that can decisively clarify the presence of chronic pain. Thus, chronic pain meets the criteria for progressive central nervous system (CNS) dysfunction with the development of pathological neuroplastic changes at the level of axons, synaptic connections, receptor complexes, neurotransmitter function, etc., and can be understood as central neurogenic pain. According to the International Association for the Study of Pain (IASP) [12], chronic pain is defined as "pain of no apparent biological value that persists after the normal expected time of tissue healing (which is usually 3 months)" [13, 14].

Unlike an acute pain, **chronic pain is a complex disease** of both central and peripheral NS with polymorphic symptoms and persistent suffering. In the process of **chronifying of acute pain**, it is important to gradually change the significance of individual **components of pain**. Raudenská states that in chronic pain, nociception relatively recedes and affective, cognitive, evaluative, and behavioral aspects, which, together with somatic ones, interact with each other gradually become more important [11]:

1. **In the somatic component**, chronic pain is characterized over time by varying intensity, localization, nature of pain (prickly, dull, burning, etc.), lowered threshold for shortening of skeletal muscles (especially neck muscles, trapezoid muscles, and others) and their failure to respond to physical release techniques, various visceral symptoms of increased sympathetic tension (cardiac, digestive) and many others.

2. **In the psychological component**, chronic pain is often manifested by insomnia, mood disorders (anxiety, depression.), anhedonia, loss of appetite, weight disproportion, loss of libido, loss of interests, energy, increased fatigue, power reduction, lack of concentration, etc. The emotional component of pain is characterized by anger, fear, anxiety, or a sad, pessimistic mood with feelings of hopelessness, that the treatment will last for the rest of life.
3. **The cognitive component** of chronic pain is represented by ideas about the origin and maintenance of pain, views on treatment and its evaluation, feelings of possible guilt (own or others), subjective feelings of inperformance, use and effect of coping strategies and more.
4. **The behavioral component** is characterized by painful behavior. We can define it as a set of psychic phenomena, subjectively felt by the sufferer himself/herself, i.e., as their experience of the situation with the subsequent and reaction to them. Objectively, then, painful behavior can be perceived as an observable activity, i.e., a specific physical activity [11]. Individual aspects of painful behavior (motor, emotional, cognitive, physiological) form a system, the components of which interact with each other. Typical painful behaviors may include limiting or avoiding activity, lying during the day, taking protective and relieving attitudes, muscle tension, grimacing, sighing, seeking social support, drug abuse, re-seeking medical care, re-hospitalizations, coercion financial and social benefits, etc. [15].

2 General Conditions Stimulating Chronic Pain

In the diagnosis and treatment of chronic pain, unfortunately, physicians usually do not know exactly what causes the chronification of acute pain in their patients. A better understanding of these processes is therefore of great importance for the prediction and subsequent prevention of pain chronification and is fully in line with the position of European Association for Predictive, Preventive, and Personalized Medicine (EPMA) in the field of PPPM [1, 16–18].

Several factors play an important role in the process of transition from acute—normal pain to chronic—pathological pain. Among them, not only the intensity and duration of acute pain dominate, but also the gradual failure of the hitherto functional segmental, descending and supraspinal pain inhibitory system.

At least **two conditions must be present for the onset of chronic pain**, which can in principle be divided into peripheral and central. Must be present:

1. Sufficiently long-term and intensive nociceptive afferent of pain impulses from the area of damage to the CNS (peripheral cause of chronic pain).
2. Predisposed, “latent” situation of sensitization of CNS structures (central cause of chronic pain).
   (a) **The persistence of pain pulse transmission** from the periphery to the Pain matrix can have several causes:
      - **Wrong diagnosis of the cause of pain** through the fault of healthcare professionals, where the source of pain is not remedied at all and the

patient is being treated for a completely different diagnosis. It can also be a delayed treatment or a poorly chosen treatment of a known cause. However, one of the most common reasons in this area is that with current treatments we are not able to causally eliminate the source of the patient's pain, i.e., we cannot cure the patient. Of course, this cannot be a reason why, even in the acute stage of the disease, we should not at least try to alleviate his pain and suffering.

- it is also quite often **patient's non-cooperation with the health care system**, e.g., such as ignoring the symptoms of the disease, not finding adequate help, not accepting the recommended treatment, etc.

(b) **Disruption of central pain processing** is the second, central condition for pain chronification. Under normal, physiological conditions, the CNS effectively filters excessive painful afferents in the event of severe acute pain, thus preventing the possibility of impairing the normal functioning of the nociceptive nervous system. However, the CNS may be in a state of disturbance of the dynamic balance of its activity, which is conditioned by disturbance of the action (synthesis, action, degradation) of neurotransmitters with the predominance of the influence of excitatory molecules over inhibitory ones. In particular, the CNS (even before an obvious harmful stimulus) may be at some degree initially very discreet "hyperexcitated," which in the clinic may not yet show significant physical or mental symptoms. Rather, we can observe only slight **signs of irritation** in the patient, both **psychological**, such as nervousness, irritability, lacrimosity, insomnia, anergy, concentration problems, etc. and on the other hand, where with a careful history and examination we can register the **physical** persistence of shortening of the neck (or other) muscles, a reduced pain threshold, but also sensory sensations (hypersensitivity to sounds, light, etc.). Various manifestations of **vegetative imbalance** are also present, such as oppression, palpitations, hypertensive disease (often drug-resistant), dyskinesia of digestive tract—including irritable bowel syndrome and reflux disease, sweating, peripheral congestion disorders, and many other manifestations of sympathetic tone predominance.

The reasons for this sensitive setting of the nervous system can be various, but in principle (as we have mentioned above) it is probably a relative predominance of secretion of excitatory neurotransmitters over inhibitory, respectively reduced synthesis of inhibitory neurotransmitters in the synaptic cleft. However, this hypersensitive, neurasthenic setting may be somewhat innate, constitutive in the patient.

At present, chronic pain is understood as a **biopsychosocial phenomenon**, as a result of the interaction between physiological, emotional, motivational, and cognitive processes. For chronic pain, the question often arises as to whether the pain is somatic or psychogenic. The dualistic model of the origin of pain is as follows: pain arises from nociception (i.e., primary tissue damage) or suffering (primary psychological damage). Both forms of pain are related to stress. During life, a number of minor stressful events also affect a person, which can contribute to the onset and maintenance of pain [11].

3 Stressful Situations as a Cause of Chronic Pain

Based on clinical experience more than 30 years of pain medicine practice we can assume that the diffuse disturbance of neurotransmitters levels described above is caused by a chronic, sufficiently intense and long-lasting stress situation, or also by acute, very intense stress. In patients with chronic pain, we most often encounter the following **stressful situations** in practice (see also Fig. 2):

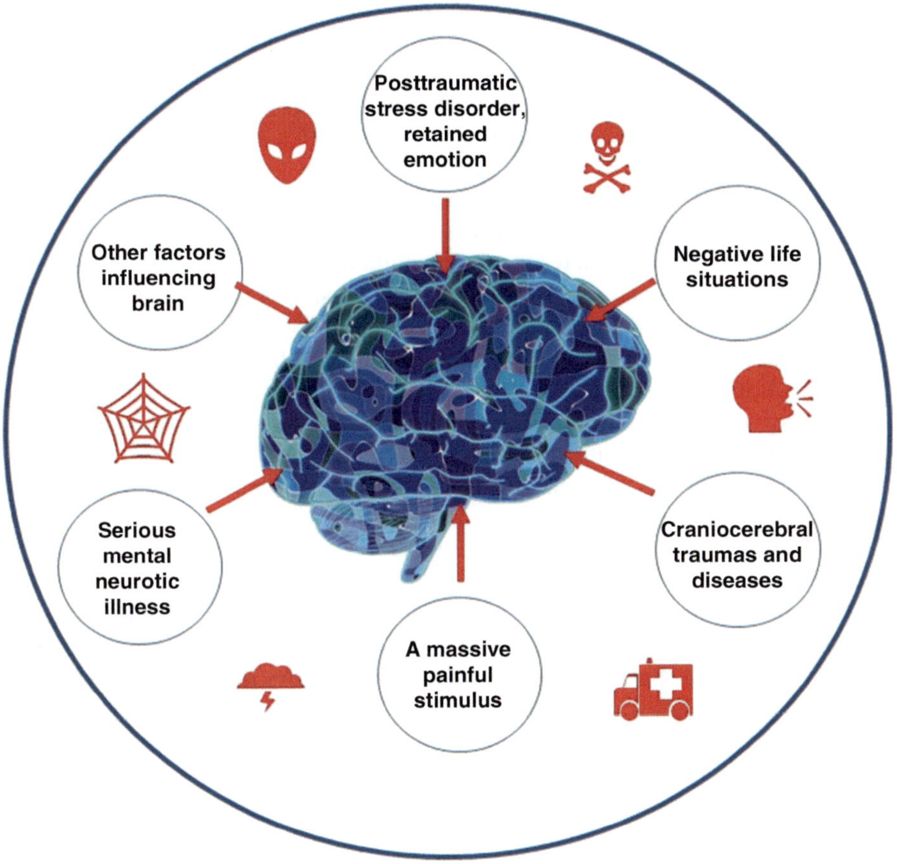

Fig. 2 An outline of particular stressful situations which may contribute to the nervous system sensitization and development of chronic pain. Not essentially all factors are named in the figure but the idea is more clear using this visualization. Our thanks go to Geralt Altmann from Pixabay for sharing his picture of the brain under Pixabay licence at the site https://pixabay.com/sk/illustrations/mozog-biol%c3%b3gia-abstraktn%c3%a9-veda-951874/

1. **Chronic post-traumatic stress disorder** is a condition in which the integration of a traumatic experience into other everyday experiences fails [19]. These are persistent **uncompensated psychotraumas** from the patient's past, usually after surviving serious life situations such as the death of a loved one, divorce, long-term suffering with a violent partner, but also sexual and other parental abuse, car accidents, natural disasters and wars and many other hardships. These often persist displaced in the patient's subconscious, usually in the form of unprocessed experiences and **retained emotions** [20] which are probably the cause of the gradually emerging imbalance of neurotransmitters at the expense of inhibitory substances (poetically called "hormones of happiness").
2. In most patients with whom we encounter in everyday pain medicine practice, the dominant etiological factors of chronic pain appear to be **less intense, but long-lasting negative life situations**. These are situations that come with everyday life and can be encountered by anyone. They do not always have the features of serious "psychotrauma," but rather they are life-uncomfortable and disruptive to the well-being and happiness of a person. Most often we can encounter long-term discomfort in the home or work environment, dissatisfaction with the social situation, the consequences of neighborhood disputes, underestimation and misunderstanding by the environment, but also chronic physical overload, burnout, e.g., for teachers, health professionals, etc.
3. **Craniocerebral traumas and diseases** with the development of chronic post-concussion syndrome as a result of either mild brain injury (coma, concussion) in about 5% of patients, or more often severe contusion brain injuries (brain contusion), or other brain damage, e.g., after a sudden stroke, brain surgery, encephalitis, etc. The result may be the development of similar chronic diffuse biochemical, metabolic brain damage, and somatic, cognitive, and psychological symptoms [21].
4. **A massive painful stimulus** of sufficient intensity and duration, usually associated with severe traumatic devastating injury, such as limb loss, etc.
5. **Serious conditions of mental illnesses**, poorly responding, even resistant to adequate psychiatric treatment, the most common anxiety-depressive mood disorders, generalized anxiety disorder, etc.

The common denominator of the above conditions is the **stress stimulus of excessive intensity**, which acts on the central nervous system. Subsequently, the **disruption of the dynamic balance of excitatory and inhibitory neurotransmitter levels** arises and further deepens with a reduction in the production of inhibitory mediators and an increase in excitatory mediators. The reason may be the need for the neuromatrix, often for a long time (months and years) to calm, suppress or inhibit stress-induced excessive irritation of the brain, which is a very metabolically demanding process. The result can be a significant decrease, even depletion of stocks of building materials and energy reserves for the synthesis of the necessary receptor complexes, neurotransmitters and other membrane and cytosolic structures of neurons with inhibitory function. Subsequent progressive irritation affects the sensitive and motor functions of the nervous system, including the vegetative system (with a predominance of sympathetic activity) and the associated hormonal imbalance.

However, these observations would deserve further, more detailed clinical research, as there is not enough relevant data in the literature and the situation may in fact be different. Such a status of patient's health can be easily described as being far from optimal yet we suppose that it can be reversible under early preventive and truly personalized measures. That is why we see the potential of combination of the tools for suboptimal health status assessment [22–25], and tools for determination of chronic pain predisposition as suggested further.

Based on the above information, we can imagine the **process of chronification of pain** in such a way that practically the entire nervous system is latently sensitized, excited and ready, waiting for a suitable trigger moment. It can also be, for example, a physiological pain in an uncomplicated operation, injury, or disease with a normal course. Although the intensity of this initiating pain may not be significant, it is sufficient that it is relatively excessive to overwhelm a poorly functioning nociceptive (transmission, perceptual, and modulatory) system, which can then relatively quickly (during several weeks) to develop a state of sensitization. This begins the process of developing changes that lead to chronic pain.

4 Stages of Chronic Pain

According to the above model of acute pain chronification, we can distinguish the following three stages in the development of chronic pain [1, 4, 18]:

1. **Latent stage**, the stage of neuromatrix sensitization in which the conditions for the development of chronic pain are already prepared, non-specific symptoms of sensitization of NS are present, but the pain is not yet present.
2. **Prodromal stage**, at the beginning of which the initiating normal painful stimulus (operation, injury, painful illness) is intense enough to overcome the disturbed pain inhibitory mechanisms, which starts a cascade of further progression of functional and structural changes nociceptive system. The present pain persists despite the healing of its cause, it intensifies, pain begins to limit the affected person's activities, the first signs of modified pain behavior appear.
3. **Manifested stage** is characterized by more or less fully developed symptoms of chronic pain with an individual combination of somatic and psychological symptoms with painful behavior, in the somatic area the pain usually manifests in a weakened area or system of the body (the so-called locus minoris resistentiae).

5 The Most Common Clinical Characteristics of Chronic Pain

Chronic pain is manifested by a set of symptoms on a somatic, mental, and social level. In clinical practice, we usually meet them with each patient in an individual combination. However, some symptoms are present in most patients, some of which we have already mentioned in the previous text.

At the **somatic level**, we often observe easier shortening of skeletal muscles, predominantly in the neck, trapezoid muscles, reduced pain threshold, but also sensory sensations (hypersensitivity to sounds, light, and other), as well as imbalance of the **autonomic nervous system** and subsequently also the functions of the visceral organs of the gastrointestinal tract (GIT), urogenital tract (UGT), cardiovascular system (CVS), etc. (in terms of excitation, spasms), e.g., palpitations, hypertension, GIT dyskinesia—including reflux disease and irritable bowel syndrome, sweating, peripheral circulatory disorders, and many more. It is also common not to respond to standard medical procedures (e.g., to appropriately selected analgesics) and to a paradoxical worsening of pain after therapy (e.g., after well-indicated physical therapy, prehabilitation, rehabilitation, etc.).

In the **psychological field**, patients with chronic pain regularly encounter various degrees of mood disorders, especially in the form of anxiety-depressive disorder, which itself can further worsen the experience of chronic pain. We also see a wide range of emotional changes, such as various fears, phobias, anger and aggression, a negative worldview and hopelessness, but also panic, psychosensitive irritability, self-blame, catastrophic tendencies, sleep disorders, anergy, etc. The patient's personality type (e.g., hypochondriac, neurotic, anxiety, and others) can also affect pain perception and experience.

In the **social field**, chronic pain significantly affects the patient's life, especially by limiting his work, social and cultural habits. On the contrary, the patient's social environment can significantly affect his attitude to experience chronic pain. Chronic patients often use their suffering for personal gain in the company of their loved ones. The so-called Rentier syndrome in an effort to obtain inadequate relief and financial benefits. It is well known that there are significantly fewer patients with chronic pain from the environment of managers and self-employed people with higher education than in the group of unemployed and with lower education.

6 Pathological Processes in Chronic Pain: Nervous System Sensitization

Chronic pain is characterized not only by its duration, but above all by clinical characteristics resulting from a complex of dynamic pathophysiological changes in the nervous system. These pathological changes in function and later in structure not only characterize chronic pain, but it also directly creates and provides its maintenance and progression. The preconditions for the development of changes in the nervous system, which characterized chronic pain, are, in particular, persistent nociceptive transmission, which may precede or immediately follow the gradual development of **sensitization of the nervous system**. It is mainly based on the development of pathological neuroplastic changes in Pain Matrix.

Pathological changes in various neuronal nociceptive structures relate initially to functional and later also to structural neuroplasticity. Changes in functional plasticity are at the molecular, synaptic and cellular levels up to changes in the function of the neural network, when more cell groups respond synchronously to harmful stimuli by increasing the generation of impulses by the spinal neural network with the emergence of the so-called **wind-up phenomenon**. Changes in structural plasticity are manifested mainly by an increase in the size and density of synaptic spines. The neural axons can respond to persistent nociceptive activity in two ways: by sprouting and producing of new connections (sprouting), or by degeneration. Neurocytes, which can also proliferate (e.g., microglia and astrocytes) or atrophy (e.g., loss of inhibitory interneurons), react similarly [1, 26].

Peripheral tissue damage or nerve injury often leads to various conditions of pathological pain, such as spontaneous pain, hyperalgesia, and allodynia, which can persist for years to decades after the healing of the injured tissues has ended. Although peripheral neuronal mechanisms (such as nociceptor sensitization and neuroma formation) also contribute to the development and maintenance of pathological pain, current evidence also points to an important role for changes in central neuronal functions [14]. Due to the processes of central sensitization, harmful stimuli can cause chronic pain, respectively misinterpretation of harmless stimuli (secondary hyperalgesia and allodynia).

Thus, the **pathological neuroplastic changes** associated with chronic pain affect to some extent all structures of both peripheral and central nervous system, especially synaptic connections, receptor membrane complexes, neurotransmitters production, as well as changes in the shape and number of neuronal axons and dendrites. Chronic irritation of nociceptive pathways mainly results in changes in the functional sensitization of membrane ion channels with subsequent gene expression (C-fos gene) and changes in the function of perisynaptic region receptors (their types, structures, affinities) and neurotransmitter levels (e.g., increased substance P synthesis, calcitonin gene related peptide—CGRP—on Aβ fibers and neurons of dorsal spinal horns). The penetration of Aβ fibers into the gelatinous substance and the formation of synaptic connections to C fibers in this area, the expansion of neuronal reception areas and the extinction of inhibitory interneurons occur. The pain is chronifying [27, 28].

As a result of these dysregulating neuroplastic changes, **NS sensitization** (represented by the "wind-up" phenomenon), functional and anatomical changes in the neural structures of the pain pathway with impaired pain transmission and inhibition and long-term changes in neuronal functions arise. The most important changes in neuronal functions in the chronification of pain include increased sensitivity and neuronal excitability of the afferent part of spinal neurons, decreased activity of inhibitory mechanisms facilitating painful transmission, increased excitability of posterior root ganglion cells, but also the development of ectopic activity on damaged or neuroplastic altered neurons and glia activation. In the clinical picture, these changes condition the development of the mentioned allodynia, hyperalgesia, spontaneous pain, and hyperpathia (with an increased response to painful stimuli).

7 Potential Markers for the Prediction and Prevention of Chronic Pain in the Context of Suboptimal Health Status

On the basis of our long-term clinical experience with Chronic Pain Management, as well as published global clinical research [1, 4, 18, 29], we can assume that chronic pain conditions are most common due to chronic, sufficiently intense, individual and long-lasting stressful situations and influencing factors as outlined in Fig. 2. These factors, together with a set of clinical signs of sensitization, as discussed further, can serve as **specific predictors** of pain chronification from the point of view of PPPM, as well as objects of interest in targeted prevention in specific individuals. Here again we want to emphasize the important relation between pain chronification and **suboptimal health status** (SHS). According to the definition the SHS is a physical state between health and disease, and is characterized by the perception of health complaints, general weakness, low energy, decline in vitality within a period of 3 months and it is regarded as a subclinical, reversible stage of chronic disease [22–25]. We suggest that particular conditions for pain chronification may very well be understood as belonging or creating the conditions for suboptimal health status and should be taken into consideration in a complex application of PPPM principles in future healthcare as we outline in the other chapter dealing with "prehabilitation" as a practical application of prediction, prevention and personalized attitude in a hospital.

Just as in the case of SHS, the most basic method for assessing individual patient assumptions for pain chronology is a form of well-designed **questionnaire**, combined with substantiated theoretical and practical **diagnostic methods**. The chronic post-traumatic stress disorder mentioned above can serve as an example of such a condition, but also the less intense, but long-lasting negative life situations, which make life-uncomfortable, reduce the level of well-being and happiness of a person. We must also mention the recent global preventive measures taken to combat the COVID-19 pandemic, which undoubtedly also cause mental, social, and physical stress. We reiterate that craniocerebral trauma with chronic post-seizure syndrome is also a common cause of CNS sensitization. In these cases, it is not only a brain and spinal cord injury, but also other brain damage, e.g., sudden stroke, encephalitis, intoxication, and other CNS disorders.

8 Clinical Symptoms of CNS Sensitization

An essential element of primary and secondary prevention, as well as of the treatment of chronic pain, is the identification of the presence of individual clinical signs of CNS sensitization. The most important of them are as follows:

1. facilitated skeletal (neck) muscle shortening,
2. the absence of objective findings despite polymorphic subjective difficulties,

3. manifestations of excessive sympathicotonia—hypertensive disease and/or tachycardia unresponsive to pharmacotherapy, spasms, and imbalance of gastrointestinal motility,
4. failure to respond to standard medical procedures,
5. paradoxical deterioration after rehabilitation and after invasive therapeutic procedures,
6. polymodal pharmacotherapy intolerance,
7. chronic fatigue syndrome,
8. excessive meteosensitivity,
9. condition after craniocerebral trauma of the CNS—of both, less serious nature (fall on the back), and of serious nature (head injury, brain surgery, coma, contusion, acute stroke, etc.)
10. reporting "whole body pain",
11. lacrimosity,
12. sleep disorders,
13. depressive—anxiety disorder,
14. rating your pain intensity on a 10-point Visual Analogue Scale (VAS) as "10 or more";
15. neurasthenic behavior,
16. persistent dissatisfaction with current treatment,
17. consequences of serious negative life situations (psychotraumas),
18. discomfort and dissatisfaction at home (broken relationships, loneliness, etc.)
19. discomfort and dissatisfaction at work (burnout, bullying),
20. purposeful action with an effort for material or social benefits from the present disease (the so-called Rentier syndrome).

9 Laboratory and Epigenetic Markers of Chronic Pain Can Complement the Markers of Nervous System Sensitization

Although older studies found that **biochemical markers** are not specific for chronic pain [30, 31], the more recent publications summarize quite a lot of interesting and promising markers like, among others, in urine it is methylmalonic acid, xanthurenic acid, homocystein, matrix metalloproteinases MMP-9, also neutrophil gelatinase-associated lipocalin (NGAL), vascular endothelial growth factor (VEGF), in serum there are pro inflammatory cytokines such as interleukines (IL-4, IL-6, IL-8, IL-10, IL-17, IL-21), tumor necrosis factor alpha (TNF-α), hs-CRP, in blood the level of T_H17 lymphocytes, in cerebrospinal fluid it is arginin vasopressin, somatostatin, tumor necrosis factor beta (TNF-β), endotelin 3, and other [32–34].

While many of the mentioned markers correlate with severity of pain and inflammation rather than with the predictive potential, and, as generally known, prolonged inflammation can cause various chronic painful disorders [34], still the early determination of their levels before the surgery, or medical procedure, may very well be combined with the information about potential neural system sensitization in the particular patient. And it may as well be combined with assessment of the suboptimal health status which takes into consideration also a psychological status that is affected by the same external factors, for example, long-lasting stressful situations that may cause neural sensitisation [22, 24, 25].

Moreover, some of these biochemical markers, many of them related to the diet and lifestyle, are routinely measured in the clinical labs and offer a possibility for targeted preventive actions within the process of prehabilitation which can further be supported by nutrition profiling that would include particular markers. Among such markers that can be relatively easily monitored in the clinical laboratory there are: vitamin D, vitamin B12, vitamin B6, coenzyme Q10, glutathione, homocysteine, n-3 PUFA (linoleic acid, EPA, DHA), zinc, selenium, magnesium, 4-hydroxynonenal (4-HNE), malondialdehyde (MDA), whose early determination prior to the planned surgery can contribute to the prediction of pain chronification as well as it can help in personalized therapy and monitoring after the surgical/medical procedure undergone by the patient [32, 34–37].

There are also studies which link chronic pain to the **epigenetic factors** influencing particular methylation sites at concrete regions of human DNA [38]. Other studies show that DNA methylation markers in T cells could serve as "predictors" of pain sensitivity and potentially chronic pain [39]. This kind of analysis, however, is rather complicated for being implemented in the routine processes of healthcare at the current state of the technology in the vast majority of hospital laboratories. Although the predictive potential for pain chronification on the basis of specific epi/genetic analyses (DNA methylation, histone acetylation, mi RNA, etc.) is, undoubtedly, very high, we don't expect that these tests will become a routine in the near future so that we propose more feasible way of pain chronification prediction which would proceed from the specific questionnaire with combination of measurement of biochemical markers. Moreover, the very factors (see Fig. 2) which the questionnaire is focused on to identify, may contribute to chronification of pain via changing particular genes' expression [38] thus causing pain hypersensitivity in the patient who may possibly be early identified on the basis of well-designed predictive questionnaire.

10 Role of Mitochondrial Health in Prediction of Chronic Pain

In the context of another chapter of this book dedicated particularly to the mitochondrial health and its role for PPPM/3 PM here we want to emphasize the interrelations between the topics. The mitochondrial dysfunction has been linked to chronic pain through several mechanisms mediated via mitochondrial electron transport chain, mitochondrial permeability transition pore, apoptotic pathways, calcium homeostasis, reactive oxygen species. It was suggested that mitochondrial energy generating system and mitochondrial reactive oxygen species play important roles in the pathogenesis of chronic pain [40, 41]. We want to stress that monitoring of mitochondrial health may serve as yet another marker since the improper function of mitochondria in the cells of a patient indicate that there is the potential for pain chronification. Moreover, this knowledge provides the tools and strategies for personalized therapies and interventions based on dietary supplements. Antioxidants such as vitamin C and vitamin E show additive antinociceptive (pain reducing) effects after peripheral nerve injury [34, 35].

Numerous studies have also reported that polyphenols, biologically active phytochemicals with flavonoids being among them, have antioxidant and anti-inflammatory properties and ability to activate sirtuin 3 (SIRT3), a mitochondrial protein directly or indirectly controlling antioxidant enzymes such as manganese superoxide dismutase (MnSOD). Other findings also demonstrate that restoring mitochondrial functions and protecting activity of sirtuin 3 by natural antioxidants such as mentioned polyphenols, could be beneficial during oxidative-stress-induced allodynia and hyperalgesia. Besides, re-establishing the activity of SIRT3 by polyphenolic fractions of particular plant extracts may serve as a new target in therapeutic intervention for the management and rehabilitation of pain-suffering patients [36, 42, 43].

11 Role of Microbiome in the Personalized Prediction and Prevention of Pain Chronification

Although this topic goes far beyond the scope of our chapter, we cannot omit yet another possibility for complex intervention in the case of predicting and preventing chronic pain through the particular mechanisms of the gut–brain axis. The studies show various links between pain, inflammation, immunity, and gastrointestinal microbiota. Thus preventive action in pain chronification may also lead, in parallel to other preventive actions, to supporting healthy microbiome via well-designed personalized diet based on the analysis of nutritional status and patient's gut microbiome [34, 37, 44–47]. Such an attitude is well in agreement with prehabilitation process, as discussed in the particular chapter of this book, and with practical application of PPPM in the procedures of future healthcare.

12 Standard Prevention of Chronic Pain

By understanding the pathophysiological characteristics of thc pain chronification process, we are able to identify this condition in the patient and recognize risk factors for each stage of chronic pain. As a result, we are able to identify and apply at each stage an individually selected combination of preventive and therapeutic approaches to minimize suffering associated with chronic pain and subsequently to mitigate the socio-economic impact of chronic pain.

In clinical practice, we can distinguish two types of **chronic pain prevention**:

1. **primary prevention**: it is an effort to prevent the development of chronic pain, i.e., that the chronification process of acute pain does not even start. As these

measures should be performed at the latent or early prodromal stage of chronification, they are non-standard for the pain specialists and rather concern the work of general practitioners and specialists in the treatment of acute pain in individual specialties. In any case, they relate to the influence of the peripheral component of pain, which can be influenced by effective preemptive and postoperative analgesia, infiltration of the surgical incision, etc., as well as the central component of pain, when it is necessary to identify or predict or therapeutic procedures, planned operation, etc.

2. **secondary prevention**: it is aimed primarily at reducing the spectrum and reducing the intensity of progression of chronic pain symptoms, as well as alleviating the consequences and complications of the manifest stage of chronic pain. This is already mostly in the hands of the pain specialists.

13 Chronic Pain Pharmacotherapy Algorithm

The success of the treatment of chronic pain lies in understanding the pathophysiological changes associated with sensitization of the nervous system and in deploying the right combination of drugs individually for the patient. When striving for complexity and purposefulness of the therapeutic procedure, it is necessary to influence the central and peripheral component of chronic pain and at the same time to time the individual therapeutic steps correctly. This process of complex treatment of chronic pain is structurally illustrated by the so-called **Chronic pain pharmacotherapy algorithm**, which emphasizes the need to combine pharmacists from different groups influencing several levels of the nervous system that are involved in the development of pain [1]:

1. **Stimulation of damaged and failing central pain inhibition.** In pain medicine practice, it is often necessary firstly to stimulate and stabilize impaired pain inhibition mechanisms (segmental, descending, and central), usually by using an appropriate antidepressant (from the group of Tricyclic antidepressants (TCA), Selective serotonin reuptake inhibitors (SSRIs), and Serotonin norepinephrine reuptake inhibitors (SNRIs)), administered for a long time (on average 1 year) in a low dose once a day, but also transcutaneous electrical nerve stimulation (TENS), but also others.
2. **Stabilization of the present CNS sensitization.** N-methyl-D-aspartate (NMDA) receptor antagonists (e.g., ketamine, nonsteroidal anti-inflammatory drugs—NSAIDs), transient receptor potential V channel (TRPV) agonists (capsaicin) and potassium channels (flupirtine), as well as antidepressants (TCAs, SSRIs, SNRIs) as an antinociceptives or "antisensitising" drugs, that stimulate central inhibitory mechanisms, or opioids, anxiolytics, neuroleptics, calcium channel blockers and many others. There is, too, possible to use some non-pharmacological procedures (such as psychotherapy, autogenous training, targeted motivation, TENS), and others.

3. **Reduction of nociceptive peripheral afferentation.** In addition to strengthening the central component of pain, we must also secure the reduction of excessive nociceptive afferentation from the periphery in different ways. This is either.
   (a) by reducing the generation of pain impulses (the so-called pain generator) either by **controlling sterile inflammation** at the site of tissue damage by applying anti-inflammatory drugs (NSAIDs, corticoids) or,
   (b) by trying to **reduce ectopic excitation** by anticonvulsants (pregabalin, gabapentin, carbamazepine) and on the one hand,
   (c) by **reducing painful transmission** by applying regional anesthesia techniques at the level of the spinal cord, nervous plexus, and peripheral nerves (by local anesthetics in the role of Na^+ channel blockers).

   Depending on the patient's condition, we can apply them either at the same time as the pharmacotherapy is started, or only after the effect of this treatment. In clinical practice, it is really interesting to see how a few hours of limiting the supply of painful impulses coming from the point of origin to the spinal cord can allow to reconstruct segmental and supraspinal "defense" (inhibitory mechanisms) of the central nervous system with consequent improvement in patient pain and suffering.
4. **Ensuring current analgesia.** In addition to the above-mentioned therapeutic interventions, we strive to ethically ensure quality up-to-date analgesia according to the principles of the analgesic ladder with the application of non-opioid and opioid analgesics, adjuvant drugs, non-pharmacological procedures, etc.

14 Suggested Strategy for Prevention of Chronic Pain from the PPPM Point of View: Creating a Questionnaire as a Research Tool for Pain Chronification Prediction and Its Relation to the Assessment of the Suboptimal Health State and the Possibilities of Photobiomodulation Therapy in Management of Chronic Pain

In the previous text we hypothesized that the above spectrum of pathognomonic symptoms, typical of the presence of CNS sensitization and usually leading to chronic pain, can be used to predict the risk of pain chronification in the context of PPPM as well as in the context of established SHS assessment. Based on these assumptions, we believe that from a PPPM perspective, these symptoms may serve as specific predictors of pain chronification. The most basic method for assessing the patient's individual assumptions for pain chronification is the form of a suitably designed **questionnaire**, combined with substantiated theoretical and practical scientific diagnostic methods.

Creating a questionnaire as a sophisticated research tool is a relatively complex professional activity, but even so, it is the most frequent research method in biomedical research. Questionnaire research is a good choice as it provides us with a wide range of information from a large number of respondents and may very well extend the information potentially acquired by analyzing particular biomarkers of chronic pain, inflammation, malnutrition, and SHS.

In addition to the prediction of pain chronification, from the PPPM/3 PM point of view we must emphasize also preventive therapy and management of chronic pain by particular diet as outlined in the literature [34, 36, 37, 42, 43] and non-phamacological interventions using modern photobiomodulation therapy (PBMT), formerly known as low level laser light therapy (LLLT) [48] which has effect on the mitochondrial processes, apoptosis, inflammation, and other which may be linked to pain at different levels [49–53].

15 Risk of Pain Chronification Questionnaire

The questionnaire we are currently working on is named "**Risk of Pain Chronification Questionnaire**" (RPCQ). It is designed the way that will allow a patient to fill it him/herself—usually before the first, initial algesiological examination. Thematically, it touches the level of somatic or unspecified mental attributes. It further examines the anxiety and depression of the patient. The topics of questions complement each other in order to achieve the main goal—to detect risk factors, predictors of pain chronification, or to reveal the occurrence of predictive factors that can detect and especially quantify the risk of transition of acute pain to chronic. The scoring system identifies the degree of **risk of pain chronification**. Based on the total score obtained, we will be able to determine the degree of risk of acute pain chronification (ranging from none to clearly present signs of chronic pain). The questionnaire is currently undergoing the validation process in our hospital and will be published to share the experience with worldwide scientific community.

16 Practical Significance of the Questionnaire for the Prehabilitation Processes in the Future Healthcare Set Up in the Context of PPPM

The questionnaire has two potential benefits. On one hand, it is the detection of the degree of sensitization in the patient, the detection of risk factors that could lead to the process of transition from acute pain to chronic pain but eventually it can reveal the presence of chronic pain as the disease itself, if not properly and early managed ahead of the medical procedure.

The second important significance of this questionnaire lies in the fact that it is able to detect the risk of surgery failure due to the existence of CNS irritation and sensitisation in the preoperative period. In clinical practice, we sometimes encounter a situation where, despite the standard preoperative and perioperative course, the result of the operation did not turn out well. The patient is dissatisfied, constantly complaining of pain in the surgical wound, suffers from insomnia, mood disorders, and develops persistent postoperative pain. This situation leads to various misunderstandings between the surgeon and the patient, and it is usually the patient who ends up with, at best, being labeled as "maladapted patient." Thus, the key question is not if we can, even in the preoperative period, predict whether and in whom such a postoperative complication can occur but rather how we should do it the most feasible and effective way to prevent it from happening.

In the field of planned surgical procedures in the preoperative and perioperative period—the use of the concept of **Enhanced Recovery After Surgery** (ERAS) [54] is known in healthcare. ERAS is a multimodal perioperative care designed to achieve early recovery in patients undergoing major surgery. ERAS represents a paradigm shift in perioperative care in two directions. First, it re-examines traditional practices and, where necessary, replaces them with evidence-based best practices. Second, it is complex in its scope and covers all areas of the patient's pathway through the surgical process which is well in an agreement with complex attitude of PPPM.

It is known that the key factors that keep patients in the hospital after surgery and prevent them from rapidly returning home, include the need for parenteral analgesia or the need for intravenous fluids, e.g., in intestinal dysfunction. Central elements of the ERAS pathway address these key factors and help elucidate how they interact to influence a patient's recovery. In addition, ERAS provides advice to all those present and involved in the perioperative care process and helps them work as a well-coordinated team in providing the best care. ERAS minimizes the occurrence of complications, leads to a faster recovery, shortens the hospital stay. It consists of various interventions, whether preoperative, perioperative or postoperative.

In the context of the principles and visions of PPPM/3 PM it is very important to emphasize the role of the preoperative period that is essential for preoperative optimization and prehabilitation—the common intention is compensation of comorbidities. In the field of prehabilitation, particular approaches are implemented that are crucial for the best outcome of the medical procedure. For example, well prepared patient (prehabilitated) should undergo evaluation of the nutritional status and consequent improvement of this status on the basis of particular laboratory tests if necessary. Furthermore, it is psychological grounding, suboptimal health status assessment, pain chronification questionnaire, and other evaluations of the factors having influence on the particular medical procedure. The essence is that it is no longer possible to achieve the optimal functional capacity of the patient or his/her optimal psychological/physical/nutritional status postoperatively, which is too late, and only 40% of patients regain their initial functional status postoperatively.

And it is in this preoperative period, within ERAS and prehabilitation that the immense potential of the well-designed questionnaire that is currently, as described above, being under validation process in our hospital, and its predictive power will rise even more in synergy with the suboptimal health status assessment [22–25] In practice, the patient pre-operatively completes a questionnaire, which is then evaluated by an ERAS specialist.

- If none or the first risk level (level 0 or 1) of pain chronification is detected, prehabilitation continues, the operation is recommended to the patient.
- If a low risk of chronification (level 2) is detected after completing the questionnaire, the patient must undergo a psychological examination and, based on the

psychological examination, the operation is recommended or postponed—then the patient must undergo a psychological intervention.
- If, after completing and evaluating the questionnaire, the third or fourth risk degree of chronification is classified (i.e., high risk of chronification or chronic pain is present)—the operation is postponed, psychological examination follows and the patient's sensitization must be treated.

We anticipate the completion of the validation process for predicting the risk of pain chronification by the end of 2022. After the validation, we plan to apply it in the clinical practice of several workplaces of pain specialists, surgeons, general practitioners and other specialists, especially within the ERAS system. Expected benefits of the questionnaire implementation for prediction of pain chronification in clinical practice we plan to share through scientific publications and we also plan to share the experience and facilitate implementation of PPPM in the hospital environment in cooperation with other institutions worldwide.

17 Conclusion and Recommendations

The need for determination of risk factors or predictors that support and/or describe the process of pain chronification follows from our long-term experience in daily routine practice in the field of Pain medicine as well as it is emerging from the scientific knowledge accumulated to date.

Nervous system sensitization plays a key role in the transition from acute to chronic pain. The occurrence of certain factors, predictors, is clearly associated with the phenomenon of pain chronification. Recognizing, identifying, and using them as predictive markers plays a key role in preventing chronic pain as well as providing targeted and personalized treatment. Therefore, the detection of these factors, which are directly related to the phenomenon of pain chronification, plays a key role not only in pain medicine but also in the practical implementation of the concept of predictive, preventive, and personalized medicine, where by detecting these factors we can prevent suffering from pain and reduce the risks of surgery or other medical procedures.

In the context of the main topic of the whole publication, "PPPM from Bench to Bedside," here we propose that the strategies of suboptimal health status assessment, prehabilitation procedures that include nutrition profiles assessment, mitochondrial health, and assessment of the health status for pain chronification prediction should all be combined into one complex attitude under the PPPM/3 PM strategy in the future system of healthcare worldwide. In our hospital we are working on the practical implementation of all particular attitudes benefiting primarily our individual patients as well as the whole society. An international collaboration may substantially speed up the process and catalyze the essential changes that are needed to transform the current systems of healthcare into the new, perspective, sustainable, science-and-common-sense-based system of future healthcare.

References

1. Martuliak I (2020) Patofyziológia bolesti pre klinickú prax, 2nd edn. Martimed s r.o, Banská Bystrica, p 344; ISBN 978-80-971753-2-0
2. Zimmermann M (2004) Basic physiology of pain perception. In: Lautenbacher S, Fillingim RB (eds) Pathophysiology of pain perception. Plenum series in rehabilitation and health. Springer, Boston, MA, pp 1–24. https://doi.org/10.1007/978-1-4419-9068-6_1
3. McMahons SB, Koltzenbrug M, Tracey I, Turk DC (2013) Wall & Melzack's textbook of pain, 6th edn. Elsevier Health Sciences, Saunders, Philadelphia, PA, p 1184; ISBN: 978-0-7020-4059-7
4. Morlion B, Coluzzi F, Aldington D, Kocot-Kepska M, Pergolizzi J, Mangas AC, Ahlebeck K, Kalso E (2018) Pain chronification: what should a non-pain medicine specialist know? Curr Med Res Opin 34(7):1169–1178. https://doi.org/10.1080/03007995.2018.1449738
5. Van Griensven H, Strong J, Unruh A (2013) Pain—a textbook for health professionals, 2nd edn. Churchill Livingstone, London, p 448; ISBN: 978-0-7020-3478-7
6. Loeser JD (1982) Concepts of pain. In: StantonHicks M, Boas R (eds) Chronic low back pain. Raven Press, New York, NY, p 146
7. Neradílek F (2006) Bolest jako syndrom. In: Rokyta R et al (eds) Bolest: monografie algeziologie, 1st edn. Tigis, Praha, pp 22–26; ISBN 80–903750–0-6
8. Bonica JJ (1980) Pain. Raven Press, New York, NY, p 391; ISBN 0890043760
9. Turk DC (2001) Pain terms and taxonomies. In: Loeser JD et al (eds) Bonica's management of pain, 3rd edn. Lippincott Williams & Wilkins, Philadelphia, PA, pp 18–25; 2067–2079, ISBN 0-683-30462-3
10. Ševčík P, Čumilivski R (2006) Akutní bolest. In: Rokyta R et al (eds) Bolest: monografie algeziologie, 1st edn. Praha, Tigis, pp 202–225; ISBN 80-903750-0-6
11. Raudenská J (2012) Biopsychosociální model chronické nenádorové bolesti. In: Paliatívna medicína a liečba bolesti, vol 5(1), pp 27–29; ISSN 1337–6896
12. IASP. https://www.iasp-pain.org/. Accessed 8 Aug 2022
13. Bubnov RV (2012) Evidence-based pain management: is the concept of integrative medicine applicable? EPMA J 3:13. https://doi.org/10.1186/1878-5085-3-13
14. Coderre TJ, Katz J, Vacarrino AL, Melzack R (1993) Contribution of central neuroplasticity to pathological pain: review of clinical and experimental evidence. Pain 52(3):259–285; ISSN 0304–3959
15. Raudenská J, Javůrková A (2003) Kognitivně behaviouralni terapie deprese, generalizované úzkostné poruchy a panické úzkostné poruchy u chronicke bolesti. Bolest 1:8–16; ISSN 1212–0634
16. EPMA. https://epmanet.eu. Accessed 8 Aug 2022
17. Martuliak I (2019) Farmakoterapia bolesti pre lekárov a farmaceutov. Martimed s ro, Banská Bystrica, p 302; ISNB 978-80-971753-1-3
18. Apkarian AV, Baliki MN, Farmer MA (2013) Predicting transition to chronic pain. Curr Opin Neurol 26(4):360–367. https://doi.org/10.1097/WCO.0b013e32836336ad
19. Tucker W (1998) Recognition and management of posttraumatic stress disorder: approaches for the practitioner. J Pract Psychiatry Behav health 4(1):20–27; ISSN 1076–5417
20. Hašto J, Vojtová H (2012) Posttraumatická stresová porucha, bio-psycho-sociálne aspekty EMDR a autogénny tréning pri pretrvávajúcom ohrození: prípadová štúdia, 1st edn. Univerzita Palackého v Olomouci, Olomouc, p 186; ISBN 978-80-244-2944-1
21. Sivák Š, Nosá V, Kurča E (2013) Súčasné názory na problematiku ľahkého mozgového poranenia. In: Neurológia pre prax, vol 14(2), pp 74–77; ISSN 1335–9592
22. Yan YX, Liu YQ, Li M, Hu PF, Guo AM, Yang XH, Qiu JJ, Yang SS, Wang W (2009) Development and evaluation of a questionnaire for measuring suboptimal health status in urban Chinese. J Epidemiol 19(6):333–341
23. Wang W, Tan X (2020) Suboptimal health status and cardiovascular deficits. In: Golubnitschaja O (ed) Flammer syndrome. Advances in predictive, preventive and personalised medicine, vol 11. Springer, Cham, pp 287–315. https://doi.org/10.1007/978-3-030-13550-8_17

24. Zhu J, Ying W, Zhang L (2020) Psychological symptoms in Chinese nurses may be associated with predisposition to chronic disease: a cross-sectional study of suboptimal health status. EPMA J 11:551–563. https://doi.org/10.1007/s13167-020-00225-y
25. Wang W, Yan Y, Guo Z, Garcia M, Tan X, Anto EO, Mahara G, Zheng Y, Li B, Kang T, Zhong Z, Wang Y, Guo X, Golubnitschaja O (2021) All around suboptimal health—a joint position paper of the suboptimal health study consortium and European association for predictive, preventive and personalised medicine. EPMA J 12:403–433. https://doi.org/10.1007/s13167-021-00253-2
26. Li J, Simone DA, Larson AA (1999) Windup leads to characteristics of central sensitization. Pain 79(1):75–82. https://doi.org/10.1016/s0304-3959(98)00154-
27. Gold MS, Gebhart GF (2010) Nociceptor sensitization in pain pathogenesis. Nat Med 16(11):1248–1257. https://doi.org/10.1038/nm.2235
28. Farinelli I, Dionisi I, Martelletti P (2011) Rehabilitating chronic migraine complicated by medication overuse headaches: how can we prevent migraine relapse? Intern Emerg Med 6:23–28. https://doi.org/10.1007/s11739-010-0410-9
29. Golubnitschaja O, Baban B, Boniolo G, Wang W, Bubnov R, Kapalla M, Krapfenbauer K, Mozzafari M, Costigliola V (2016) Medicine in the early twenty-first century: paradigm and anticipation–EPMA position paper 2016. EPMA J 7:23. https://doi.org/10.1186/s13167-016-0072-4
30. Lucas HJ (2006) Fibromyalgia-new concepts of pathogenesis and treatment. Int J Immunopathol Pharmacol 19(1):5–10; ISSN: 0394-6320
31. Russell IJ (2004) The fibromyalgia syndrome: a clinical case definition for practitioners. CRC Press, Boca Raton, FL, p 140; ISBN 978-0789025746, (Journal of Musculosceletal Pain)
32. Gunn J, Hill MM, Cotten BM, Deer TR (2020) An analysis of biomarkers in patients with chronic pain. Pain Physician 23(1):E41–E49; https://www.proquest.com/openview/b0eb368948ba36af477f6f2daeca07f7/1?pq-origsite=gscholar&cbl=5453642
33. Hagedorn JM, Gunn J, Budwany R, D'Souza RS, Chakravarthy K, Deer TR (2021) How well do current laboratory biomarkers inform clinical decision-making in chronic pain management? J Pain Res 14:3695–3710. https://doi.org/10.2147/JPR.S311974
34. Rondanelli M, Faliva MA, Miccono A, Naso M, Nichetti M, Riva A, Guerriero F, De Gregori M, Peroni G, Perna S (2018) Food pyramid for subjects with chronic pain: foods and dietary constituents as anti-inflammatory and antioxidant agents. Nutr Res Rev 31(01):131–151. https://doi.org/10.1017/s0954422417000270
35. Lu R, Kallenborn-Gerhardt W, Geisslinger G et al (2011) Additive antinociceptive effects of a combination of vitamin C and vitamin E after peripheral nerve injury. PLoS One 6:e29240
36. Ilari S, Giancotti LA, Lauro F, Gliozzi M, Malafoglia V, Palma E, Tafani M, Russo MA, Tomino C, Fini M, Salvemini D, Mollace V, Muscoli C (2020) Natural antioxidant control of neuropathic pain—exploring the role of mitochondrial SIRT3 pathway. Antioxidants 9(11):1103. https://doi.org/10.3390/antiox9111103
37. Philpot U, Johnson MI (2019) Diet therapy in the management of chronic pain: better diet less pain? Pain Manag 9(4):335–338. https://doi.org/10.2217/pmt-2019-0014
38. Ren K, Bai G (2019) An overview of epigenetic correlates of human chronic pain conditions. epigenetics of chronic pain. In: Bai G, Ren K (eds) Translational epigenetics, epigenetics of chronic pain, vol 7. Academic Press, pp 183–228. https://doi.org/10.1016/B978-0-12-814070-3.00011-9; ISBN 9780128140703
39. Massart R, Dymov S, Millecamps M et al (2016) Overlapping signatures of chronic pain in the DNA methylation landscape of prefrontal cortex and peripheral T cells. Sci Rep 6:19615. https://doi.org/10.1038/srep19615; https://www.nature.com/articles/srep19615
40. Sui B, Xu T, Liu J, Wei W, Zheng C, Guo B, Wang Y, Yang Y (2013) Understanding the role of mitochondria in the pathogenesis of chronic pain. Postgrad Med J 89(1058):709–714. https://doi.org/10.1136/postgradmedj-2012-131068

41. Koklesova L, Mazurakova A, Samec M, Kudela E, Biringer K, Kubatka P, Golubnitschaja O (2022) Mitochondrial health quality control: measurements and interpretation in the framework of predictive, preventive, and personalized medicine. EPMA J 13:177–193. https://doi.org/10.1007/s13167-022-00281-6
42. Mazurakova A, Koklesova L, Samec M, Kudela E, Kajo K, Skuciova V, Csizmár SH, Mestanova V, Pec M, Adamkov M, Al-Ishaq RK, Smejkal K, Giordano FA, Büsselberg D, Biringer K, Golubnitschaja O, Kubatka P (2022) Anti-breast cancer effects of phytochemicals: primary, secondary, and tertiary care. EPMA J 13:315–334. https://doi.org/10.1007/s13167-022-00277-2
43. Kubatka P, Mazurakova A, Samec M, Koklesova L, Zhai K, Al-Ishaq R, Kajo K, Biringer K, Vybohova D, Brockmueller A, Pec M, Shakibaei M, Giordano FA, Büsselberg D, Golubnitschaja O (2021) Flavonoids against non-physiologic inflammation attributed to cancer initiation, development, and progression—3PM pathways. EPMA J 12:559–587. https://doi.org/10.1007/s13167-021-00257-y
44. Pusceddu MM, Gareau MG (2018) Visceral pain: gut microbiota, a new hope? J Biomed Sci 25(1):73. https://doi.org/10.1186/s12929-018-0476-7
45. Probert L, Quintana FJ, Bar-Or A (2020) Editorial: update on translational neuroimmunology—research of ISNI 2018. Front Immunol 11:11. https://doi.org/10.3389/fimmu.2020.02012
46. Jogia T, Ruitenberg MJ (2020) Traumatic spinal cord injury and the gut microbiota: current insights and future challenges. Front Immunol 11:704. https://doi.org/10.3389/fimmu.2020.00704
47. Cady N, Peterson SR, Freedman SN, Mangalam AK (2020) Beyond metabolism: the complex interplay between dietary phytoestrogens, gut bacteria, and cells of nervous and immune systems. Front Neurol 11:11. https://doi.org/10.3389/fneur.2020.00150
48. Anders JJ, Lanzafame RJ, Arany PR (2015) Low-level light/laser therapy versus photobiomodulation therapy. Photomed Laser Surg 33(4):183–184. https://doi.org/10.1089/pho.2015.9848
49. Tomazoni SS, Costa LOP, Joensen J, Stausholm MB, Naterstad IF, Leal-Junior ECP, Bjordal JM (2019) Effects of photobiomodulation therapy on inflammatory mediators in patients with chronic non-specific low back pain: protocol for a randomized placebo-controlled trial. Medicine (Baltimore) 98(15):e15177. https://doi.org/10.1097/MD.0000000000015177
50. Tripodi N, Feehan J, Husaric M, Kiatos D, Sidiroglou F, Fraser S, Apostolopoulos V (2020) Good, better, best? The effects of polarization on photobiomodulation therapy. J Biophotonics 13:e201960230.1–e201960230.9. https://doi.org/10.1002/jbio.201960230
51. Salehpour F, Mahmoudi J, Kamari F, Sadigh-Eteghad S, Rasta SH, Hamblin MR (2018) Brain photobiomodulation therapy: a narrative review. Mol Neurobiol 55(8):6601–6636. https://doi.org/10.1007/s12035-017-0852-4
52. Jahani- Sherafat S, Mokmeli S, Rostami-Nejad M, Razzaghi Z, Rezaei Tavirani M, Razzaghi M (2020) The effectiveness of photobiomudulation therapy (PBMT) in COVID-19 infection. J Lasers Med Sci 11(suppl 1):S23–S29. https://doi.org/10.34172/jlms.2020.S4
53. Bjordal JM, Lopes-Martins RAB, Joensen J, Iversen VV (2010) The anti-inflammatory mechanism of low level laser therapy and its relevance for clinical use in physiotherapy. Phys Ther Rev 15(4):286–293. https://doi.org/10.1179/1743288x10y.0000000001
54. ERAS. https://erassociety.org/. Accessed 8 Aug 2022

Prevention and Prediction of Body Posture Defects in Children Aged 5–6 Years

Barbara Cieślik

Abbreviations

BMI	Body Mass Index
N	Number of children tested
p	P value
PPPM	Predictive, preventive, and personalized medicine
WHO	World Health Organization

1 Introduction

The prevalence of postural defects in children and adolescents has been of concern to those concerned with the development of the younger generation for years [1]. Posture is called the way an individual hold themselves in a free-standing position, and the external manifestation of this is the mutual spatial arrangement of the various parts of the body and the silhouette of a person. Posture is similar but not identical in all people—it is an individual trait [2]. Posture according to Kasperczyk's definition, is the arrangement of individual body parts, not affected by pathological changes, providing optimal stability of the body requiring minimal muscular effort and "creates conditions for optimal positioning of internal organs" [3]. By abnormal posture we mean one in which, due to the occurrence of a defect, deformities have occurred in the formation of the spine, chest, pelvis, lower limbs or feet [4]. The greatest risk of developing abnormal posture is during the period of rapid growth,

B. Cieślik (✉)
Faculty of Health and Physical Culture Sciences, Witelon Collegium State University, Legnica, Poland

H. Podbielska, M. Kapalla (eds.), *Predictive, Preventive, and Personalised Medicine: From Bench to Bedside*, Advances in Predictive, Preventive and Personalised Medicine 17, https://doi.org/10.1007/978-3-031-34884-6_6

i.e., between the ages of 5 and 7, and adolescence, i.e., between the ages of 12 and 16 [5]. However, it should be noted that some deviations from normal posture are physiological for a certain age. Until about age 6, lumbar hyperlordosis is present, and the formation of spinal curvatures occurs at age 7. The ontogeny of the development of the lower extremities is distinguished by greater variability. Up to the age of 3 years, the characteristic feature is the scoliosis of the knees. At the age of 4–6 years, physiological valgus of the knees occurs [6]. Schildt showed that the changes that occur in the musculoskeletal system at the age of 5–7 are genetically determined, while external factors (including the influence of physical activity) have a significant impact along with the improvement of the function of the musculoskeletal system [4]. According to Prof. Wiktor Dega, a postural defect is a set of postural errors defined as a small single deviation from normal posture that can be corrected with appropriate passive and active exercises [6].

Data from the Center for Health Information Systems shows that spinal deformities were diagnosed in 17.14% of children and adolescents aged 0–18 and in 9.7% of those aged 2–9. Changes in skeletal elements directly related to the spine (thorax, pelvis) and disorders of the upper and lower extremities account for 45–55% of all postural defects [2, 6].

Factors that contribute to postural defects include: poorly chosen learning positions, inappropriate positions during rest, genetic diseases, bad dietary habits leading to overweight and obesity, overtiredness, vision and hearing defects, and low levels of physical activity [6, 7]. Overweight parameters are as follows: for females, body mass index (BMI) 25–30 and for males, BMI 26–30. Obesity parameters are as follows: class I—BMI 30–35; class II—BMI 35–40; class III—BMI > 40. According to the World Health Organization (WHO), in 2016, 50 million girls and 74 million boys around the globe were registered as being obese [8]. In Germany approx. 1.9 million children and adolescents are overweight, and among these 800,000 are obese. In the USA the number increased from around 5% in the 60 s/70 s to 17% in 2003/04. In Europe approx. Five percent of the children aged 5–17 year are concerned [9]. Pubertal gender dichotomy of girls accumulating fat vs. boys losing fat and growing muscles and height illustrates an obesity-related aspect of gender differential adaptation to scarcity and women's advantage [10]. Posture can also be affected by age, gender, race, somatic structure of joints, bones and muscles, mental state, including stress, and sports practiced [11, 12]. Nowadays, the increasing prevalence of postural defects seems to be most influenced by low levels of physical activity and the rising rates of overweight and obesity observed in the population of preschool and school-aged children. This is primarily due to a sedentary lifestyle associated with low physical activity and a tendency to spend leisure time in front of the computer or television. Undoubtedly, the occurrence of postural defects is related to the lifestyle. Lifestyle is a term to describe the way individuals, family circles, and societies live and which behavior they manifest in coping with their physical, psychological, social, and economic environments on a day-to-day basis. Lifestyle is expressed by daily work and leisure profiles, including activities, attitudes, interests, opinions, values, and allocation of income. From a psychological point of view lifestyle derives from people's self-image or self-concept (the way they see themselves and believe they are seen by the others), including self-esteem and self-efficacy [13]. Overall results reported in 2008 by the National Institute of Public Health indicate that physical activity in Poles is too low, and activity in children and adolescents is declining in older age groups [14]. Table 1 illustrates the characteristics of normal posture and faulty posture. Abnormal posture in childhood carries consequences in adulthood, such as reduced cardiorespiratory and lung capacity, pain in the spine and related structures, and displacement of internal organs [15].

Postural defects are any deviation from normal posture. They are fixed changes in the skeletal apparatus that cause various types of dysfunction. Tadeusz Kasperczyk says that postural defects are deviations from the generally accepted characteristics of normal posture, appropriate for a given age group, gender or physique. Postural defects are various types of deformities in the organs of locomotion, such as chest defects, back defects or defects of the lower extremities [7]. **The most common posture defects in children and adolescents are as follows:**

- **Round back** is characterized by excessive backward curvature of the spine. This defect is located in the thoracic region, it is known as hyperkyphosis or deepened thoracic kyphosis. In the round back, the muscles of the back are weakened and stretched: rhomboid, trapezius, neck muscles and extensors of the back, the dysfunction of which causes the torso to tilt forward, spread the shoulder blades, and put the shoulders forward. The muscles that are strained and excessively contracted are: the muscles of the thorax, the serratus and intercostal muscles.
- **Concave back** is characterized by a deepening of the lumbar lordosis, an increase in the anterior tilt of the pelvis, a protruding abdomen and a protrusion of the buttocks. In the concave back, the muscles that are excessively stretched and contracted are the straight thigh muscle, the iliac-lumbar muscle, the quadratus

Table 1 Characteristics of normal posture and faulty posture [7]

Normal posture	Faulty posture (acc. to Kasperczyk)
• Straight head alignment, • The spine is physiologically curved in the sagittal plane, and straight in the frontal plane, • Arched chest, which is the most forward part of the body, • The pelvis is supported by the heads of the femurs, • The lower limbs are straight, and the feet are properly arched	• Head protruded forward or to the side, • Chest flat, sunken or distorted, • Shoulders protruded forward, • Abdomen protuberant, protruding forward or flabby, sagging, • Back raked, rounded, and the pelvis has too much inclination, • Feet flat

lumborum muscle, and the lumbar extensor muscle of the back. Excessively stretched muscles are: gluteal muscles, ischiofemoral muscles, abdominal muscles.

- **Concave-round** back is a postural defect in which both round and concave back symptoms are present. The characteristic features of this defect are increased lumbar lordosis and deepened thoracic kyphosis. In a child with a concave back, the head is forward, not projecting onto the sternum, the chest is flattened, the shoulders are protruded, the shoulder blades are outstretched and protruding from the chest, the abdomen is flabby, the buttocks are accentuated.
- **Flat back** is a postural defect characterized by a flattening of both physiological curvatures of the spine. The reduction of physiological curvatures reduces the strength of the spine, whose normal shape—with retained curvatures—has 17 times greater strength. Untreated flat back can lead to scoliosis and inversion of the physiological curvatures.
- **Scoliosis,** known as lateral curvature of the spine, is a postural defect involving a multiplanar deviation of the spinal line from normal. This deviation occurs in the planes:
  - Frontal—the spine bends to the side, right or left,
  - Sagittal—lordotic and kyphotic bending deepens,
  - Transverse—there is rotation of the vertebrae, which leads to the formation of a hump.
- **Funnel chest** is characterized by a collapse of the sternum in the region of the xiphoid process. Here the chest is flat and flattened, the abdominal and back muscles are weakened, causing the shoulders to protrude.
- **Pigeon chest** is characterized by the fact that the sternum along with the adjacent parts of the ribs protrude significantly forward, while the distal parts of the ribs are collapsed at the sides. This defect is caused by disorders of the ossification processes.
- **Cross-knees**, this defect is characterized by an X-shaped medial alignment of the knees. The axis of the lower leg forms an outward open angle with the axis of the thigh. The peripheral segment, which is the shank, is located in abduction. We speak of cross-knees when the distance between the medial ankles exceeds 4–5 cm when the knees are compact and straightened.
- **Bow-legs**, are characterized by an inward twisting of the limb. Bow knees are diagnosed when the distance between the knees is greater than 4–5 cm (the legs take the shape of the letter "O") with the feet together. The most common cause of this defect is rickets caused by vitamin D3 deficiency, overweight children, and adolescents and prolonged sitting in a cross-legged position [7].

In Fig. 1 the relationship between risk factors, assessment of body posture, and the consequences of untreated disorders is shown.

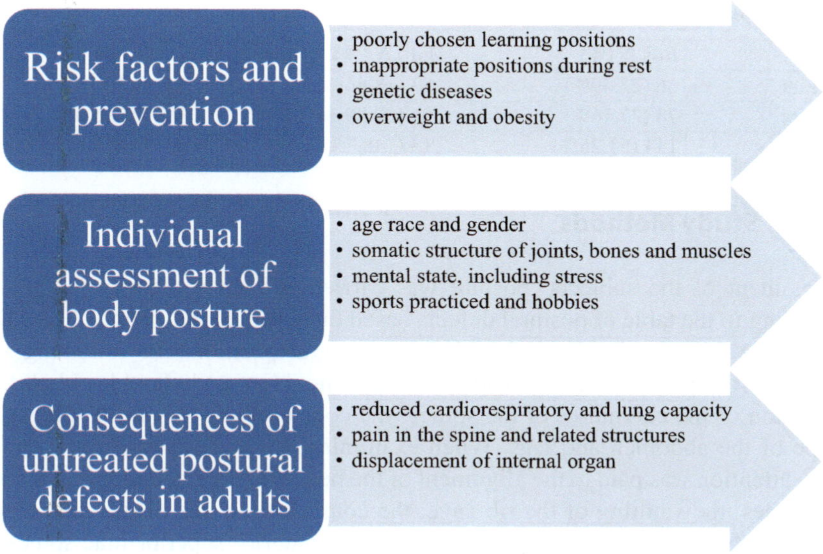

Fig. 1 Risk factors, assessment of body posture, and consequences in adulthood

Being aware of the above-mentioned problems and the predictive and preventive potential of the PPPM attitude toward the health of children, the aim of this study was to assess posture in boys and girls aged 5–6 years attending kindergartens in the city of Jawor, Poland as an example of the potential mentioned.

2 Study Group and Research Methods

The tests were conducted as part of the preventive posture testing program implemented by the Jawor District Clinic. The tests were aimed at children aged 5–6 who attend kindergarten in the Jawor municipality. Children from four public kindergartens and one non-public kindergarten were assessed. The study lasted from October 2018 to January 2019. Written consent from a parent or legal guardian was obtained for each child's participation in the study. Each parent or guardian of a child participating in the study received an examination card describing the child's posture and recommendations for further management, in case of the presence of a postural defect.

2.1 Study Group

The study group consisted of 281 children aged 5–6 years. 119 (42.35%) children were 5 years old and 162 (57.65%) were 6 years old. The majority of the study group were boys 144 (51.25%). The characteristics of the study group are given in Table 2.

Table 2 Characteristics of the study group

Age	Boy *N* (%)	Girl *N* (%)	Total *N* (%)
5 years	66 (23.49%)	53 (18.86%)	119 (42.35%)
6 years	78 (27.76%)	84 (29.89%)	162 (57.65%)
Total	144 (51.25%)	137 (48.75%)	281 (100%)

2.2 Study Methods

Assessment of the subjects' posture was carried out using the viewing method according to the table of postural defects based on modified criteria of Wiktor Dega (see Table 3) [16, 17]. In each child, in a lateral position, the following were observed: the position of the head and neck, shoulders and shoulder blades, the formation of the curvatures of the spine—the course of lordosis and kyphosis, the shape of the abdomen and legs. When examining the posture from the front and back, attention was paid to the alignment of the head and neck, shoulders and shoulder blades, the vaulting of the rib cage, the course of the line of the spinous processes of the spine, the triangle of the waist, the anterior superior iliac spines, the knees (crossed, bowed), the structure of the foot (foot: flat, valgus, inflexed). During the examination of the course of the spinal line, the child—standing with his or her back to the examiner—was instructed to perform a loose forward bend of the trunk (feet slightly apart, head and upper limbs loose). The examiner, by running the index and middle finger along the spinous processes of the spine, was able to determine (after the child returned to an upright position) whether the child had a scoliotic posture or not. List of postural defects based on Wiktor Dega's criteria:

- Head.
- Shoulders.
- Pigeon chest.
- Funnel chest.
- Hyperkiphosis.
- Scoliotic posture.
- Scoliosis.
- Hyperlordosis.
- Pelvis.
- Abdomen.
- Flat back.
- Cross-knee.
- Bow-legs.
- Flat foot.
- Valgus foot.
- Contractures:
  - Shoulder joint.
  - Hip joint.
  - Knee joint [11, 12].

Table 3 Assessment of the severity of postural defects in the children studied

Grouping variable	No defect *N* (%)	Slight defect *N* (%)	Severe defect *N* (%)
Age			
5 years	79 (28.11%)	38 (13.52%)	2 (0.71%)
6 years	107 (38.08%)	54 (19.22%)	1 (0.36%)
Gender			
Boy	84 (29.89%)	58 (20.64%)	2 (0.71%)
Girl	102 (36.30%)	34 (12.10%)	1 (0.36%)
Study population			
Total	186 (66.19%)	92 (32.74%)	3 (1.07%)

In addition, the children examined were classified into one of the three groups based on the severity of the postural defect. These groups included children without a defect, children with a mild defect that is subject to correction with corrective gymnastics and other physiotherapeutic measures, and subjects with a severe postural defect in whom surgical intervention to correct the defect should be considered.

2.3 Statistical Analysis

The obtained results of the study were subjected to statistical analysis using Statistical version 13.1 software. Normality of distribution of the studied variables was assessed using the Shapiro-Wilk test ($p = 0.50$), and homogeneity of variance was assessed using the Levene's test ($p = 0.00$). The Student's t-test for independent variables was used to evaluate differences in the incidence of postural defects by age and gender. Spearman's rank order correlation was used to evaluate the relationship between the incidence of postural defects and age and gender. The p-values were considered statistically significant for $p \leq 0.05$.

3 Results

No postural defect was found in 186 (66.19%) of the children studied. A slight defect was found in 92 (32.74%) children, and a severe defect was found in 3 (1.07%) subjects (see Table 3). The most common postural defects in the study group were asymmetry and forward tilt of the shoulders in 30 (10.68%) children, flat feet in 16 (5.69%) subjects, lower limb shortening in 11 (3.91%), and scoliosis in 14 (4.98%). It should be noted that the above-mentioned postural errors were often observed simultaneously in a single child, further increasing the prevalence. Lower limb shortening and shoulder girdle asymmetry co-occurred in 2 (0.71%) subjects, scoliosis and shoulder girdle asymmetry were observed in 13 (4.63%) children, and flat feet and shoulder girdle asymmetry were observed in 4 (1.42%) subjects (see Table 4). Statistical analyses conducted indicate differences between the prevalence of postural defects and gender ($p = 0.00$), while no such relationship was shown for age ($p = 0.30$). The majority of girls were characterized by normal

Table 4 Prevalence of postural defects in the children studied

Postural defects	Gender		Age		Total population
	Boy *N* (%)	Girl *N* (%)	5 years *N* (%)	6 years *N* (%)	*N* (%)
Normal posture	84 (29.89%)	102 (36.30%)	79 (28.11%)	107 (38.08%)	186 (66.19%)
Scoliosis	8 (2.85%)	6 (2.14%)	7 (2.49%)	7 (2.49%)	14 (4.98%)
Asymmetry and anteflexion of the shoulders	16 (5.69%)	14 (4.98%)	14 (4.98%)	16 (5.69%)	30 (10.68%)
Shortening of the lower limb	8 (2.85%)	3 (1.07%)	6 (2.14%)	5 (1.78%)	11 (3.91%)
Asymmetry of the head	1 (0.36%)	0 (0%)	0 (0%)	1 (0.36%)	1 (0.36%)
Lower limb shortening and shoulder girdle asymmetry	0 (0%)	2 (0.71%)	0 (0%)	2 (0.71%)	2 (0.71%)
Scoliosis and shoulder girdle asymmetry	8 (2.85%)	5 (1.78%)	6 (2.14%)	7 (2.49%)	13 (4.63%)
Flat feet and shoulder girdle asymmetry	4 (1.42%)	0 (0%)	1 (0.36%)	3 (1.07%)	4 (1.42%)
Pigeon/funnel chest	2 (0.71%)	0 (0%)	0 (0%)	2 (0.71%)	2 (0.71%)
Flat feet	11 (3.91%)	5 (1.78%)	6 (2.14%)	10 (3.56%)	16 (5.69%)
Hyperlordosis	1 (0.36%)	0 (0%)	0 (0%)	1 (0.36%)	1 (0.36%)
Cross-knee	1 (0.36%)	0 (0%)	0 (0%)	1 (0.36%)	1 (0.36%)

posture, while boys were more likely to have postural defects, the differences were statistically significant ($p \leq 0.05$).

4 Discussion

4.1 The Occurrence of Postural Defects and Correct Posture in Children

The growing number of postural defects is a significant social problem [18]. However, in the study presented here, the majority of the study population had normal posture. It should be borne in mind that the preschool age is characterized by a large inter-individual variation. This is not only due to the different rates of the development of basic somatic characteristics, but also to the variation in body structure and posture [16]. Similar results were obtained by Wilczyński [14], in whose study there was also a preponderance of children with normal posture, with 71.0% of the subjects, 15.0% of the subjects had concave backs, and 13.0% had flat backs. Also in the study by Drzał-Grabiec et al. [9] children with normal posture predominated, a small percentage of faulty postures (7%) was found, and no poor postures were found. Different results were observed in a pilot study conducted by Janiszewska et al. [4] where the presence of postural defects was found in as many as 93.2% of the children studied. Specific postural abnormalities of the studied population of children occur with similar frequency in both girls and boys. The most common postural abnormalities include: foot defects (78.4%), thoracic and lumbar scoliosis—combined (73.9%) and malaligned shoulder blades (59.5%).

4.2 Type and Frequency of Posture Defects

In the present study, the most common postural defects were asymmetry and anteflexion of the shoulder girdle, scoliosis, flat feet, and lower limb shortness. A similar study was conducted by Andrzejewska and Grabarczyk [19], whose goal was to demonstrate postural abnormalities in children from Wroclaw.

The authors obtained the following results: Among the analyzed postural abnormalities of children, trace scoliosis occurred in boys in an average of 36%, typical scoliosis in 3% at the age of 7–15 years. In girls, trace scoliosis and typical scoliosis were revealed in a similar percentage as in boys—37% and 3%, respectively. Shoulder asymmetry was the most common of all the postural defects analyzed, averaging 55% in boys, with more than 70% in subjects aged 8 and 15. In girls, the asymmetry averaged 56%, with the highest number of subjects with shoulder asymmetry (about 70%) registered among 7- and 14-year-old children. Among abnormalities in knee alignment, cross-knees were observed primarily among both boys and girls. In the evaluation of foot arches, flattening of the feet was found to be the most common defect. More than 35% of boys aged 9 and 11 and girls aged 8 and 10 had this defect. Flat feet were found less frequently, with the exception of 7-year-old boys (40%). There were also defects in the arches of only one of the feet. In a study by Macialczyk-Paprocki et al. [16] the most common abnormalities in the table of errors according to W. Dega concerned the foot (48.2%) and shoulders (37.2%).

The most common abnormalities were flat feet and plano valgus, as well as shoulder malalignment, which occurred significantly more often in boys, compared to girls. Cross-knees were more common in boys than in girls; the differences were not statistically significant. Bow-knees were observed in only about 3% of boys; this defect did not occur in girls. Scoliotic posture was detected in 24.7% of boys and in 20.8% of girls.

4.3 Relationship Between Posture Defects and Overweight and Obesity

The purpose of the study by Wilczynski et al. [20] was to evaluate the relationship between the anteroposterior shape of spinal curvatures and body composition in school-aged children. The study included 257 children aged 11–12 years. Normal spinal curvatures were present in 106 (41.08%) subjects. The other types of abnormalities were: decreased kyphosis and normal lordosis—40 subjects (15.50%), normal kyphosis and decreased lordosis—24 subjects (9.30%), increased kyphosis and normal lordosis, 17 subjects (6.59%), normal kyphosis and increased lordosis, 22 people (8.53%), decreased kyphosis and decreased lordosis, 32 patients (12.40%), decreased kyphosis and increased lordosis, 4 people (1.55%), increased kyphosis and increased lordosis, 13 participants (5.04%).

Another study by Maciałczyk-Paprocki et al. in 2017 [21] assessed the epidemiological prevalence of abnormal posture in overweight and obese children and adolescents residing in Poznań (Poland). The study population consisted of a representative group of children and adolescents aged 3–18 years randomly selected from dozens of kindergartens (3–6 years), elementary schools (7–12 years), and middle and high schools (13–18) in Poznań. The duration of the study was 2 years. In the entire study population (2732 subjects), postural defects were found in 67.9% of the subjects (918 boys and 938 girls). In obese children, the prevalence of postural defects was significantly higher than among normal-weight children ($p = 0.001$) and overweight children ($p = 0.0046$). Among girls and boys with excessive body weight (overweight and obese), the percentage of postural defects was highest in the group of children 7–12 years old. Despite the fact that girls with excessive body weight aged 7–12 as well as 13–18 had a higher number of postural defects than boys, the difference was not statistically significant ($p > 0.05$). The prevalence of abnormal posture in all obese boys was found to be 1.5 times higher than among normal-weight boys, but the difference was not statistically significant. In obese girls, the prevalence rate of postural abnormalities was twice that of the normal-weight group, and this difference was found to be significant ($p = 0.004$). In children aged 3–6 years, obesity and overweight do not increase the likelihood of postural defects In the group of students aged 7–12 years, the likelihood of postural defects was significantly higher in obese than in normal-weight students, both in boys ($p = 0.042$) and in girls ($p = 0.007$). Only overweight boys aged 13–18 had a significantly lower number of foot defects than their normal-weight peers ($p = 0.021$).

4.4 Foot Defects in Children

Foot defects are a common phenomenon especially in children and are a serious medical and social problem. Feet, more than other parts of the musculoskeletal system, are exposed to adverse effects of the external environment. The most important moment of foot formation is the preschool period [22]. In the present study, flat feet were present in 16 (5.69%) of the children studied, but more often in boys, i.e., in 11 cases (3.91%). The study conducted by Klimczak et al. [18] shows that among the children studied, 48% had normal feet, 25% had flat feet, and 28% had hollow feet in relation to the plantocontourogram with patterned foot types. Rykała et al. [23] observed that in loading the feet with their own body weight, as the children grew older they were characterized by worse transverse arches, while better longitudinal arches of the feet. In a study by Skowron et al. [24], 30% of children had a properly arched foot, 30% had a flattened foot, and 40% had a flat foot.

It should be emphasized that in recent years most studies on the assessment of body posture in children have been conducted by senders from Poland. This situation is evident in the research results cited above.

5 Conclusion and Recommendations

On the basis of our study we conclude and recommend for the practical application of PPPM principles the following:

1. **Normal posture** was present in 186 (**66.19%**), and **postural defects** were found in 95 (**33.81%**) of the children studied.
2. The most common postural defects were asymmetry and anteflexion of the shoulder girdle, scoliosis, flat feet, and lower limb shortening.
3. Postural defects were more common in boys, while normal posture was more common in girls.
4. The age of the children studied did not affect the prevalence of postural defects.
5. **Preventive screening of posture in children and adolescents should become a routine procedure for assessing a child's health, at each stage of development, which will help to avoid serious health consequences in the future.**
6. The use of **visual assessment of children's posture is a simple and effective method of capturing postural abnormalities and referring the child for further diagnosis and treatment.**
7. The criteria for correct posture cannot be constant and unambiguous for everyone; on the contrary, they should undergo changes depending on the child's developmental period. In this assessment, **factors such as constitutional type, sports disciplines, and forms of recreation cannot be ignored.**

References

1. Pokrywka J, Fugiel J, Posłuszny P (2011) Prevelance of postural disorders in children from copper basin in Poland. Fizjoterapia 19(4):3–10. https://doi.org/10.2478/v10109-011-0025-3
2. Górecki A, Kiwerski J, Kowalski IM, Marczyński W, Nowotny J, Rybicka M et al (2099) Profilaktyka wad postawy u dzieci i młodzieży w środowisku nauczania i wychowania—rekomendacje ekspertów. Pol Ann Med 16(1):168–177
3. Zmyślna A, Żurawski AŁ, Śliwiński G, Śliwiński ZW, Kiebzak WP (2021) Assessment of body posture of children with chest pain. Front Pediatr 9:704087. https://doi.org/10.3389/fped.2021.704087
4. Janiszewska R, Tuzinek S, Nowak S, Ratyńska A, Biniaszewski T (2009) Nieprawidłowości postawy ciała u dzieci 6-12 letnich—uczniów szkół podstawowych z Radomia—badania pilotażowe. Problemy Higieny i Epidemiologii 90(3):342–346
5. Ziętek M, Machniak M, Wójtowicz D, Chwałczyńska A (2022) The incidence of body posture abnormalities in relation to the segmental body composition in early school-aged children. Int J Environ Res Public Health 19(17):10815

6. Wawrzyniak A, Tomaszewski M, Mews J, Jung A, Kalicki B (2017) Wady postawy u dzieci i młodzieży jako jeden z głównych problemów w rozwoju psychosomatycznym. Pediatria i Medycyna Rodzinna 13(1):72–78. https://doi.org/10.15557/PiMR.2017.0007
7. Rosa K, Muszkieta R, Zukow W, Napierała M, Cieślicka M (2013) The incidence of defects posture in children from classes I to III elementary school. J Health Sci 3(12):107–136
8. Golubnitschaja O, Liskova A, Koklesova L, Samec M, Biringer K, Dietrich Büsselberg D et al (2021) Caution, "normal" BMI: health risks associated with potentially masked individual underweight—EPMA position paper 2021. EPMA J 12:243–264. https://doi.org/10.1007/s13167-021-00251-4
9. Graf C (2011) Preventing and treating obesity in pediatrics through physical activity. EPMA J 2:261–270. https://doi.org/10.1007/s13167-011-0091-0
10. Shapira N (2013) Women's higher health risks in the obesogenic environment: a gender nutrition approach to metabolic dimorphism with predictive, preventive, and personalised medicine. EPMA J 4:1; http://www.epmajournal.com/content/4/1/1
11. Wyszyńska J, Podgórska-Bednarz J, Drzał-Grabiec J, Rachwał M, Baran J, Czenczek-Lewandowska E et al (2016) Analysis of relationship between the body mass composition and physical activity with body posture in children. Biomed Res Int 2016:1. https://doi.org/10.1155/2016/1851670
12. Drzał-Grabiec J, Snela S (2012) The infuence of rural environment on body posture. Ann Agric Environ Med 19(4):846–850
13. Trovato GM (2012) Behavior, nutrition and lifestyle in a comprehensive health and disease paradigm: skills and knowledge for a predictive, preventive and personalized medicine. EPMA J 3:8; http://www.epmajournal.com/content/3/1/8
14. Permoda-Białozorczyk A, Olszewska-Karaban M, Permoda A, Zajt J, Wiecheć M, Żurawski A (2022) Evaluation of the functional status of the posture control system in children with detected disorders in body posture. Int J Environ Res Public Health 19(21):14529. https://doi.org/10.3390/ijerph192114529
15. Rusek W, Baran J, Leszczak J, Adamczyk M, Baran R, Weres A et al (2021) Changes in children's body composition and posture during puberty growth. Child 8(4):288. https://doi.org/10.3390/children8040288
16. Maciałczyk-Paprocka K, Krzyżaniak A, Kotwicki T, Kałużny Ł, Przybylski J (2011) Postawa ciała dzieci w wieku przedszkolnym. Problemy Higieny i Epidemiologii 92(2):286–290
17. Maciałczyk-Paprocka K, Krzyżaniak A, Kotwicki T, Sowińska A, Stawińska-Witoszyńska B, Krzywińska-Wiewiorowska M et al (2012) Występowanie błędów w postawie ciała u uczniów poznańskich szkół podstawowych. Problemy Higieny i Epidemiologii 93(2):309–314
18. Wilczyński J (2006) Najczęściej występujące wady postawy u chłopców w wieku 13–16 lat badanych komputerową metodą Moiré. Med Pr 57(4):347–352
19. Andrzejewska J, Grabarczyk M (2005) Charakterystyka postawy ciała dzieci wrocławskich. Słupskie Prace Biologiczne 1:7–10
20. Wilczyński J, Lipińska-Stańczak M, Wilczyński I (2020) Body posture defects and body composition in school-age children. Child 7(11):204. https://doi.org/10.3390/children7110204
21. Maciałczyk-Paprocka K, Stawińska-Witoszyńska B, Kotwicki T, Sowińska A, Krzyżaniak A, Walkowiak J et al (2017) Prevalence of incorrect body posture in children and adolescents with overweight and obesity. Eur J Pediatr 176(5):563–572. https://doi.org/10.1007/s00431-017-2873-4
22. Klimczak K, Kochański B, Kałużny K, Plaskiewicz A, Smuczyński W, Ratuszek-Sadowska D et al (2014) Analiza występowania wad stóp u dzieci w wieku 6-10 lat. J Health Sci 4(2):29–38
23. Rykała J, Snela S, Drzał-Grabiec J, Podgórska J, Nowicka J, Kosiba W (2013) Ocena wysklepienia podłużnego i poprzecznego stóp w warunkach odciążenia i obciążenia masą własną u dzieci w wieku 7–10 lat. Przegląd Medyczny Uniwersytetu Rzeszowskiego i Narodowego Instytutu Leków w Warszawie 2:183–193
24. Skowron N, Malak R, Mojs E, Samborski W (2015) Foot arch condition in comparison with the muscular balance of lower limbs in children at school age of 6–14 years. J Med Sci 2(84):85–89. https://doi.org/10.20883/medical.e21

A Powerful Paradigm: Predictive, Preventive, and Personalized Medicine with Multiomics of Human Pituitary Adenomas

Dominic M. Desiderio and Xianquan Zhan

Abbreviations

2DGE	Two-dimensional gel electrophoresis
3 PM	Predictive, preventive, personalized medicine
ACTH	Adrenocorticotropin hormone
AKT	Protein kinase B
ARE	Antioxidant response element
BMI	Body mass index
Capzb	F-actin capping protein subunit beta
CAT	Catalase
COX6B1	Cytochrome c oxidase subunit 6b1
CT	Computed tomography
DEP	Differentially expressed protein
EpRE	Electrophile response element
ERK	Extracellular signal regulated kinase
FSH	Follicle-stimulating hormone
GH	Growth hormone
GHP	Growth hormone proteoform
GHRH	Growth hormone-releasing hormone
hGH	Human growth hormone

D. M. Desiderio (✉)
Department of Neurology, The University of Tennessee Health Science Center, Memphis, TN, USA
e-mail: ddesiderio@uthsc.edu

X. Zhan
Medical Science and Technology Innovation Center, and Gastroenterology Research Institute and Clinical Center, Shandong First Medical University, Jinan, Shandong, China

H. Podbielska, M. Kapalla (eds.), *Predictive, Preventive, and Personalised Medicine: From Bench to Bedside*, Advances in Predictive, Preventive and Personalised Medicine 17, https://doi.org/10.1007/978-3-031-34884-6_7

HSP	Heat shock protein
iTRAQ	Isobaric tag for relative and absolute quantification
Jak STAT	Janus kinase signal transducer and activator of transcription proteins
Jnk	c-Jun N-terminal kinase
Keap	Kelch-like ECH associated protein
LC-MS	Liquid chromatography-mass spectrometry
LH	Luteinizing hormone
MAPK	Mitogen-activated protein kinase
M_r	Relative molecular mass
MRI	Magnetic resonance imaging
MS	Mass spectrometry
MS/MS	Tandem mass spectrometry; MS^2
NADH	Nicotinamide adenine dinucleotide
ncRNA	Non-coding RNA
NDUFS8	NADH: ubiquinone oxidoreductase core subunit s8
NF	Non-functional
NFPA	Non-functional pituitary adenoma
Nrf-2	NF-E2-related factor 2 (nuclear factor, erythroid 2)
PET	Positron emission tomography
pI	Isoelectric point
PI3K	Phosphatidylinositol 3-kinase
PitNET	Pituitary neuroendocrine tumor
PPPM	Predictive, preventive, personalized medicine
PRL	Prolactin
PRLP	Prolactin proteoform
PTM	Post-translational modification
PVDF	Polyvinylidene difluoride
RNS	Reactive nitrogen species
ROS	Reactive oxygen species
SOD	Superoxide dismutase
SS	Somatostatin
STAT3	Signal transducer and activator of transcription 3
USD	U.S.A. dollar
UV	Ultraviolet
WHO	World Health Organization

1 Introduction

We introduce a new research paradigm that involves PPPM in conjunction with multiomics to study human pituitary adenomas [1]. The goal is to clarify differences between proteins in controls versus adenomas. This research is performed within the framework of predictive, preventive, and personalized medicine (PPPM; 3 PM). Multiomics collects the variety of new methodologies developed over the past

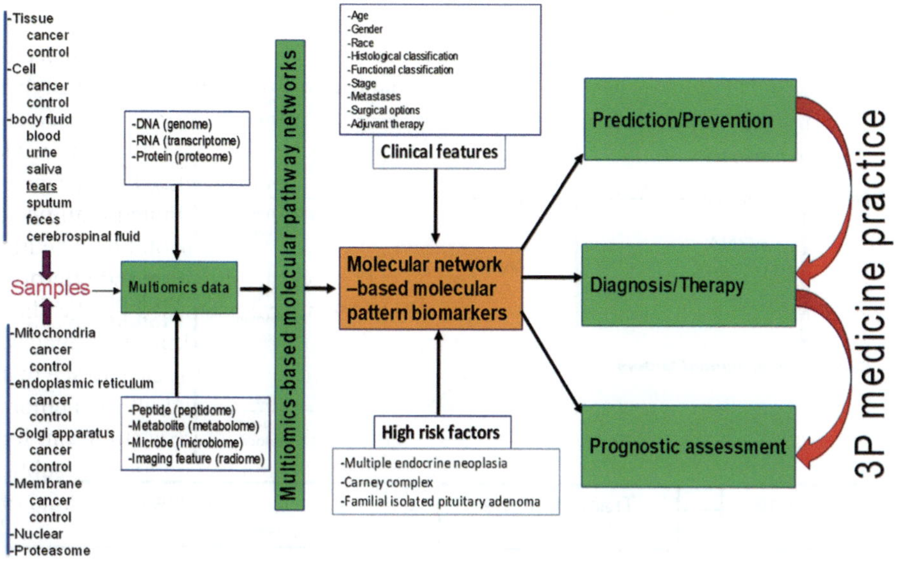

Fig. 1 The basic process of multiomics in pituitary adenomas. (Modified from Li N, Desiderio DM, and Zhan X (2021) [1], copyright permission from Wiley publisher, copyright 2021. Modified from X. Zhan, Zhou, et al. (2019) [2], copyright permission from IntechOpen publisher open-access book chapter, copyright 2019)

several years, and includes transcriptomics, genomics, proteomics, etc. (Fig. 1). We focus here primarily on the proteome and proteoforms of adenomas.

The adenohypophysis (anterior pituitary) contains corticotrophs, gonadotrophs, somatotrophs, thyrotrophs, and lactotrophs [3]. Those anterior pituitary cells are tightly regulated throughout the multiple hypothalamic-pituitary-target axes. Hypothalamic-releasing hormones transit to the pituitary to release the individual hormones from corresponding cells, and the pituitary hormones travel to their target organs. Tumors are a common disease that occurs in the anterior pituitary to affect the hypothalamic-pituitary-target axis systems and affect an individual's health. Many omics studies, especially proteomics and transcriptomics, were performed in this research to reveal the molecular changes and signaling pathway alterations in pituitary adenomas, and to discover effective biomarkers for PPPM practice.

Recently, the concept of proteome has been further developed. The traditional concept was that the canonical protein was the basic unit of a proteome. However, after a protein amino acid sequence is synthetized in a ribosome, it must be translocated to a specific location and form a spatial conformation that interacts with its surrounding molecules to form a complex to exert its final function. In the translocation process, many post-translational modifications (PTMs) form; they are important factors that yield the diversity of a canonical protein. The final structural and functional format of a gene or a canonical protein is termed a proteoform, which is the basic unit of a proteome. The estimate of the number of proteoforms is in the billions. The term "canonical protein" includes multiple proteoforms derived from

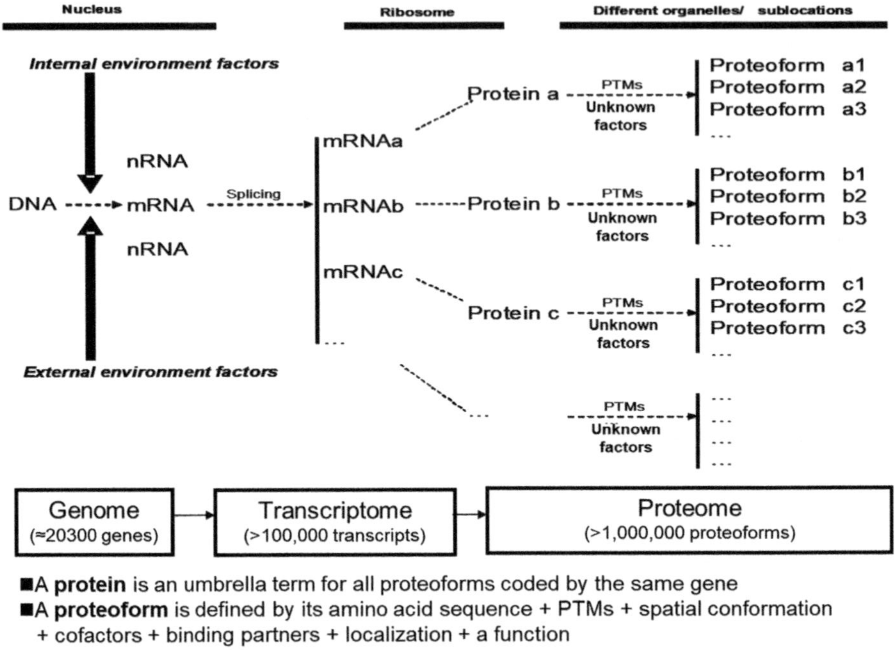

Fig. 2 Relationship of proteoform, protein, and proteome. (Modified from Zhan et al. (2018) [4], with permission from Hapres publisher open access publication, copyright 2018; and reproduced from Zhan, Li et al. (2019) [5], with permission from MDPI publisher open access publication, copyright 2019). *mRNA* messenger RNA, *nRNA* noncoding RNA, *PTM* post-translational modification

the same gene. Each proteoform has its individual isoelectric point (p*I*) and relative molecular mass (M_r). Proteoforms derive from alternate splicing, PTM, proteolysis, etc. The term "protein" collects a number of individual molecular species: precursor to the protein, amino acid sequence, PTMs, conformation, cofactors, binding partners, receptor (which is a protein with its associated proteoforms, PTMs, etc.), localization, and function of that complex (Fig. 2). Complexity increases rather than decreases as we gather more basic structural information.

This book chapter will primarily discuss the proteome changes of adenomas, and proteoforms of two anterior pituitary hormones—growth hormone (GH) from somatotrophs and prolactin (PRL) from lactotrophs.

2 Current Achievements in Pituitary Adenoma Multiomics

Approximately 20% of all intracranial tumors are pituitary adenomas; most are benign (~65%) some are invasive (~35%), and a few (~0.2%) become malignant carcinomas [6]. Some adenomas are macroadenomas (>10 mm) and some are microadenomas (<10 mm). Some are hormone-secreting, and some are non-secreting. The World Health Organization (WHO) developed a new classification system to include transcription factors in addition to immunohistochemistry and hormone secretion.

We have studied neuropeptidergic systems in human adenomas since 1985 [7, 8]. Those studies include non-functional pituitary adenomas (NFPA), invasive NFPAs, control pituitaries, and secreting adenomas (GH-, PRL-, and ACTH-secreting) [9]. A wide range of methods was used: quantitative transcriptomics (DEGs), quantitative proteomics (DEPs), proteomic mapping, nitroproteomics, phosphoproteomics, proteoformics, and metabolomics.

We have discovered in human pituitary tissues 149 new proteins, 46 GH proteoforms, nine nitroproteins, six prolactin variants, 108 ubiquitinated proteins, 56 differentially expressed proteins (DEPs), 26 phosphoproteins, and two differential peptides. As we delve deeper into the basic molecular chemistry of the pituitary, we continue to uncover more structure-rich information.

We will rationalize in the following sections these experimental data of pituitary adenomas within the PPPM framework.

3 Pituitary Hormone Proteoforms of Pituitary Adenomas Within the PPPM Framework

Human pituitary hormones such as GH and PRL are the important message factors in the hypothalamic–pituitary–target axis systems in the human endocrine system, and any changes (structural; quantitative) could significantly affect human health. The traditional opinion is that quantity changes of these hormones (GH and PRL) are the main reasons that cause GH- or PRL-related diseases. However, our recent studies based on two-dimensional gel electrophoresis in combination with mass spectrometry (2DGE-MS) discovered many proteoforms of GH and PRL, which significantly clarified and expanded our knowledge about the structure and functions of hormones, including GH and PRL.

3.1 Human Growth Hormone Proteoforms (GHPs)

GH is biosynthesized in the acidophilic somatotrophs in the anterior pituitary. We discovered 24 GHPs in our 2DGE-MS analysis of pituitaries. GH is released from the pituitary under strict regulation from hypothalamic GH-releasing hormone (GHRH). GH interacts with its receptors in the liver, free fatty acid depot, and, via a long feedback loop, the somatotropin-release inhibiting factor (somatostatin = SS) neuron in the paraventricular nucleus. SS, in turn, downregulates the release of GHRH. Tight regulation of this system is critical. If too much GH is released, then gigantism or acromegaly might occur; too little might lead to stunted growth [10].

We discovered 46 GHPs that were ubiquitinated, acetylated, phosphorylated, and deaminated. It is not known which one (or several, or many) of the GH proteoforms is released from the anterior pituitary in the GH system. Clearly, more data are needed to resolve these important clinical questions.

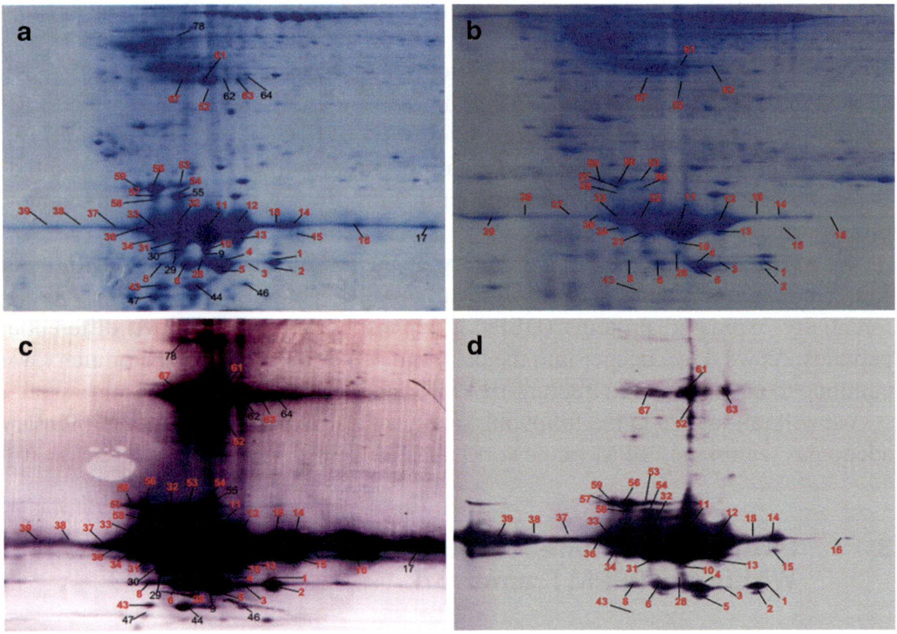

Fig. 3 2DGE-based western blot of growth hormone proteoforms (GHPs) in GH-secreting pituitary adenoma and control pituitary tissues. (**a**) Coomassie blue-stained 2D gel image (46 GHPs) in the GH-secreting pituitary adenoma tissue. (**b**) Coomassie blue-stained 2D gel image (35 GHPs) in the control pituitary tissue. (**c**) 2DGE-based western blot image of GHPs in the GH-secreting pituitary adenoma tissue. (**d**) 2DGE-based western blot image of GHPs in the control pituitary tissue. (Reproduced from Li B, et al. (2021) [13], copyright permission from Springer open access article, copyright 2021)

The GH receptor exists in an inactive homodimeric, parallel form before GH binding. After GH binding, the receptor shifts to a left-handed crossover configuration [11].

3.1.1 GHP Pattern Changes in Pituitary Adenomas

2DGE-separation, GH antibodies, mass spectrometry (MS), and MS/MS were used to characterize GHPs. In addition, three selected GHP PTMs were studied: phosphorylated (with 6-plex iTRAQ), ubiquitinated (with an anti-N_{ε}-acetyl-lysine antibody), and acetylated (with an anti-K-GG-antibody) proteomics [12]. MS and MS/MS were used to characterize each GHP and to locate each modification site. The 2D gel, after protein separation and Coomassie staining, contained ~1000 spots. After transfer to a PVDF membrane, GHPs were detected with a GH antibody and characterized with MS (Fig. 3).

3.1.2 Special Note on 2DGE

Many researchers would rather use LC-MS rather than 2DGE because 2DGE is labor-intensive. However, it is crucial that any quantitative LC-MS data demonstrate a high level of reproducibility (>96%) of LC peak retention times; similar to 2DGE spot volume and spot position data.

2DGE provides several important experimental factors: (1) a "bird's eye view" of a pituitary proteome; (2) a very high level (>96%) of within-gel and between-gel reproducibility of spot volume and spot position; and (3) most importantly, an archival storage for precious human tissue and separated proteins. The latter point is important because, whenever MS improves sufficiently, one can revisit those gels to detect and characterize low-copy number proteins.

Even more important is that significant improvements in 2DGE resolution have been published by Zhan et al. [14], who predict a 2DGE resolution of 500,000 protein species. That quantum improvement in 2DGE will impact significantly onto PPPM, and will allow the separation and characterization of proteins with a very low-copy number.

3.1.3 Discovery of 46 GHPs

We found 46 GHPs in GH-secreting pituitary adenomas and 35 GHPs in control pituitaries. Those 35 GHPs in controls were a subset contained within the 46 GHPs in pituitary adenomas. Eleven GHPs were found only in pituitary adenomas [13]. Such an extensive metabolic re-shuffling of that number of GHPs between pituitary controls and adenomas is quite significant, and leads to an important question: what metabolic dysfunction(s) occurred to create so many extensive alterations? That question requires further research.

3.1.4 Significant PTMs of GHPs

The four types of PTMs found in GHPs [13] include the following:

1. *Phosphorylation* at Ser 77, Ser 132, Ser 134, Thr 174, and Ser 176. Phosphorylation could indicate a potentially new regulatory system. Phosphorylation adds a negative charge at physiological pH. Differential phosphorylation patterns occurred between pituitary controls and adenomas.
2. *Ubiquitination* at Lys 96 was found in pituitary adenomas, but not in controls. Ubiquitination could lead to protein degradation and/or modulate a protein's metabolic activity.
3. *Acetylation* (removes a positive charge) was found at Lys 171.
4. *Deamination* (adds a negative charge) was found at Asn 178.

Again, all of those diverse, multiple PTM data indicate that extensive differential remodeling and PTM formation occur between controls and adenomas. Those differential GHP data lead to a question: What role do these multiple and diverse PTMs play in a wide range of clinically important mechanisms that include GH receptor binding/interactions, signaling pathways, homeostasis, and pathologies?

Removal of a positive charge and addition of a negative charge in GHPs could play a significant role in protein: protein interactions such as in protein: receptor interactions. For example, in the COVID-19 delta variant spike protein, Pro-681 was replaced with Arg near the furin cleavage site. Also, the omicron

MATGSRTSLLLAFGLLCLPWLQEGSAFPTIPLSRLFDNAMLRAHRLHQLAFDTYQE

FEEAYIPKEQKYSFLQNPQT-pS-LCFSESIPTPSNREETQQ-ubiK-SNLE

L L R I S L L L I Q S W L E P V Q F L R S V F A N S L V Y G A - p S - D - p S -

NVYDLLKDLEEGIQTLMGRLEDGSPRTGQIFKQTYS–acK-FDpT-N-pS-H-N*-

D D A L L K N Y G L L Y C F R K D M D K V E T F L R I V Q C R S V E G S C G F

T+S = 31 (5 were phosphorylated. S77; S122, S134, S176, T174).

N+Q = 10 (N*-178 deaminated).

K = 7 (96-ubi; 171-acetyl).

Fig. 4 GH amino acid sequence. 217 amino acids. Signal peptide 1–26 (underlined). Isoform 1 (191 amino acids; MW = 24,847 kDa)

variant has ~50 modifications in several critical binding regions. Profound biologic activity changes might also occur from these charge modifications of pituitary proteins.

Another question: what role do these PTMs play in GH receptor binding, protein interactions, and signaling pathways? Changes in the charge of particular amino acids could increase or decrease the strength of protein: protein binding.

All of these protein data are substantiated with MS/MS amino acid sequence data, which are assembled via tryptic peptide analysis, and incontrovertibly identify each protein. When we use the name of a protein, that means that we know the protein. *No other analytical method provides critical amino acid sequence information of a protein at endogenous biological levels.*

Furthermore, it is quite helpful to illustrate the location of each amino acid modification that we found in GHP. Figure 4 highlights in different colors the modified K, N, T, and S amino acid residues that we discovered during our recent studies. It is clear that the amino acid sequences contained within the region residues 171–178 constitute a highly modified region. GH contains two anti-parallel alpha-helices that, most probably, contribute to the access of those particular residues to modification mechanisms.

3.1.5 Signalomics of GHPs

All GHPs (except for one GHP, T46) found in this study derived from mature GH; that finding means the signal peptide 1–26 was removed from the GH prehormone. These significant data indicate that a potential regulatory system, or a dysregulated system, might participate in the formation of pituitary adenoma.

3.1.6 Splicing Variants of GHPs

Alternative splicing is an important factor to produce protein diversity. Human GH has four splicing variants [15] that include: splicing variant 2 (removal of amino acid sequence 58–72); splicing variant 3 (removal of amino acid sequence 111–148); and splicing variant 4 (removal of amino acid sequence 117–162); all from the normal GH (GH variant 1) [16]. We found that two GHPs were splicing variant 2, one GHP was splicing variant 3, 43 GHPs were splicing variant 1 (normal GH), and no splicing variant 4, in GH-secreting pituitary adenomas. Three GHPs were splicing variant 2, 32 GHPs were splicing variant 1 (normal GH), and no splicing variants 3 and 4 were found in control pituitaries [13]. Those multiple, diverse, and significant differential splicing variant patterns found between pituitary adenomas and controls reflect differential biosynthetic patterns that were significantly altered between controls and adenomas. More-detailed knowledge of the basic molecular, enzymatic, and PTM mechanisms that produce those differential patterns might help to clarify the pathophysiology of pituitary adenomas.

3.1.7 Rationale for Different GHPs

Several factors that contribute to the different amounts and structures of the GHPs include:

1. *Certain genes*. STAT3 induces GH-secreting pituitary adenoma cell growth. Genes bind specifically to the hGH promoter to induce transcription to further promote GH secretion.
2. *Alterations* in cell-cycle regulation and growth-factor signaling; epigenetic changes (DNA methylome; histone modification) lead to gene mutations for GH hypersecretion.
3. *Mis-translation*: source of great diversity.
4. *PTMs* that impact structure and function of proteins include glycosylation, phosphorylation, acetylation, ubiquitination, deamidation, nitration, plus others. Those PTMs allow for an exponential increase in the number of proteoforms.

3.1.8 Strengths, Weaknesses, and Future GHP Studies. An Important Question for PPPM: Which GHP Interacts with the GH Receptor?

The *strengths* of this GH study include solid experimental protocols and the unambiguous amino acid sequence data that elucidated the molecular basis of differential GHP patterns. The *limits* of this study are the small sample size and the need for more tissue samples. However, it is difficult to obtain pituitary controls (post-mortem) and adenomas (post-surgery).

Future studies include several important factors: (1) serum GH proteoform patterns, which could be an effective biomarker for PPPM to treat GH-secreting pituitary adenomas and GH-related diseases; (2) GHP interactions with its GH receptors; and (3) include other PTMs.

A very difficult, theoretical, but extremely fruitful, goal would be to develop "chrono-pan-omics" experimental strategies to monitor over time all of the ongoing changes in all of the pertinent pituitary proteoforms.

Moreover, when we state that a pituitary "protein" hormone interacts with its receptor, specifically which "protein (GHP)" do we mean out of the dozens of GHPs? That same question exists for any pathology, and is an important question for PPPM studies and clinical practice.

3.2 Human Prolactin Proteoforms (PRLPs)

We discovered six PRLPs in pituitary adenomas [17]. Those six PRLPs had a significantly different distribution pattern among the five groups of pituitary adenomas: NF^-, FSH^+/LH^+, FSH^+, LH^+, and PRL^+ (Fig. 5). The proportional ratio of those PRLPs in the adenoma subtypes demonstrates striking differences that result from a variety of dysfunctional metabolic pathways. Apparently, rich sub-molecular mechanistic pathways occur in PRL-secreting pituitary adenomas, and it is important to elucidate the multiple molecular pathways that participate in those pathways.

Bioinformatic analysis of these PRLPs predicted that all six PRLPs derive from deamidation, phosphorylation, N-glycosylation, and O-glycosylation. Interestingly, in contradistinction to GHPs, all PRLPs derived from the PRL prohormone, and not from the mature PRL [17]. They retain the signal peptide. The GH and PRL data are different and indicate that signalomics is a novel concept that apparently plays a significant role within GH and PRL adenomas, and that could provide an effective diagnostic PPPM tool for those adenomas.

It is again important to know which PRLP interacts with its receptor, and what are the effects of the different PRLPs on the signaling pathways. PRL interacts with either the short PRL receptor or the long PRL receptor. The short PRL receptor activates the PI3K/AKT system, and the long receptor activates the Jak STAT signaling pathway [17]. At this time, we do not know which one of the six PRLPs interacts with which receptor, and thus we do not know the effect on the two separate pathways. Further studies are needed on those crucial molecular pathways.

Proportion ratio of prolactin proteoforms of five subtypes in pituitary adenomas

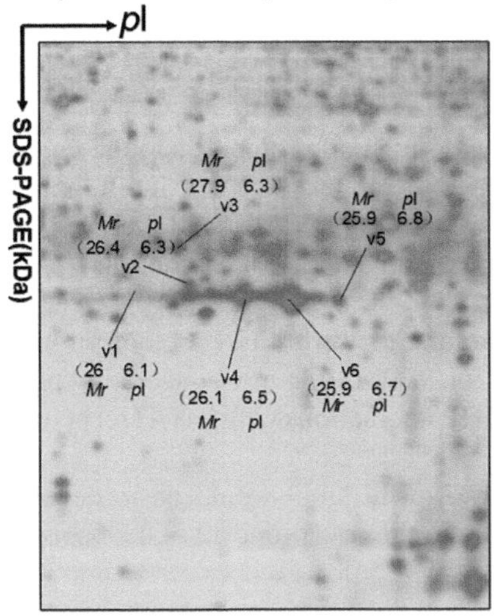

Proportion ratio of PRL variants amount of five subtypes in pituitary adenomas

Varinat No.	NF-	FSH+/LH+	FSH+	LH+	PRL
V1	2.64%	53.34%	24.24%	9.45%	40.48%
V2	1.56%	2.03%	0.52%	3.08%	11.90%
V3	0.31%	6.57%	7.66%	19.65%	11.91%
V4	31.83%	10.14%	9.18%	15.08%	11.90%
V5	31.83%	10.52%	52.47%	27.53%	11.91%
V6	31.83%	17.40%	5.93%	25.21%	11.90%
Total	100%	100%	100%	100%	100%

*χ^2=360.606, P= 0.000<0.005, amount of five subtypes of pituitary adenomas

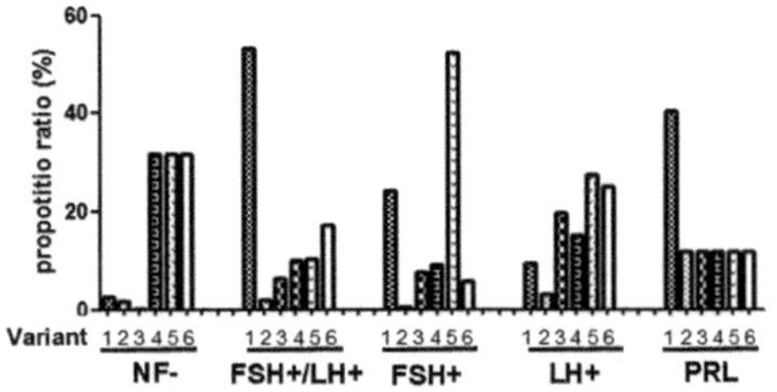

Fig. 5 2DGE image of prolactin proteoforms (PRLPs) in human pituitary tissues and its proportion ratio among five subtypes of pituitary adenomas. (Modified from Qian S, et al. [17], copyright permission from Frontiersin publisher open access article, copyright 2018)

4 Multiomics of Pituitary Adenomas in the Framework of PPPM

4.1 Comparative Proteomics of Pituitary Adenomas

We also studied the detailed comparative proteomics of eight control and 15 macroadenoma pituitary tissue samples [12, 16, 18–22]. We rigorously demonstrated the experimental reproducibility (gel spot volume and spot position) within each gel set, and synthesized a master gel for controls. When we compared each individual adenoma gel to that master gel, we accurately located differentially expressed proteins (DEPs).

Those comparative 2DGE data can be rationalized readily within a 7-dimensional space (five dimensions for protein abundance; one for protein name; one for protein: protein interactions). Protein abundances either increased (10- or 100-fold), did not change, or decreased (10- or 100-fold). Those significant differential abundance data were the first glimpse into the extensive variety of protein changes within a pituitary adenoma, and led to many subsequent studies. Interaction analysis linked how those proteins interacted with each other and yielded a rich interaction network that involved GH, PRL, CAPZB, cytochrome c, Jnk, ERK, among many other proteins. Modified proteins were found in mitochondrial complex 1 (NADH dehydrogenase ubiquitinone Fe-S protein, NDUFS8) and in complex four (cytochrome c oxidase, COX6B1). Those modified proteins might play a role to generate reactive oxygen species (ROS).

Other studies contributed to those comparative proteomics data. Lu, et al. listed several sites of potential pharmacology treatment for pituitary adenomas in the MAPK signaling pathway [23] (Fig. 6). The ERK-MAPK signaling, p38-MAPK signaling, and JNK signaling all play important roles in pituitary adenomas. For the MAPK signaling system in pituitary adenomas, the activation of ERK signaling is generally thought to promote cell proliferation and growth, whereas the activations of p38 and JNK signaling are generally thought to promote cell apoptosis [23]. Some therapeutic drugs exert anti-tumor effects by targeting one of these pathways or all three pathways at the same time. MAPK signaling is a very complex network, and always interacts with other pathways such as the PI3K and cAMP pathways to affect tumor progression. The latest development of MAPK signaling in pituitary adenomas and the related anti-tumor drugs that target MAPK signaling pathways would provide new insights into critical pituitary adenoma pathogenic mechanisms and pre-clinical data for effective treatment [23].

The Nrf-2-mediated oxidative stress response signaling pathways are important and offer potential targets for personalized medicine of pituitary adenomas [9, 24] (Fig. 7). Oxidative stress is sensed by this Nrf2 system. Oxidative stress derives from a rich variety of sources: heavy metals, drugs, xenobiotics, UV radiation, etc.

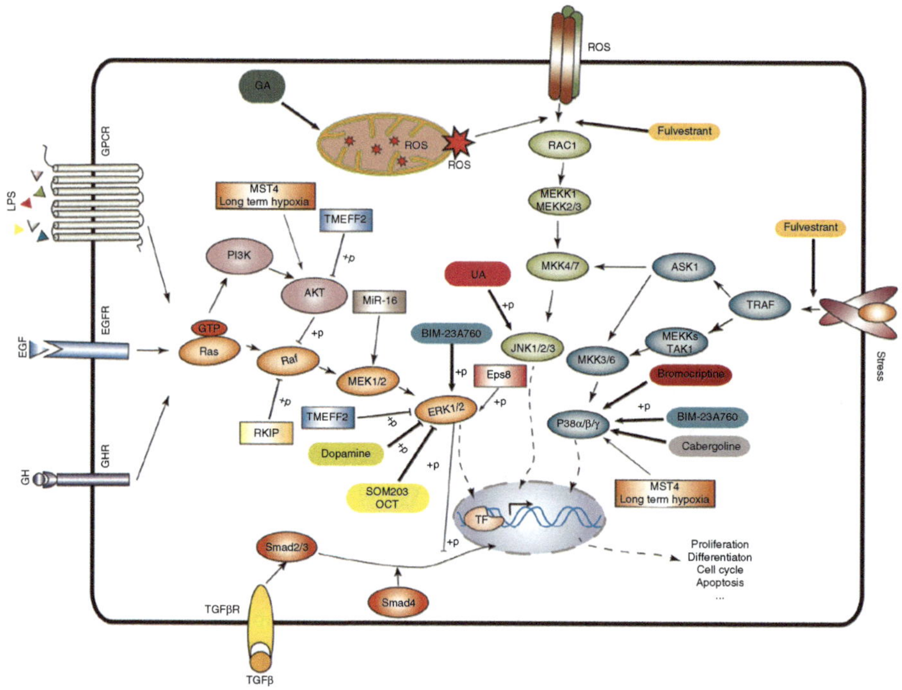

Fig. 6 MAPK signaling pathways and the potential therapeutic targets. In p38 signaling, TRAF activates ASK1, TAK1 or MEKK1, which activates MKK3/6, which subsequently phosphorylates p38 isoforms. In the ERK signaling, Ras activates the serine/threonine protein kinase Raf to activate MEK1/2; then MEK1/2 phosphorylates the ERK1/2. In JNK signaling, RAC1 activates MEKK1 or MEKK2/3 to activate MKK4/7; and then MKK4/7 phosphorylates JNK1/2/3. The ASK1 in the p38 signaling also activates MKK4/7 to crosstalk with JNK signaling. *ROS* reactive oxygen species, *GA* 18β-glycyrrhetinic acid. BIM-23A760 is a dopamine–somatostatin chimeric compound. *OCT* octreotide. SOM230 and OCT are somatostatin analogs. Rectangle denotesmeans the potential drug targets. (Reproduced from Lu et al. (2019) [23], with permission from Frontiersin publisher open-access article, copyright 2019)

That oxidative stress is transferred into the cytoplasm to produce electrophiles [reactive oxygen species (ROS), and reactive nitrogen species (RNS)] that alter multiple cytoplasm pathways and the Nrf2/Keap1 complex. Phosphorylated Nrf2 separates and transfers into the nucleus to interact with the antioxidant-response element (ARE)/electrophile-response element (EpRE). Thereafter, multiple systems are activated: ubiquitination; chaperone and stress response; phase 1 and 2 detoxification and reactive metabolites; phase III detoxifying proteins; and antioxidant proteins. Our comparative proteomics studies found many of the molecules discussed here (HSPs, CAT, SOD, etc.)

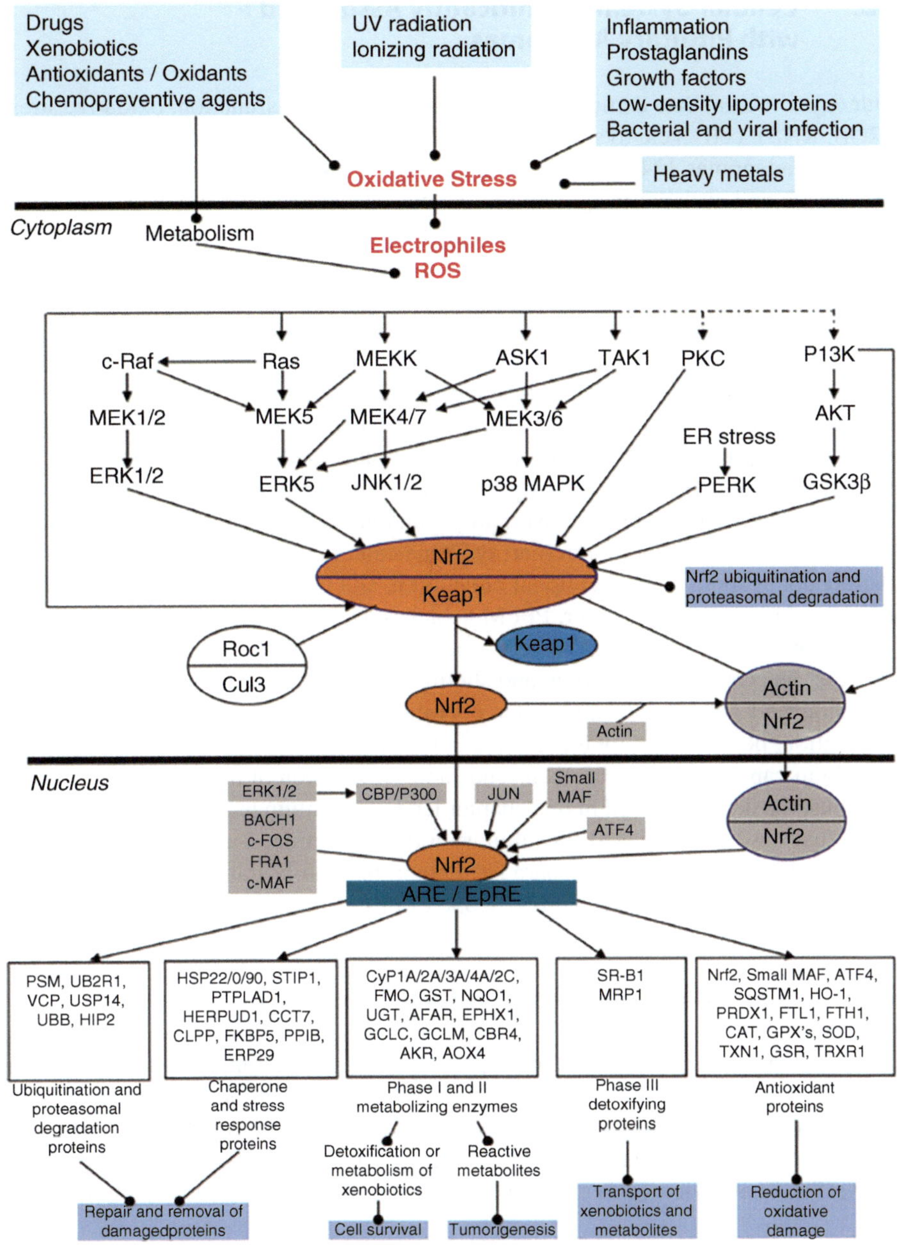

Fig. 7 Nrf2-mediated oxidative stress response signaling pathways in human pituitary adenomas. (Modified from Zhan & Desiderio (2010) [24], with permission from BioMed Central publisher open-access article, copyright 2010; modified from Long et al. (2019) [25], with permission from Frontiersin publisher open-access article, copyright 2019; and reproduced from Zhan et al. (2021) [9], with permission from Frontiersin publisher open-access article, copyright 2021)

4.2 Cellular Systems Significantly Associated with Pituitary Adenomas

Our experimental data demonstrate that mitochondrial dysfunction, oxidative stress (ROS; RNS), cell-cycle dysregulation, and MAPK signaling associate with human pituitary adenomas [24, 25]. Those signaling pathway system changes provide a systematic and in-depth insight into molecular mechanisms, and indicate the effective biomarkers and therapeutic targets for PPPM of pituitary adenomas.

4.3 Quantum Improvements in PPPM of Pituitary Adenomas

The diverse experimental data discussed in this chapter can be readily assembled into a coherent, focused synopsis of their significance and of their roles in PPPM. For example, the pituitary adenoma proteome can be accessed via two separate branches: the tissue proteome and/or the body-fluid proteome/peptidome [26].

For the body-fluid branch, CSF and plasma are used to elucidate pattern variations with protein/antibody microarrays. One can readily and accurately assess the therapeutic response, interventional prevention, and predictive diagnosis for a high-risk population. In this manner, PPPM achieves a very high level of accuracy [26].

For the tissue proteome branch, one detects proteome variations in protein expression, protein modification, and slicing. Those data lead to modality of protein variation and an accurate molecular classification that is used for interventional prevention, personalized treatment, and personalized patient care [26]. Overall, this paradigm can lead to halt the occurrence and progression of tumors.

Thus, the data described in this chapter led to a quantum level of PPPM improvement that has been achieved for pituitary tumor detection, analysis, and treatment. Clearly, the basics of this new paradigm could be readily translated to many other human pathologies within the broad scope of PPPM.

4.4 Omics Biomarkers for Pituitary Tumors

An excellent review demonstrated graphically the omics biomarkers that have been published in the literature of pituitary tumors [27]. The authors correlated 171 different biomarkers with associated pituitary neuroendocrine tumor (PitNET) subtypes (lactotrophs, somatotrophs, corticotrophs, NF-PitNET, null cell, and varied PitNETs). That review is an excellent source for pituitary adenoma biomarkers.

4.5 Differential Patterns and PPPM

Similar to a cell, we can now organize all of the various omics into one coherent differential pattern. For example, all of the patterns obtained from DNA, RNA, proteins, etc. can be distilled into one "cell-like" "meta-omics" system to accurately reflect the metabolism in normal cells in order to clarify the dysfunctional systems within a pathology [28]. The biomarker patterns that are under study in many laboratories can be assembled into an integrated pattern that, at a "birds-eye view" level, reflects the metabolism and pathology that occurs within a cell [29] (Fig. 8). For example, a DNA marker pattern derives from genomics data (mutation, loss, inserts, fusion); an RNA biomarker pattern from transcriptomics (splicing, ncRNA); protein biomarker patterns from proteomics (PTMs, variants, proteoforms); metabolite biomarker pattern from metabolomics (control and tumor metabolites); and image-texture features from radiomics (PET-CT, MRI, CT) [28–30]. After all of those individual patterns are combined, a clearer, more-accurate picture of the pathology emerges that occurs within an adenoma. The rapid improvements in experimental paradigms, instrumentation, and application in each contributing field provide a dramatically improved ability in our ability to monitor basic molecular events that occur in human control and pathological tissues. PPPM, in turn, improves at a rapid, significant, and more-accurate pace to improve the individual health care of each patient.

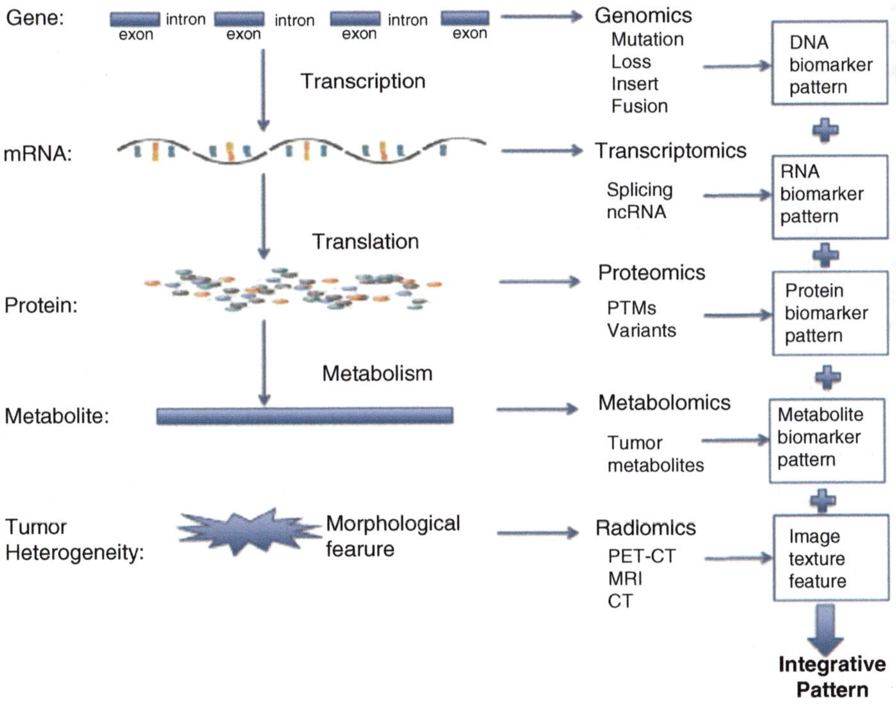

Fig. 8 Multiomics-based integrative pattern biomarkers. (Reproduced from Cheng and Zhan (2017) [29], with permission from Springer publisher open access article, copyright 2017)

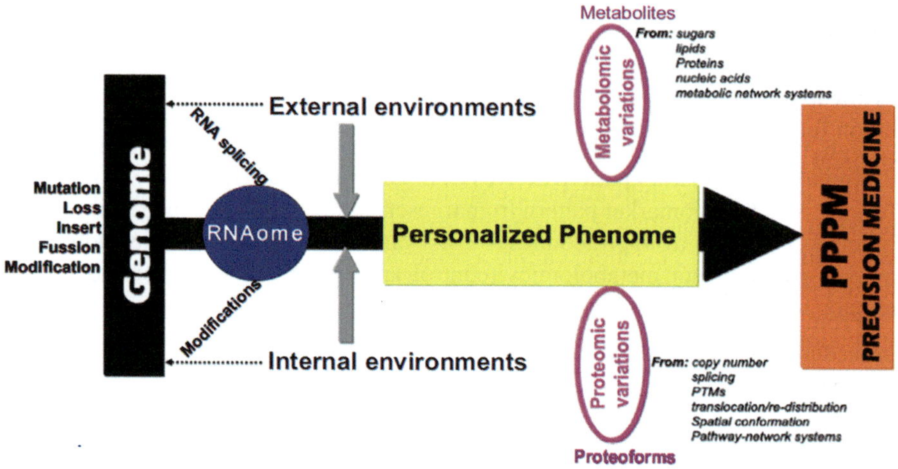

Fig. 9 The contribution of mulltiomics to pituitary adenoma clinical practice. (Modified and upgraded from Zhan et al. (2018) [15], with permission from Elsevier publisher, copyright 2018. Reproduced from Li N, Desiderio DM, and Zhan X (2021) [1], copyright permission from Wiley publisher, copyright 2021)

4.6 Improved PPPM Practice in Pituitary Adenomas

The amount of novel data accumulated in recent pituitary adenoma research provides a quantum leap in our ability to improve accurate PPPM in practice. For example, multiomics data plus biomarker data lead to improved prediction/prevention, diagnosis/therapy, and prognostic assessment [26, 28, 30]. Those improvements derive from several factors. The combination of multiomics data (genome, transcriptome, proteome, peptidome, metabolome, microbiome, and radiome) with molecular network-based pattern biomarkers (age, gender, race, histology classification, functional classification, stage, metastases, surgical options, adjuvant therapy, multiple endocrine neoplasia, Carney complex, familial isolated pituitary adenoma) leads effectively to improved prediction/prevention, diagnosis/therapy, and prognostic assessment [26]. As a result, PPPM improves significantly.

In sum, PPPM is moving from the genome, via the RNAome, to the personalized phenome and PPPM high-precision medicine [1, 15] (Fig. 9).

4.7 PPPM of the Personal Phenome

Along that long route, several components play a significant role. The genome incorporates mutations, losses, inserts, fusion, and modifications [1, 15] (Fig. 9). The RNAome involves RNA splicing and modifications [1]. External and internal environments impact on the genome, RNAome, and personalized phenome [15]. Variations in the metabolome and proteome impact on the phenome [15]. In sum, the cell (normal; tumor) results from the delicate interplay among a wide variety of molecular components.

It is the goal of this research program to elucidate (as many as possible) the molecular components in those systems to improve significantly PPPM.

5 PPPM-Related Aspects in Pituitary Adenomas

5.1 Literature Analyses of BMI, Pituitary, Adenomas, Carcinomas, and Neoplasias

The recent EPMA position paper 2021 that focused on "normal" BMI is very important (via a serendipitous circuitous route) to our study of pituitary adenomas [31]. The section on prostate cancer was significant to DMD, and circuitously prompted the question: "what effect does BMI have on the pituitary." A literature search found two pertinent papers that expanded on that question [32, 33]. One paper discussed malignant transformation in a non-functional pituitary adenoma—NFPA (pituitary carcinoma) [32], and a second paper discussed increased incidence of neoplasia in patients with pituitary adenomas [33]. Those papers are striking, and suggest that one must consider *all* of the molecular mechanisms and dysfunctional systems that lead from a control, to an adenoma, and on to a neoplasia. It is quite clear that something (that we do not yet know- but is very important) happens in those special cases, and warrants further study. All of these intertwined pieces of information point to potential future studies on pituitary carcinomas.

5.2 Economics of Acromegaly Care

It is quite helpful to place this research into proper perspective, and therefore to also analyze the economic aspects of pituitary adenomas.

The U.S.A. population is ~3.3×10^8, and acromegaly patients total ~ 4/million (330 million × 4/million = 1320 acromegaly patients.). It has been estimated that 25 years of acute care costs for an acromegaly patient are ~1000,000 USD. Therefore, the estimated total cost to the U.S.A. healthcare system is 1320 × 1000,000 USD, or 1.3 billion USD over 25 years.

Correspondingly, for a world population of 7.9 billion, costs for acromegaly patients (total ~ 31,300) equal $31{,}300 \times 10^6$, or 31.3 billion USD over 25 years.

All of those total costs increase further when all of the other pituitary hormones and associated adenomas are included.

5.3 Guiding Principle of this Research Program

The greatest level of understanding of any human disease always derives from an in-depth and accurate analysis of the molecules that are involved in that disease. That concept means that the structural elucidation of a molecule- and the amino acid sequence determination of each peptide, protein, PTM, proteoform, etc. must always be rigorously established in order to secure the highest confidence and the most-accurate PPPM care of a pituitary adenoma patient. These concepts apply to all human pathologies.

6 Conclusions and Expert Recommendations for PPPM in Pituitary Adenomas

Multiomics is an effective approach to resolve the complex pituitary adenomas in the framework of 3P medicine (PPPM) [1, 15]. However, an individual phenome (especially proteome and metabolome) is a bridge to link the genome to PPPM practice [15]. Phenome-centered multiomics is a trend for PPPM practice in pituitary adenomas [1]. Metabolomics and proteomics are equally important to provide insight into phenomic variations to discover effective biomarkers and therapeutic targets for pituitary adenomas [1, 15]. Moreover, biomolecular modifications, including DNA modifications, RNA post-transcriptional modifications, protein PTMs, and RNA alternative splicing are important factors that produce proteoforms [34]. A proteoform is the basic unit of a proteome, which is the final structure and functional format of a canonical protein or a gene [5]. Therefore, proteoformics is the future direction of next-generation proteomics. In this study, significant multiomics-based signaling pathways, biomarkers, and therapeutic targets [13, 17, 23–25, 27] were found for pituitary adenomas in the framework of PPPM.

We recommend an emphasis on multiomics-driven PPPM for pituitary adenomas in the following three aspects:

1. Predictive approach. Pituitary adenomas are an intracranial, very complex, chronic, and whole-body disease, with high-level heterogeneity, and involve a series of molecular changes in the levels of DNA, RNA, protein, and metabolite. Multiomics-based body-fluid biomarkers (for example, from CSF and serum) are an effective approach to predict high-risk person who might develop pituitary adenomas, or prognostically assess the therapeutic effects [26]. In this aspect, serum peptidomics and metabolomics might offer important roles.
2. Targeted prevention. For targeted prevention, multiomics based on pituitary adenoma tissues can offer significant signaling pathway changes to discover important hub molecules. Those important signaling pathway changes, and the corresponding hub molecules, would elucidate the molecular mechanisms of

pituitary adenomas and discover novel therapeutic targets for targeted prevention [1, 26]. Another aspect, invasive behavior, is a very challenging clinical problem. Multiomics analysis of invasive vs. noninvasive pituitary adenomas can uncover invasiveness-related molecules for targeted prevention of invasive behavior.

3. Personalized medical services. Pituitary adenomas are highly heterogenous, and include different subtypes and invasive vs. noninvasive subtypes. Multiomics analysis can discover effective biomarkers to stratify different subtypes of pituitary adenoma patients for personalized treatments [35, 36]. For example, we can establish serum growth hormone proteoform pattern biomarkers to discriminate the invasive vs. noninvasive pituitary adenoma patients for personalized therapy [13]. If the patient is stratified into invasive group, then this patient will receive radiation therapy and even drug therapy in addition to neurosurgery. If the patient is stratified into the noninvasive group, then this patient will only receive neurosurgery, which would be fine.

Acknowledgements This work was supported by the Shandong First Medical University Talent Introduction Funds (to X.Z.), the Shandong Provincial Natural Science Foundation (ZR202103020356/ZR2021MH156 to X.Z.), the National Natural Science Foundation of China (82172866), NIH grants (NS 42843, DA 08924, RR 14593, 10522, and 16679, to DMD), and NSF grants (DBI 9604633, to DMD).

References

1. Li N, Desiderio DM, Zhan X (2021) The use of mass spectrometry in a proteome-centered multiomics study of human pituitary adenomas. Mass Spectrom Rev 41:1–50. https://doi.org/10.1002/mas.21710
2. Zhan X, Zhou T, Cheng T, Lu M (2019) Recognition of multiomics based molecule-pattern biomarker for precise prediction, diagnosis and prognostic assessment in cancer. In: Samadikuchaksaraei A (ed) Bioinformatics tools for detection and clinical interpretation of genomic variations. InTech-Open Science Publisher, London
3. Batt J, Asa S, Fladd C, Rotin D (2002) Pituitary, pancreatic and gut neuroendocrine defects in protein tyrosine phosphatase-sigma-deficient mice. Mol Endocrinol 16(1):155–169. https://doi.org/10.1210/mend.16.1.0756
4. Zhan X, Li N, Zhan X, Qian S (2018) Revival of 2DE-LC/MS in proteomics and its potential for large-scale study of human proteoforms. Med One 3:e180008
5. Zhan X, Li B, Zhan X, Schlüter H, Jungblut PR, Coorssen JR (2019) Innovating the concept and practice of two-dimensional gel electrophoresis in the analysis of proteomes at the proteoform level. Proteomes 7(4):36. https://doi.org/10.3390/proteomes7040036
6. Ezzat S, Asa SL, Couldwell WT, Barr CE, Dodge WE, Vance ML, McCutcheon IE (2004) The prevalence of pituitary adenomas: a systematic review. Cancer 101(3):613–619. https://doi.org/10.1002/cncr.20412
7. Desiderio DM, Cezayirli RC, Fridland G, Robertson JT, Sacks H (1985) Metabolic profiling of radioreceptor-assayable opioid peptides in a human pituitary ACTH-secreting tumor. Life Sci 37(19):1823–1828. https://doi.org/10.1016/0024-3205(85)90225-5

8. Kusmierz JJ, Sumrada R, Desiderio DM (1990) Fast atom bombardment mass spectrometric quantitative analysis of methionine-enkephalin in human pituitary tissues. Anal Chem 62(21):2395–2400. https://doi.org/10.1021/ac00220a026
9. Zhan X, Li J, Zhou T (2021) Targeting Nrf2-mediated oxidative stress response signaling pathways as new therapeutic strategy for pituitary adenomas. Front Pharmacol 12:565748. https://doi.org/10.3389/fphar.2021.565748
10. Marks DL, Butler AA, Turner R, Brookhart G, Cone RD (2003) Differential role of melanocortin receptor subtypes in cachexia. Endocrinology 144(4):1513–1123. https://doi.org/10.1210/en.2002-221099
11. Dehkhoda F, Lee CMM, Medina J, Brooks AJ (2018) The growth hormone receptor: mechanism of receptor activation, cell signaling, and physiological aspects. Front Endocrinol 9:35. https://doi.org/10.3389/fendo.2018.00035
12. Desiderio DM, Zhan X (2003) The human pituitary proteome: the characterization of differentially expressed proteins in an adenoma compared to a control. Cell Mol Biol (Noisy-le-Grand) 49(5):689–712
13. Li B, Wang X, Yang C, Wen S, Li J, Li N, Long Y, Mu Y, Liu J, Liu Q, Li X, Desiderio DM, Zhan X (2021) Human growth hormone proteoform pattern changes in pituitary adenomas: potential biomarkers for 3P medical approaches. EPMA J 12(1):67–89. https://doi.org/10.1007/s13167-021-00232-7
14. Zhan X, Yang H, Peng F, Li J, Mu Y, Long Y, Cheng T, Huang Y, Li Z, Lu M, Li N, Li M, Liu J, Jungblut PR (2018) How many proteins can be identified in a 2DE gel spot within an analysis of a complex human cancer tissue proteome? Electrophoresis 39(7):965–980. https://doi.org/10.1002/elps.201700330
15. Zhan X, Long Y, Lu M (2018) Exploration of variations in proteome and metabolome for predictive diagnostics and personalized treatment algorithms: innovative approach and examples for potential clinical application. J Proteome 188:30–40. https://doi.org/10.1016/j.jprot.2017.08.020
16. Zhan X, Giorgianni F, Desiderio DM (2005) Proteomics analysis of growth hormone isoforms in the human pituitary. Proteomics 5(5):1228–1241. https://doi.org/10.1002/pmic.200400987
17. Qian S, Yang Y, Li N, Cheng T, Wang X, Liu J, Li X, Desiderio DM, Zhan X (2018) Prolactin variants in human pituitaries and pituitary adenomas identified with two-dimensional gel electrophoresis and mass spectrometry. Front Endocrinol 9:468. https://doi.org/10.3389/fendo.2018.00468
18. Zhan X, Desiderio DM (2003) Spot volume vs. amount of protein loaded onto a gel: a detailed, statistical comparison of two gel electrophoresis systems. Electrophoresis 24(11):1818–1833. https://doi.org/10.1002/elps.200305375
19. Zhan X, Desiderio DM (2003) Differences in the spatial and quantitative reproducibility between two second-dimensional gel electrophoresis systems. Electrophoresis 24(11):1834–1846. https://doi.org/10.1002/elps.200305389
20. Zhan X, Desiderio DM (2003) Heterogeneity analysis of the human pituitary proteome. Clin Chem 49(10):1740–1751. https://doi.org/10.1373/49.10.1740
21. Zhan X, Desiderio DM (2005) Comparative proteomics analysis of human pituitary adenomas: current status and future perspectives. Mass Spectrom Rev 24(6):783–813. https://doi.org/10.1002/mas.20039
22. Zhan X, Evans CO, Oyesiku NM, Desiderio DM (2003) Proteomics and transcriptomics analyses of secretagogin down-regulation in human non-functional pituitary adenomas. Pituitary 6(4):189–202. https://doi.org/10.1023/b:pitu.0000023426.99808.40
23. Lu M, Wang Y, Zhan X (2019) The MAPK pathway-based drug therapeutic targets in pituitary adenomas. Front Endocrinol (Lausanne) 10:330. https://doi.org/10.3389/fendo.2019.00330
24. Zhan X, Desiderio DM (2010) Signaling pathway networks mined from human pituitary adenoma proteomics data. BMC Med Genet 3:13. https://doi.org/10.1186/1755-8794-3-13
25. Long Y, Lu M, Cheng T, Zhan X, Zhan X (2019) Multiomics-based signaling pathway network alterations in human non-functional pituitary adenomas. Front Endocrinol 10:835. https://doi.org/10.3389/fendo.2019.00835

26. Zhan X, Desiderio DM (2010) The use of variations in proteomes to predict, prevent, and personalize treatment for clinically nonfunctional pituitary adenomas. EPMA J 1(3):439–459. https://doi.org/10.1007/s13167-010-0028-z
27. Aydin B, Caliskan A, Arga KY (2021) Overview of omics biomarkers in pituitary neuroendocrine tumors to design future diagnosis and treatment strategies. EPMA J 12(3):383–401. https://doi.org/10.1007/s13167-021-00246-1
28. Hu R, Wang X, Zhan X (2013) Multi-parameter systematic strategies for predictive, preventive and personalised medicine in cancer. EPMA J 4(1):2. https://doi.org/10.1186/1878-5085-4-2
29. Cheng T, Zhan X (2017) Pattern recognition for predictive, preventive, and personalized medicine in cancer. EPMA J 8(1):51–60. https://doi.org/10.1007/s13167-017-0083-9
30. Lu M, Zhan X (2018) The crucial role of multiomic approach in cancer research and clinically relevant outcomes. EPMA J 9(1):77–102. https://doi.org/10.1007/s13167-018-0128-8
31. Golubnitschaja O, Liskova A, Koklesova L, Samec M, Biringer K, Büsselberg D, Podbielska H, Kunin AA, Evsevyeva ME, Shapira N, Paul F, Erb C, Dietrich DE, Felbel D, Karabatsiakis A, Bubnov R, Polivka J, Polivka J Jr, Birkenbihl C, Fröhlich H, Hofmann-Apitius M, Kubatka P (2021) Caution, "normal" BMI: health risks associated with potentially masked individual underweight-EPMA position paper 2021. EPMA J 12(3):1–22. https://doi.org/10.1007/s13167-021-00251-4
32. Lenders N, McCormack A (2018) Malignant transformation in non-functioning pituitary adenomas (pituitary carcinoma). Pituitary 21(2):217–229. https://doi.org/10.1007/s11102-017-0857-z
33. Popovic V, Damjanovic S, Micic D, Nesovic M, Djurovic M, Petakov M, Obradovic S, Zoric S, Simic M, Penezic Z, Marinkovic J (1998) Increased incidence of neoplasia in patients with pituitary adenomas. The pituitary study group. Clin Endocrinol (Oxf) 49(4):441–445. https://doi.org/10.1046/j.1365-2265.1998.00536.x
34. Zhan X, Li J, Guo Y, Golubnitschaja O (2021) Mass spectrometry analysis of human tear fluid biomarkers specific for ocular and systemic diseases in the context of 3P medicine. EPMA J 12(4):1–27. https://doi.org/10.1007/s13167-021-00265-y
35. Liu D, Li J, Li N, Lu M, Wen S, Zhan X (2020) Integration of quantitative phosphoproteomics and transcriptomics revealed phosphorylation-mediated molecular events as useful tools for a potential patient stratification and personalized treatment of human nonfunctional pituitary adenomas. EPMA J 11(3):419–467. https://doi.org/10.1007/s13167-020-00215-0
36. Wang Y, Cheng T, Lu M, Mu Y, Li B, Li X, Zhan X (2019) TMT-based quantitative proteomics revealed follicle-stimulating hormone (FSH)-related molecular characterizations for potentially prognostic assessment and personalized treatment of FSH-positive non-functional pituitary adenomas. EPMA J 10(4):395–414. https://doi.org/10.1007/s13167-019-00187-w

Critical Role of Telemedicine as a Platform for Predictive, Preventive, and Personalized Diabetes Care During the COVID-19 Pandemics

Ivica Smokovski, Marija Jovanovski Srceva, Lidija Petkovska, and Olga Golubnitschaja

Abbreviations

3P	Predictive, preventive, and personalized
ARDS	Acute respiratory distress syndrome
BGM	Blood glucose meter
BMI	Body mass index
CGM	Continuous glucose monitor
DBP	Diastolic blood pressure
DPP-4	Dipeptidyl peptidase-4
EHR	Electronic healthcare record

I. Smokovski (✉)
University Clinic of Endocrinology, Diabetes and Metabolic Disorders, Skopje, Republic of North Macedonia

Faculty of Medical Sciences, University Goce Delcev, Stip, Republic of North Macedonia
e-mail: ivica.smokovski@ugd.edu.mk

M. J. Srceva
University Clinic of Anesthesia, Reanimation and Intensive Care, Skopje, Republic of North Macedonia

Medical Faculty, University Ss Cyril and Methodius, Skopje, Republic of North Macedonia

L. Petkovska
Medical Faculty, University Ss Cyril and Methodius, Skopje, Republic of North Macedonia

University Clinic of Toxicology and Emergency Medicine, Skopje, Republic of North Macedonia

O. Golubnitschaja
3P Medicine Research Unit, University Hospital, Rheinische Friedrich-Wilhelms Universität Bonn, Bonn, Germany

H. Podbielska, M. Kapalla (eds.), *Predictive, Preventive, and Personalised Medicine: From Bench to Bedside*, Advances in Predictive, Preventive and Personalised Medicine 17, https://doi.org/10.1007/978-3-031-34884-6_8

GLP-1	Glucagon-like peptide-1
HbA1c	Glycated hemoglobin A1c
ICU	Intensive care unit
NeHS	National e-Health System
PwD	People with diabetes
SBP	Systolic blood pressure
SGLT2	Sodium glucose cotransporter 2
USD	United States dollars
WHO	World Health Organization

1 The Rising Diabetes Prevalence Has a Huge Impact on the Healthcare Systems

Diabetes mellitus has been reaching pandemic proportions as it has been estimated that 537 million adults were living with diabetes worldwide in 2021 [1, 2]. The vast majority, over 75% of people with diabetes (PwD), are living in middle or low-income countries having already limited resources allocated for diabetes care [1, 3]. In addition, diabetes is among the top causes of mortality in the adult population, responsible for 6.7 million deaths in 2021 [1]. Diabetes related expenditures have increased by more than three times in the last 15 years, estimated at 966 billion USD in 2021 [1].

Diabetes drivers, such as prediabetes, might result in even higher diabetes prevalence in the future. Current estimates suggest 541 million people worldwide have impaired glucose tolerance, a form of prediabetes, and a huge number of them would eventually be diagnosed with diabetes in near future [1]. The number of PwD is, unfortunately, predicted to further rise to 643 million by 2030 and 783 million by 2045 [1]. Due to the very high and rising prevalence, it is one of the biggest healthcare challenges humanity has ever faced.

The Republic of North Macedonia is a developing country with one of the highest diabetes prevalence in Europe [1, 3–6]. The increasing prevalence of type 2 diabetes in the past three decades has been alarming and had a significant impact on the healthcare system in the country [3]. The estimated total diabetes prevalence, of both diagnosed and undiagnosed cases, in the Republic of North Macedonia was approximately 80,000 people in 2004 [3–5]. Diabetes prevalence has more than doubled in the last 15 years, and the estimate of total diabetes prevalence was 175,100 in 2019, with national diabetes prevalence of 11.2% (20–79 years), and age-adjusted comparative prevalence of 9.3% [3–6].

Such high national diabetes prevalence has been explained by similar dietary habits and lifestyle to Turkey, having the highest diabetes prevalence in Europe, i.e., food abundant in wheat flour, bread, pastry, lots of sweets, and high-fat meals [3–5]. Total caloric intake in the country per person per day increased by almost 50% from 1993 to 2011, which in combination with inadequate physical activity has resulted in 53% of the population being overweight and 20% obese [3–5].

Another factor contributing to the high increase of diabetes prevalence has been the psychosocial stress associated with the so-called transitional economy, i.e., a transition from planned economy with job security in the past to market economy with unprecedented rise in unemployment and associated stress, especially among the middle-aged population [3–5]. Additionally, the country has been in the top 10 countries in smoking prevalence worldwide [3–5]. The first stratified analysis of diabetes prevalence in the country found a difference in the place of living, with the population living in rural areas having higher diabetes prevalence [3–5].

2 COVID-19 Infection in People with Diabetes: A Perfect Storm

Another pandemic, an infectious one, COVID-19 has been an ongoing public health crisis, with over 557,917,904 confirmed cases globally, including 6,358,899 deaths, as reported to the World Health Organization (WHO) as of 15-July-2022 [7]. The Republic of North Macedonia has also been strongly affected by the COVID-19 pandemics with 317,634 confirmed cases of COVID-19 and 9,337 deaths, reported to the WHO as of 15-July-2022 (Fig. 1) [7]. The country has been ranked fifth worldwide in terms of COVID-19 mortality rate, as of 15-July-2022 [7, 8].

Recent meta-analysis has demonstrated that diabetes is significantly associated with increased odds of severe COVID-19, increased acute respiratory distress syndrome (ARDS) rate, mortality, and need for mechanical ventilation in hospitalized patients [9]. The estimated overall pooled prevalence of diabetes has been 31% in hospitalized COVID-19 patients [9].

The co-existence of COVID-19 and diabetes has been labeled as a perfect storm [10]. The COVID-19 infection is associated with acute inflammatory response and

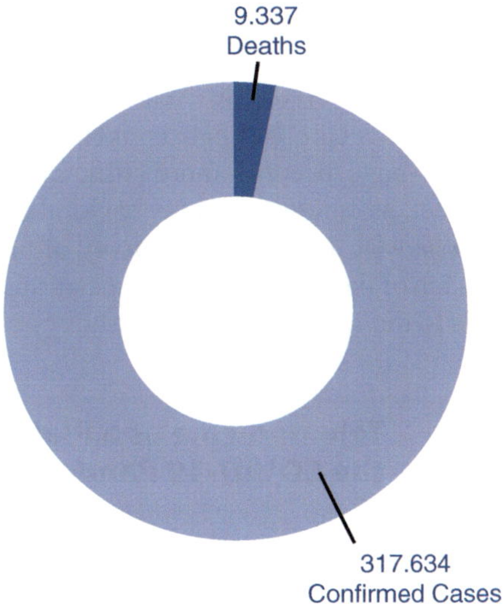

Fig. 1 Adapted from the WHO data for COVID-19 (confirmed cases and deaths) for the Republic of North Macedonia, as of 15-July-2022 [7]

cytokine storm, acute tissue damage, acute coronary ischemia, acute kidney injury, ARDS, hyperglycemic surges, hypercoagulability, endothelial function, and fibrosis [10]. On the other hand, diabetes is associated with chronic, low-grade inflammatory response and insulin resistance, slowly progressing tissue damage, cardiovascular disease, chronic kidney disease, neuropathy, brain changes, glucose variability, hypercoagulability, endothelial dysfunction, and fibrosis [10]. Despite the marked difference in the duration of inflammation, both COVID-19 and diabetes ultimately share the same pathway resulting in glucose disturbances, hypercoagulability, endothelial dysfunction, and fibrosis [10].

Diabetes mellitus has been the most common co-occurring chronic disease in patients with multi-morbidity testing positive for COVID-19 [11]. In addition, diabetes has been the second most prevalent co-morbidity, after hypertension, in people with COVID-19 admitted to hospital [12]. It has already been emphasized that PwD were predicted to have increased risk of severe form of COVID-19 pneumonia and hospitalization [9, 12].

Of those hospitalized, people with type 1 diabetes were predicted to have approximately three times higher risk of in-hospital mortality, whereas people with type 2 diabetes were predicted to have approximately two times higher risk of in-hospital mortality compared to matched controls [13]. It has been demonstrated that poor glycemic control increases the mortality of PwD hospitalized due to COVID-19 as early as within 28 days after admission [14].

Furthermore, hazard ratio for all-cause mortality was higher in patients with higher values of fasting plasma glucose among COVID-19 patients even without known diabetes, when adjusted for age, sex, smoking, systolic blood pressure and total cholesterol [15]. A meta-analysis has demonstrated a high proportion of newly diagnosed diabetes in COVID-19 patients [16]. Newly diagnosed diabetes has been associated with higher risk of mortality than known diabetes in hospitalized patients with COVID-19 [15]. In addition, the post-discharge rate of new-onset diabetes was elevated in hospitalized COVID-19 patients compared with matched controls [17].

Public health crises, such as COVID-19, pose risks to people with diabetes, in terms of their (1) Outcomes, as PwD experience worse outcomes than the general population; (2) Access to care and management, as PwD experience reduced access to diabetes care and management; (3) Adherence to treatment, as long-term treatments have become more difficult for PwD to maintain; and (4) Psychosocial impact, as emotional and behavioral changes are increasing for PwD in response to a crisis [18, 19]. A global survey of healthcare professionals has listed diabetes on the top of the list of chronic diseases and comorbidities most impacted by COVID-19 due to the reduction in care [20].

3 Telemedicine as a Platform for 3P Diabetes Care During the COVID-19 Pandemics

Taking into consideration the magnitude of the healthcare challenge of co-existence of diabetes and COVID-19, application of Predictive, Preventive, and Personalized (3P) Medicine approach in diabetes care during COVID-19 pandemic has been of critical importance, with Predictive Medicine covering the predicted risk of related morbidity and mortality, Preventive Medicine covering the prevention of micro- and macrovascular complications, and Personalized Medicine covering personalized monitoring and treatment (Fig. 2) [21].

Diabetes has been one of the major risk factors for COVID-19 morbidity and mortality [22]; on the other hand, COVID-19 has resulted in an increase of diabetes prevalence, including iatrogenic diabetes due to corticosteroids used for its treatment [23]. Our response has been swift when it comes to infectious pandemic such as COVID-19 infection; however, when we have to deal with another pandemic developing more insidiously over years, such as diabetes, our action has not been so effective [3].

The introduction of the National e-Health System (NeHS) in the Republic of North Macedonia on 01-July-2013 was an immense step in the monitoring and improving the performance of the national healthcare system [3]. The comprehensive, national Electronic Healthcare Record (EHR) system covered all citizens across the three healthcare levels: primary care provided by family physicians, secondary care provided by specialists in general and regional hospitals, and tertiary care provided by university clinics. Implementation of the NeHS has been praised internationally as a key platform for improving the performance of the national healthcare system [3, 24].

Since the beginning of 2015, the diabetes care module in the NeHS has been upgraded with the possibility to record diabetes treatment, metabolic parameters, and diabetes complications [3, 24]. In that way, the NeHS has enabled for monitoring the prevalence of morbidities and mortalities, prescribed medications, referrals across the system, and metabolic control in one of the worst affected populations in Europe [3, 24]. Furthermore, NeHS has become an essential platform for 3P diabetes care, covering the total population of the Republic of North Macedonia [3, 24].

The concept of 3P medicine has emerged as the focal point of efforts in healthcare aimed at controlling the prevalence and management of non-communicable chronic diseases, including diabetes [3, 24–28]. The management of diabetes and the critical role of 3P medicine in modernization of healthcare have been acknowledged as priorities by global and regional organizations and health-related

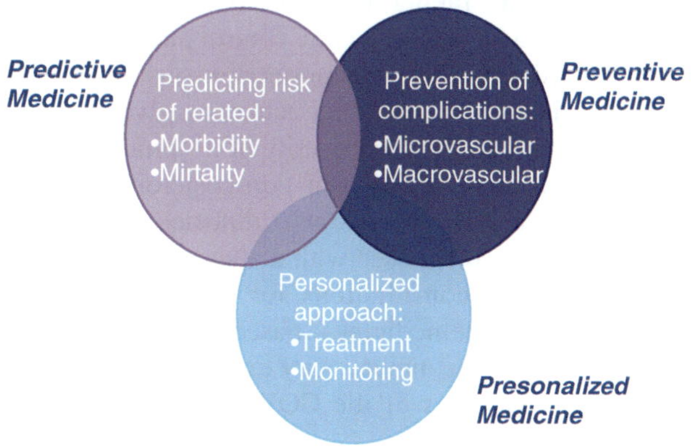

Fig. 2 Applying 3P medicine approach in diabetes care during COVID-19 pandemic

Table 1 Use of the NeHS as a telemedicine platform for 3P diabetes care during COVID-19 pandemics

#	The roles of telemedicine platform for 3P diabetes care during COVID-19 pandemics
1.	Monitoring metabolic control and comorbidities
2.	Resupply of insulin and other antidiabetic treatment
3.	Monitoring of COVID-19 status (tests, hospitalizations, vaccinations) in PwD

institutions such as the Organization of the United Nations, the European Union, and the National Institutes of Health [3, 24–28].

The role of the NeHS as a telemedicine platform for 3P diabetes care has been of utmost importance during the COVID-19 pandemics through its use for (1) monitoring metabolic control and comorbidities, (2) resupply of insulin and other antidiabetic treatment, and (3) monitoring of COVID-19 status (tests, hospitalizations, vaccinations) in PwD (Table 1) [3, 24].

4 Monitoring Metabolic Control and Comorbidities

In order to avoid unnecessary physical visits of PwD at out-patient clinics, the NeHS has been used as a telemedicine platform for 3P diabetes care for monitoring metabolic control through evaluation of uploaded laboratory reports, blood glucose monitor (BGM) and continuous glucose monitor (CGM) reports (Fig. 3).

By reviewing the recorded data in the NeHS, it was possible for the clinicians to provide necessary treatment recommendations. In addition, the NeHS diabetes module allows recording of metabolic parameters, such as HbA1c, glycemic profile, systolic blood pressure (SBP), diastolic blood pressure (DBP), Body Mass Index (BMI), and diabetes complications—retinopathy, nephropathy, neuropathy, peripheral artery disease, coronary artery disease, cerebrovascular disease, diabetic foot. Monitoring metabolic parameters and diabetes complications has been the cornerstone of the 3P diabetes care concept.

The NeHS as a telemedicine platform for 3P diabetes care for monitoring metabolic control and comorbidities has been essential for the PwD hospitalized due to COVID-19, or for those who have developed new-onset diabetes during COVID-19 hospitalization. Taking into consideration the above elaborated close relation between the adequate glycemic control and COVID-19 outcomes, there has been a need for frequent diabetes consultations as most of the hospitalized patients were receiving insulin treatment for achieving glycemic control. In order to alleviate the acute cytokine storm, the majority of hospitalized patients were administered pulse treatment with high doses of corticosteroids resulting in hyperglycemic surges increasing the risk of new-onset diabetes, or worsening the glycemic control of patients already diagnosed with diabetes.

All diabetes consultations for hospitalized COVID-19 patients have been done through telemedicine—based on the information recorded in the NeHS, thus preventing the unnecessary exposure of the clinicians/healthcare professionals in the red zones of the COVID-19 departments where COVID-19 patients

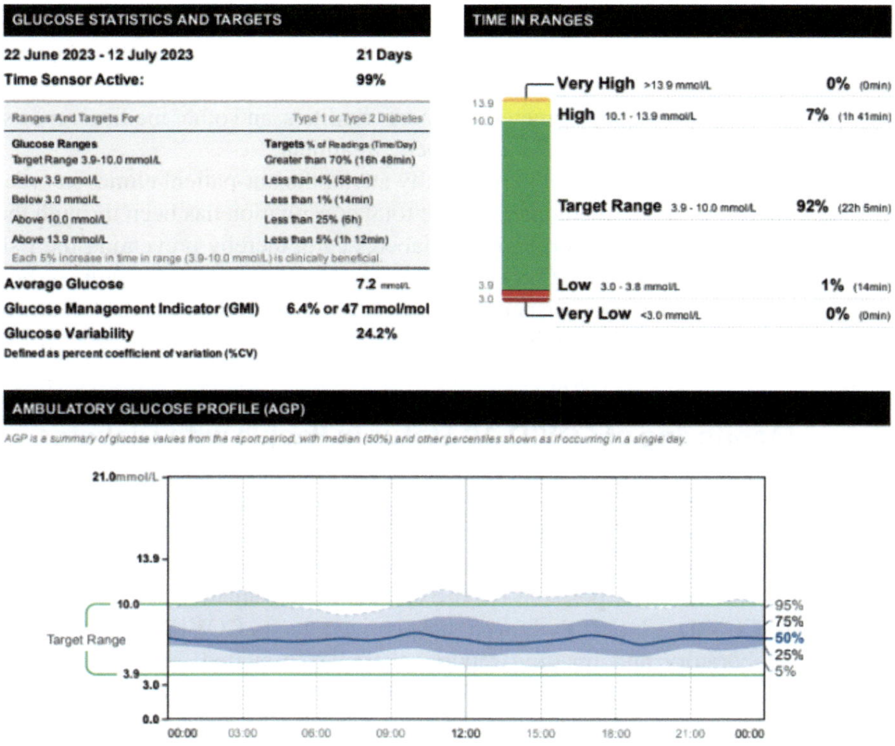

Fig. 3 The NeHS—telemedicine platform for 3P diabetes care: monitoring metabolic control and comorbidities

have been hospitalized. By preventing the unnecessary exposure, the risk for contracting COVID-19 infection among the healthcare professionals has been greatly reduced.

Clinicians were able to evaluate not only the glycemic profiles in order to initiate or titrate insulin therapy, but also to assess the medical reports of other specialists as well as the diabetes complications and comorbidities recorded in the NeHS. Treatment adjustments based on metabolic parameters and comorbidities have been recorded in the NeHS without any need of physical visit by the PwD who were not hospitalized due to COVID-19, thus minimizing their risk of contracting the infection.

5 Resupply of Insulin and Other Antidiabetic Treatment

As outlined in Table 1, the NeHS as a telemedicine platform for 3P diabetes care during COVID-19 pandemics has been used for the resupply of insulin and other antidiabetic treatment (SGLT2 inhibitors, GLP-1 Receptor agonists, DPP-4 inhibitors) dispensed by the insulin pharmacies. There have been 41 insulin pharmacies throughout the country integrated with the NeHS, so based on the report and prescription by the diabetologists they would dispense the adequate treatment. Diabetologists were again able to evaluate the laboratory reports, BGM or CGM reports, diabetes metabolic parameters and comorbidities, and other medical reports, and to recommend the appropriate antidiabetic treatment.

Thus, PwD were not required to physically attend the out-patient clinics in order to obtain their life-saving medicine, and the total consultation has been through the NeHS as a telemedicine platform for 3P diabetes care, thereby preventing the risk of acquiring or spreading the COVID-19 infection. Metformin, sulphonylureas, and thiazolidinediones have been dispensed through the regular (non-insulin) pharmacies, being also integrated with the NeHS.

6 Monitoring of COVID-19 Status in People with Diabetes

In addition, the use of the NeHS as a telemedicine platform for 3P diabetes care has enabled the monitoring of COVID-19 status of PwD, as COVID-19 tests, COVID-19 related hospitalizations, and immunization status have been recorded in their individual EHRs. It has been possible for the clinicians to evaluate if the PwD tested positive for COVID-19, or if PwD were hospitalized due to COVID-19 with all the necessary laboratory and imaging reports, therapies provided, or other medical reports being available through their individual EHR as part of the NeHS. It has also been possible to evaluate the vaccination status, number of doses, type of vaccine administered, date of vaccination, any reactions to vaccines, batch number and expiry date of the vaccines, place of vaccination, and physician responsible for the vaccination.

Despite the availability of the NeHS in the country and the importance of its use as a telemedicine platform for 3P diabetes care during COVID-19 pandemics, it has been reported that the Republic of North Macedonia has one of the highest COVID-19 mortality rates worldwide. One of the reasons for the high mortality rate was related to the lack of intensive care units (ICU) capacities, i.e., a lack of necessary infrastructure for severe cases (non-invasive and invasive ventilation, central monitoring stations), and lack of experienced and competent ICU healthcare personnel. Another reason could be the lack of standardized COVID-19 national treatment protocols and training of healthcare personnel and use of different treatment approaches in COVID-19 departments across the country. Delay in massive vaccination of the population, and regional differences in adoption of vaccination have also contributed to the poor general COVID-19 outcomes, with regions reporting lower vaccination rates associated with higher hospitalization and mortality rates. Inadequate transmission control might also have contributed to the higher COVID-19 mortality rates, with lack of adequate border control (entrance in the country without negative tests or vaccination certificate), and selective and inconsistent social distancing measures across the country.

7 Conclusions and Expert Recommendation in the Frame-Work of 3P Medicine

As a conclusion, the NeHS has had a critical role as a telemedicine platform for the 3P diabetes care during COVID-19 pandemics, enabling monitoring of metabolic control and comorbidities, treatment adjustment and evaluation of COVID-19 status. The insights for the role of telemedicine in delivering 3P care derived from PwD and COVID-19 could certainly be applied to other clinical areas as well.

8 Predictive Approach

The use of NeHS as a telemedicine platform has enabled the prediction of higher risk for diabetes complications, including COVID-19 morbidity and mortality, taking into consideration the poor outcomes of COVID-19 in people with diabetes.

9 Targeted Prevention

The identified higher risk by the use of NeHS as a telemedicine platform has enabled targeted prevention of COVID-19 morbidity and mortality in people with diabetes, by monitoring the metabolic control and comorbidities, adjusting and resupplying the necessary antidiabetic treatment, and monitoring of COVID-19 status.

10 Personalized Medical Services

Concurrently with the prediction of higher risk and implementation of targeted prevention, the NeHS as a telemedicine platform has enabled personalized medical services by providing individually adjusted care in people with diabetes and COVID-19 infection, based on the data recorded in the system.

11 Outlook

Diabetes associated small vessel disease and neuro-retinal changes create a vicious cycle resulting in systemic health adverse effects such excessive mitochondrial and retinal cell damage, chronic inflammation, neovascularization, and reduced visual field. To this end, proliferative diabetic retinopathy is considered an early and independent predictor of other severe diabetic complications such as ischemic stroke. A "domino effect" is highly characteristic for the cascading diabetic complications in which specifically mitochondrial health control is clinically relevant in overall disease management. Multiomic tear fluid analysis is considered instrumental for predictive and prognostic approach [28, 29].

References

1. International Diabetes Federation (2021) IDF diabetes atlas, 10th edn. International Diabetes Federation, Brussels
2. Duarte AA, Mohsin S, Golubnitschaja O (2018) Diabetes care in figures: current pitfalls and future scenarios. EPMA J 9:125–131
3. Smokovski I (2021) Managing diabetes in low income countries. Springer, Cham
4. Smokovski I, Milenkovic T, Trapp C, Mitov A (2015) Diabetes care in the Republic of Macedonia: challenges and opportunities. Ann Glob Health 81(6):792–802
5. Smokovski I, Milenkovic T, Cho HN (2018) First stratified diabetes prevalence data for the Republic of Macedonia derived from the national e-health system. Diabetes Res Clin Pract 143:179–183
6. International Diabetes Federation (2019) IDF diabetes atlas, 9th edn. International Diabetes Federation, Brussels
7. World Health Organization. WHO coronavirus (COVID-19) dashboard. Updated 15 July. https://covid19.who.int/. Accessed 15 Jul 2022
8. COVID-19 pandemics data. https://www.worldometers.info/coronavirus/#countries. Accessed 15 Jul 2022
9. Bradley S, Banach M, Alvarado N, Smokovski I, Bhaskar MMS (2022) Prevalence and impact of diabetes in hospitalized COVID-19 patients: a systematic review and meta-analysis. J Diabetes 14(2):144
10. Feldman E, Savelieff GM, Hayek SS, Pennathur S, Kretzler M, Pop-Busui R (2020) COVID-19 and diabetes: a collision and collusion of two diseases. Diabetes 69(12):2549–2565
11. Chudasama YV, Gillies LC, Appiah K, Zaccardi F, Razieh C, Davies JM, Yates T, Khunti K (2020) Multimorbidity and SARS-CoV-2 infection in UK biobank. Diabetes Metab Syndr 14(5):775–776
12. Singh KA, Gillies LC, Singh R, Singh A, Chudasama Y, Coles B, Seidu S, Zaccardi F, Davies JM, Kamlesh K (2020) Prevalence of co-morbidities and their association with mortality in patients with COVID-19: a systematic review and meta-analysis. Diabetes Obes Metab 22:1915–1924
13. Barron E, Bakhai C, Kar P, Weaver A, Bradley D, Ismail H, Knighton P, Holman N, Khunti K, Sattar N, Wareham JN, Young B, Valabhji J (2020) Associations of type 1 and type 2 diabetes with COVID-19-related mortality in England: a whole-population study. Lancet Diabetes Endocrinol 8(10):813–822
14. Zhu L, She ZG, Cheng X, Qin JJ, Zhang XJ, Cai J, Lei F, Wang H, Xie J, Wang W, Li H, Zhang P, Song X, Chen X, Xiang M, Zhang C, Bai L, Xiang D, Chen MM, Liu Y, Yan Y, Liu M, Mao W, Zou J, Liu L, Chen G, Luo P, Xiao B, Zhang C, Zhang Z, Lu Z, Wang J, Lu H, Xia X, Wang D, Liao X, Peng G, Ye P, Yang J, Yuan Y, Huang X, Guo J, Zhang BH, Li H (2020) Association of Blood Glucose Control and Outcomes in patients with COVID-19 and pre-existing type 2 diabetes. Cell Metab 31(6):1068–1077
15. Li H, Tian S, Chen T, Cui Z, Shi N, Zhong X, Qiu K, Zhang J, Zeng T, Chen L, Zheng J (2020) Newly diagnosed diabetes is associated with a higher risk of mortality than known diabetes in hospitalized patients with COVID-19. Diabetes Obes Metab 22(10):1897–1906
16. Satish T, Kapoor N, Cao Y, Tapp JR, Zimmet P (2021) Proportion of newly diagnosed diabetes in COVID-19 patients: a systematic review and meta-analysis. Diabetes Obes Metab 23(3):870–874
17. Ayoubkhani D, Khunti K, Nafilyan V, Maddox T, Humberstone B, Diamond I, Banerjee A (2021) Post-covid syndrome in individuals admitted to hospital with COVID-19: retrospective cohort study. BMJ 31(372):n693
18. Disaster Response Task Force (2007) ADA statement of emergency and disaster preparedness: a report of the disaster response task force. Diabetes Care 30(9):2395–2398
19. Kocurek B, Cryar K (2018) Information for HealthCare professionals. Switching between insulin products in disaster response situations. https://diabetesdisasterresponse.org/health-care-providers-resources. Accessed on 15 Jul 2022.

20. Chudasama YV, Gillies LC, Zaccardi F, Coles B, Davies JM, Seidu S, Khunti K (2020) Impact of COVID-19 on routine care for chronic diseases: a global survey of views from healthcare professionals. Diabetes Metab Syndr 14(5):965–967
21. Golubnitschaja O, Costigliola V (2012) General report & recommendations in predictive, preventive and personalized medicine 2012: white paper of the European Association for Predictive, preventive and personalized medicine. EPMA J 3(1):14
22. Wang LY, Cui JJ, OuYang QY, Zhan Y, Wang YM, Xu XY, Yu LL, Yin H, Wang Y, Luo CH, Guo CX, Yin JY (2021) Complex analysis of the personalized pharmacotherapy in the management of COVID-19 patients and suggestions for applications of predictive, preventive, and personalized medicine attitude. EPMA J 12:307–324
23. Centers for Disease Control and Prevention. COVID-19 information—people at increased risk. https://www.cdc.gov/coronavirus/2019-ncov/need-extra-precautions/people-with-medical-conditions.html. Accessed 15 Jul 2022
24. Smokovski I, Sadikario S, Cibisev A (2020) National eHealth System in Republic of North Macedonia—platform for preventive, predictive and personalized metabolic control in diabetes patients in Golubnitschaja O, et al. 10th Anniversary of the European association for predictive, preventive and personalized (3P) medicine—EPMA world congress supplement. EPMA J 11:2020. https://doi.org/10.1007/s13167-020-00206-1
25. Golubnitschaja O, Kinkorova J, Costigliola V (2014) Predictive, preventive and personalised medicine as the hardcore of 'Horizon 2020': EPMA position paper. EPMA J 5(1):6
26. Golubnitschaja O, Costigliola V (2011) European strategies in predictive, preventive and personalized medicine: highlights of the EPMA world congress 2011. EPMA J 2(4):315–332
27. Golubnitschaja O (2012) Time for new guidelines in advanced healthcare: the mission of the EPMA journal to promote an integrative view in predictive, preventive and personalized medicine. EPMA J 3(1):5
28. Kropp M, Golubnitschaja O, Mazurakova A, Koklesova L, Sargheini N, Vo TKS, de Clerck E, Polivka J Jr, Potuznik P, Polivka J, Stetkarova I, Kubatka P, Thumann G (2023) Diabetic retinopathy as the leading cause of blindness and early predictor of cascading complications-risks and mitigation. EPMA J 14(1):21–42. https://doi.org/10.1007/s13167-023-00314-8
29. Kropp M, De Clerck E, Vo TKS, Thumann G, Costigliola V, Golubnitschaja O (2023) Short communication: unique metabolic signature of proliferative retinopathy in the tear fluid of diabetic patients with comorbidities—preliminary data for PPPM validation. EPMA J 14(1):43–51. https://doi.org/10.1007/s13167-023-00318-4

Gut Microbiome and Liver Diseases from the Perspective of 3PM: The Predictive, Preventive, and Personalized Medicine

Lubomir Skladany, Tomas Koller, Michal Kukla, and Katarina Soltys

Abbreviations

3PM	Preventive, predictive, and personalized medicine
ACLF	Acute-on-chronic liver failure
AD	Acute decompensation of cirrhosis
AH	Alcoholic hepatitis

L. Skladany (✉)
HEGITO (Division of Hepatology, Gastroenterology and Liver Transplantation), Department of Internal Medicine of The Slovak Medical University, F. D. Roosevelt Teaching Hospital, Banská Bystrica, Slovak Republic

Department of Internal Medicine 2, Faculty of Medicine, P. J. Safarik University, Košice, Slovakia

T. Koller
Subdivision of Gastroenterology and Hepatology, 5th Department of Internal Medicine, Comenius University Faculty of Medicine, University Hospital Bratislava, Bratislava, Slovak Republic

M. Kukla
Department of Internal Medicine and Geriatrics, Faculty of Medicine, Jagiellonian University Medical College, Kraków, Poland

Department of Endoscopy, University Hospital in Kraków, Kraków, Poland

K. Soltys
Department of Microbiology and Virology, Faculty of Natural Sciences, Comenius University in Bratislava, Bratislava, Slovak Republic

Comenius University Science Park, Comenius University in Bratislava, Bratislava, Slovak Republic

H. Podbielska, M. Kapalla (eds.), *Predictive, Preventive, and Personalised Medicine: From Bench to Bedside*, Advances in Predictive, Preventive and Personalised Medicine 17, https://doi.org/10.1007/978-3-031-34884-6_9

AIH	Autoimmune hepatitis
ALD	Alcohol-associated liver disease
AUD	Alcohol use disorder
DAMPs	Damage-associated molecular patterns
ERAS	Early recovery after surgery
FFAR	Free fatty acid receptor
FGF	Fibroblast growth factor
FMT	Fecal microbial transplantation
FOBT	Fecal occult blood test
FXR	Farnesoid-X-receptor
GPR	G-protein-coupled receptor
GPS	Global positioning system
LPS	Lipopolysaccharide
MALT	Mucosa-associated lymphatic tissue (in Gut referred to as GALT)
MAMPs	Microbe-associated molecular patterns
MS	Microbiome science
NAFLD	Non-alcoholic fatty liver disease
PAMPs	Pathogen-associated molecular patterns
PBC	Primary biliary cholangitis
PPPM	The predictive, preventive, and personalized medicine
PRR	Pattern recognition receptor superfamily, including membrane and cytosolic receptors such as TLR, RLR, NOD, CLR
PSC	Primary sclerosing cholangitis
RIP	Receptor-interacting protein kinase family
SCFA	Short-chain fatty acids
SIBO	Small intestinal bacterial overgrowth
TGR5	Takeda G-protein-coupled bile acid receptor

1 Aim of the Chapter

Thanks to the exponential acceleration of a microbiome science (MS), in the near future we are about to witness the technological singularity. At the explosion, the realms of the predictive, preventive, and personalized medicine (3PM/PPPM) and microbiome research are bound to gravitate to the *mysterium coniunctionis*. Our chapter is aimed at providing the reader with an outlook on the particular topics related to the role of microbiome in liver diseases which belong to the top-ten causes of a global burden of morbidity, mortality, and cancer. And to emphasize until now hidden potential of microbiome analysis and healthy microbiome promotion in the practical application of 3PM as well as to stimulate further research expanding the visions of the next-generation healthcare.

2 Introduction

Microbes rule the world. It is that simple [1]

Microbial ecosystem is the oldest, richest, and most diverse living ecosystem on the planet hard-wired to all its vital processes [2, 3]. The approximately two-hundred thousand years old humankind of our kind with some 10,000 generations has evolved in an unimaginably diverse niche of microbes (our 719 billionth cousins-predecessors)—whose presence around-, on-, and in the body has become the necessary condition for survival [4]. Therefore, microbes in general are not to be considered enemies, but allies. **Healthy microbiome** implies healthy individual in the manner akin to the known statement "*Mens sana in corpore sano" (originally from the first century AD, a Latin phrase by Roman poet Juvenal, translated in English as* "a healthy mind in a healthy body"). Healthy microbiome is abundant, rich, diverse, and resilient—an ecosystem similar to a rainforest [5, 6]. Being at the same time an organ of the body and external environment, the microbiome of human being—**holobiome,** represents more than half the body's cells and 99% of its DNA. The main difference from the human genome is that the microbiome can be changed—consciously for 3PM, or unconsciously by just living in the modern world. Manipulation of microbiome for prediction, prevention, and personalization has become the main area of interest of the modern hepatology. Inhabitants of the Western and westernized world are living amidst the **microbiome diversity crisis.** Their microbiome is like the ecosystem of a desert – deprived of diversity, richness, and resilience [5]. Human microbiome diversity – the necessary condition for a good health – has co-evolved with humans over the same two hundred thousand years, but at a mutational pace of 20 min per one microbial generation. They were living in harmony with the human genome (open for a genetic change at a pace of 20 years per one generation) until recently. The microbiome extinction coincides with the modernization of our society lasting roughly five human generations (but 2.5 million microbial generations); therefore, it is of no surprise that human genome has been caught absolutely unprepared [5]. The resultant dysbiosis-associated microbiome/genome functional mismatch is the root cause behind the chronic endotoxemia and low-grade inflammation leading to a pandemic of a non-communicable diseases (NCD) including chronic liver diseases (CLD) [7]. **Gut** is by far the greatest, the most diverse, and the most health-influential of the human body microbiomes and, if not stated otherwise, is referred to in this chapter. Provided healthy gut microbiome is the body's intelligence agency responsible for peaceful handling of an external affairs (stressors and diet), liver - via the **gut-liver axis** - is its closest internal affairs proxy.

3 Microbiome in Historical Context and State of the Art

Apart from the Ancient China's Yellow soup for the soul—which was in all the probability the first mention of a fecal microbial transplantation (FMT) for the gut–brain axis in the history of medicine, as well as of the Ancient Greece's "Let your food be thy medicine" (Rephrased by J. F. Cryan to "Let food for your microbes be your medicine")—which was probably the first record on a prebiotic nature of the food, the modern microbiome science (MS) has begun with the technology: Antony van Loewenhoek's first-ever use of the microscope in 1683 displayed his own oral microbes, some still moving ("animalcules were in such enormous numbers that all the water... seemed to be alive"). More recently, the Nobel laureate of 1908 Elie Metchnikoff (then at the Pasteur's Institute), after leaving macrophages to their own, begun to study longevity and, as described in his book The Prolongation of Life, noticed that the oldest inhabitants of the Parsa consumed a noticeably more lactic bacteria from a fermented food. Strachan and Bloch have laid foundations to the hygienic hypothesis of a global tsunami of NCD's but, the really new era of MS exploded (according to the PubMed statistics) some 15 years ago as a consequence of advances in molecular biology and computer science. An enormous speed of—as Susan D. Lynch put it – "the enabling tools to interrogate microbial dark matter," begun with the discoveries of microbiome's: (1) **composition** via its genetic structure sequenced by 16S sRNA technology, followed by microbiome's, (2) **functional capacity** (by the shotgun metagenomics), (3) **gene expression** (metatranscriptomics / RNA), (4) **protein catalytic function** (metaproteomics), and (5) **metabolic activity** of molecules (metabolomics) [4, 8–10]. Clearly, the real MS revolution is coming now—with the microbiome structure being currently linked with its function measured by molecular inputs and outputs. This has laid the foundations for brand-new areas of research such as foodomics, personalized diets, microbiome-pharmacogenetics, phage therapy, etc. Microbiome output interacts with receptors on the nearby and distant host cells (such as GPR, FFAR, PRR, TLR, LRR, RIG-1, CTLR, CB_1, FXR, TGR5), and with nerve-endings of (e.g.) vagus nerve, and create a communication web with the distant organs and systems of the body; Emeran Mayer coined the term **connectome** [11, 12]. Its various extensions are called **gut-liver axis**, **gut–brain axis**, **gut–muscle axis**, etc. [13].

4 Understanding Microbiome Taxonomy and Function

The term **microbiome** was introduced by Joshua Lederberg in 2001 as a community of commensal, symbiotic, and pathogenic microorganisms within a body space or other environment. In this chapter, we use it as an umbrella term.

All microorganisms are given a name based on taxonomical rank-based classification. In the currently accepted scientific Classification of Life, there are three domains of microorganisms: the *Eukaryotes*, *Bacteria*, and *Archaea*. Within each domain, a several level species classifications can be found. Organized in a descending scale the *domain* level is followed by *kingdom, division/phyla, class, subclass, order, suborder, family, genus, and species*; in addition, species can involve several strains [14, 15]. In the scientific classification established by Carl von Linné, each distinct species is assigned to a genus using a two-part binary name (for example *Escherichia coli*). In 1987, Carl Woese divided the *Eubacteria* into 11 divisions based on 16S ribosomal RNA (SSU) sequences, which are—with several additions—still used today [16]. In the gut so far, dozens of bacterial *phyla* have been identified of which *Firmicutes, Bacteroidota, Proteobacteria, Actinobacteria,* and *Verrucomicrobia* are the most abundant; from the perspective of abundance, the first two phyla represent 90% of the microbiome [15]. Other *phyla* include *Fusobacteria, Chloroflexi, Flavobacteria, Sphingobacteria, Planctomycetes, Cyanobacteria, Thermomicrobia, Xenobacteria, Aquificae, Chlorobia,* and *Chrysogenetes.* The most abundant of *species* are *Enterobacterium rectale, Bacteroides vulgatus, and Escherichia coli.* Beneficial are species known for their symbiotic metabolic properties (see below) such as Akkermansia muciniphila, Roseburia spp, short-chain fatty acids-producing Bifidobacteria, Lactobacillus spp., etc. [14, 17].

The **gut microbiome** contains all the genomes of microbes inhabiting the gut including bacteria, archaea, viruses, and fungi [18]. Spurious is the categorization of phages, viruses, plasmids, prions, viroids, and free DNA. The term microbiome, as it was originally postulated, includes not only the community of the microorganisms, but also their "theater of activity" [19]. The latter involves the whole spectrum of molecules produced by the microorganisms, including their structural elements (nucleic acids, proteins, lipids, polysaccharides), metabolites (signaling molecules, toxins, organic, and inorganic molecules), and molecules produced by coexisting hosts and structured by the surrounding environmental conditions [20]. The term microbiome is also sometimes confused with the metagenome. **Metagenome,** however, is clearly defined as a collection of genomes and genes from the members of a microbiota. Microbiome - personal like a fingerprint and in adulthood relatively stable - can be characterized by bacterial clusters, grouped by some (but not all) authors to a three **enterotypes:** I. dominated by *Bacteroides*, II. by *Prevotella*, III. by *Ruminococcus* [21, 22]. Microbial community composition defined by the metagenome of a single sample can be characterized by its alpha-diversity (**α-diversity**), a numeric value summarizing the structure of the community, with respect to its richness, evenness, or both. Alpha-diversity belongs to the most validated metagenomic marker of gastrointestinal health. The loss of diversity has been linked to severity of a multitude of diseases. There is not yet a gold standard regarding α-diversity measures, even though the number of species (or Operational Taxonomic Units) and the Shannon diversity index are the two most widely used. The measure of similarity or dissimilarity of two communities is defined by **beta diversity**, which quantifies the (dis-)-similarities between communities or samples. Statistical or geometry approaches such as Bray-Curtis, Jaccard, and Jensen-Shannon divergence calculate such distances by counting the overlapped components, as well as an analysis of variance (PERMANOVA) or of similarity (ANOSIM). Finally, we can calculate **gamma-diversity** as the total observed richness of all samples within a habitat.

When reading MS literature in hepatology, it is of uppermost importance to be aware of which taxa are discussed or compared with which. Qin et al. (using HMP database) were the first to describe alterations in microbiome typical for liver cirrhosis, Bajaj *et al.* have created the numeric good–to–bad taxa ratio called cirrhosis dysbiosis ratio, and Schnabl et al. shifted the attention to the microbiome's function and precision phage therapy—all considered the pioneering endeavors opening hepatology for 3PM/PPPM [14, 23, 24].

A healthy **microbiome–host interface** as photographed by the group from the Stanford is associated with a several liver health-sustaining features [4, 25–30]. The first, as mentioned above, is that the microbiome is rich in the number and abundance of symbiotic microbial species and has low proportion of pathogenic microorganisms; this should produce a health-sustaining metabolic output, leading to eubiosis, thick mucus, and tightly sealed epithelium not penetrable to bacteria and their products such as PAMPs and DAMPs (Pathogen-Associated Molecular Patterns, and Damage-Associated Molecullar Patterns) [11, 15, 23, 27, 31–44]. On the one side, the healthy microbiome's output should be rich in the liver health-sustaining molecules or microvesicles such as: short-chain fatty acids (SCFA, butyrate, propionate, acetate); vitamins; secondary bile acids; endocannabinoids and other lipids; aryl-hydrocarbon receptor ligands such as tryptophan; psychoactive substances (called by Anderson, Cryan and Dinan psychobiotics); enterosynes; biotransformed medical drugs (PD 1—programmed cell death protein 1-based immunotherapy, digoxin, acetaminophen); etc. Of note, health-sustaining microbiome metabolic output includes also microbe-associated molecular patterns (MAMP) and pathogen-associated molecular patterns (PAMP), of which the lipopolysaccharide (LPS) is the prototype as it is needed in low levels for the proper immune function, but is harmful in higher levels. As regards the biotransformation of drugs by microbiome, relevant to hepatology are the microbiome-dependent liver toxicity of paracetamol and the possibility to overcome PD 1 resistance of tumors by FMT [45, 46]. On the other hand, healthy microbiome metabolism keeps under control the levels of pro-inflammatory cytokines and toxins such as trimethylamine N-oxide (TMAO); fructoselysine; imidazole propionate (IMP); paracetamol; etc.

5 Microbiome and the Liver

With its 10–100 trillion of symbiotic cells, up to 1500 species, dozens of millions of genes and weight up to 1.5–2 kg, gut microbiome is the richest, the most diverse and the most influential part of a holobiome [11]. Although we will not focus on the fungal microbiome and virome, their content of up to 10^{13} and 10^{15} microorganisms, respectively, is no less remarkable and certainly worth further research in hepatology [24, 47, 48]. The **vertical microbiome gradient** mirrors the health-sustaining abundances of microbes down the gastrointestinal tract from an oral cavity which contains 10^{11} bacteria, through stomach with 10^{7}, jejunum 10^{7}, ileum 10^{11}, up to colon with 10^{14} bacteria, respectively [49]. The other features connected with the vertical gradient are the luminal pH (relevant also in the horizontal gradient), transit-time (more than ten-times longer in the colon than in the small intestine), oxygen pressure, etc. [11, 13]. The two most important examples of a vertical microbiome gradient breakdown in hepatology are a small intestinal bacterial overgrowth (SIBO) and oralization of gut microbiome [50–52]. Liver health-promoting **horizontal microbiome gradient** refers to the different concentrations of hydrogen (pH), oxygen, and symbionts / pathogens close to the gut mucosa as compared to the center of the gut lumen [53]. There is no doubt that a liver-health promoting microbiome is an ecosystem rich, diverse, and resilient like a rainforest and CLD-associated dysbiosis is more like a desert with a low diversity, low abundance of symbiotic species, overgrowth of pathogens, distorted gradients, and low resilience to changes [54–57].

The gut–liver axis originally introduced in the 80s has been recently recognized as the key pathogenetic component in-, and a potential therapeutic target of-, virtually all the liver diseases [13, 58–60]. The anatomy of the axis is composed of an afferent and efferent limb, represented by the portal vein, and biliary tree, respectively. Between the two limbs lie the liver and the gut - the latter composed of microbiome and the complex intestinal barrier [61]. The healthy microbiome helps to maintain an unimpeded **integrity of a gut barrier** which, above many other tasks protects its intimate anatomical and functional proxy—the liver [28, 62, 63]. The barrier is made up of several interacting layers: (1) luminal microbiome with pathogens located far from mucus/mucosa; (2) the tightly sealed intestinal epithelium with a protective layer of (3) mucus; and (4) the sub-mucosal cells of the immune, lymphatic, nervous and blood systems [64]. Via portal circulation of 1 L/min and connectome, liver is the proxy encountering all the microorganisms and molecules traversing the gut barrier [65]. Although microbiome is considered an organ of the body, it is also an ecosystem representing the outer environment. These Janus-like properties are crucial for leveraging microbiome potential for 3PM purposes in hepatology. To approximate the merit of a **mucus layer—**one of the *sine qua non*'s of gut barrier - Erica Sonnenburg uses the proverb "Good fences make good neighbors." Intestinal mucus prevents bacterial adhesion and translocation into the intestine and is composed of two parts. One, adjacent to the intestinal mucosa and called "the de-militarized zone" for its lack of bacteria, is rich in peptidoglycans produced by Paneth cells and immunoglobulin A (IgA) by plasmatic cells [13], [60]. The second, which is in the direct contact with the luminal microbiome, is the glycocalyx produced by the goblet cells. Very rare exceptions notwithstanding, properly functioning mucus layer does not allow bacteria in the portal circulation and properly functioning microbiome governs the mucus barrier. Contact between the gut microbiome and the liver under physiological circumstances is thus relied only on the so-called postbiotics—products of microbiome. Any thinning and/or disturbed functionality of the mucus layer is the key component of the so-called **leaky gut syndrome** which has been proposed as the core pathophysiological mechanisms behind chronic liver diseases [66]. The most important global cause of thinning of a mucus layer is its consumption by dysbiotic bacteria; epitomized by Sonnenburgs as "hungry microbes eat you," lack of dietary fiber which resists absorption in proximal gut causes starvation of colonic microbiome which then turns to mucus as the preferred source of substrates and energy [62]. Penetration of endotoxins such as LPS through the leaky gut results [67] in activation of the inflammatory process and inflammasomes. Moreover, dysbiosis induces MALT via regulatory T lymphocytes (Treg) and Th17 to the synthesis of transforming growth factor beta 1 (TGF β1), interleukin 17 (IL17), which regulate adipogenesis [35] and inflammation by

Foxp3+Tregs processes—thus contributing to the development of liver inflammation and steatosis. **Tight junctions**, integral part of the barrier can be loosened by direct effect of alcohol metabolism, high-fat diet, and dysbiosis, which further accentuate leaky gut syndrome and close-up the vicious circle leading to progressive CLD [68]. Vertical microbiome gradient derangement, contributing to a leaky gut syndrome is characterized by the small intestinal bacterial overgrowth, and oralization of gut microbiome – both driven majorly by changes in bile acids [50, 69–71].

In summary, the proposed cascade of events, leading to the tsunami of CLDs has been primarily driven by the Western lifestyle-induced extinction of microbiome diversity which has taken place over just the few last generations of human evolution and therefore could not be followed by an adaptation on the side of the human host genome [5]. This disequilibrium leads to the leaky gut, translocation of bacteria and toxins to the portal blood, creating an inflamed intrahepatic milieu leading to an attack to the liver parenchyma by the reactive oxygen species, inflammatory molecules, and toxic metabolites; established is the state of chronic metabolic endotoxemia, impaired metabolic homeostasis, liver steatosis, inflammation, and fibrosis [13, 60, 72].

6 Liver Diseases and the Microbiome

6.1 General Considerations

In the Western and westernized world, the burden of CLDs has been increasing and this trend is predicted to continue [73–75]. The main drivers behind the tsunami are how we move, eat, drink, think, feel, and what we consider important and true; with a resulting 1.5 billion global cases of CLD, caused in the West mostly by ALD and NAFLD, accompanied by an autoimmune syndromes and hepatitis C [69, 70, 76, 77]. The individual and societal toll is mostly associated with the acute decompensation of cirrhosis (AD) and the syndrome of an acute-on-chronic liver failure (ACLF) [78–80]. Before AD/ACLF, the usual timeframe of CLD's progression spans over twenty plus years, leaving plenty of room for a 3PM intervention. Most, if not all, of the CLDs are to a certain extent pathogenetically linked with dysbiosis; however, in ALD, NAFLD, autoimmune etiologies, and in cirrhotic stage of all the etiologies, the dysbiosis is considered the key pathogenetic component [13, 80–84]. It is important to acknowledge that, the chicken-egg puzzle of what is damaged first—microbiome, or liver, has not yet been solved.

In any case, microbiome has become decimated and hostile by the lack of dietary fiber and gastric acid, long-term racism of sugar, tribism of ethanol, and genocide of antibiotics, xenobiotics, and psychopathic hygiene [5]. Deprived of a citizenship, multiculturalism, livelihood, manna and soma, microbiome fires weapons such as LPS, PAMPs, DAMPs, toxic bile acid cocktails, cytolysin, candidalysin, and kynurenine [14, 70, 85]. The liver receives the blow and responds with an inflammatory cytokines and more toxic bile acid cocktails; it becomes stuffed by inflammatory cells and, as a consequence, hepatocytes cease to function or die [13, 59, 68].

There is also a chaos on the border: The intestinal mucus layer has been demolished by chemicals and eaten by gut bacteria - hungry due to the lack of dietary fiber; immune cells, mediators, and reactive oxygen species are scattered widely and gut pathogens have broken the gut barrier and translocate to the host portal blood to attack the liver. the liver is injured again and responds back again. And then the gut again. Up until cirrhosis stage of CLD will have evolved and, provided no effective therapy intervenes, cirrhosis decompensates, and other failing organs step in: kidneys; brain; coagulation; lungs. And, while before the decompensation patients might have had mild or no symptoms, at the stage of AD/ACLF, they are hospitalized, often on ICU with a dramatically reduced short-term survival [70, 78, 80, 86]. The difficult task to predict and prevent decompensation or to personalize its management is being undertaken by the Microb-Predict and other consortia and laboratories and scientists; on the other hand, the core concept of 3PM/PPPM is to react to these trends and therefore, it has been integrating ACLD and MS to its nucleus for transcription, translation, and action.

6.2 Alcohol-Associated Liver Disease

In addition to the general mechanisms behind the public health—scale domino of dysbiosis—leaky gut—risk of CLD, one in five people older than 15 years also drink alcohol [87, 88]. In the region of authors, the situation is even worse as the alcohol-associated liver disease (ALD; if not stated otherwise, ALD serves as an umbrella term, encompassing all the syndrome's subtypes) is the leading cause of liver-related mortality, liver transplantation, liver morbidity, and cost to society [89, 90]. Most of the heavy drinkers will develop steatosis and, in at least one-third of them, it will progress to steatohepatitis [91–93]. However, to explain that "only" 8–20% of heavy drinkers will develop cirrhosis is the call for research into a genetic and enviromental (aggravating or protective) co-factors, of which one of the most promising is the microbiome [85, 94–96].

The main research questions in this regard are (1) can microbiome explain the extreme spectrum of ALD phenotypes in comparable drinkers; (2) can microbiome be used for the prediction of prognosis; and (3) for preventive and/or therapeutic interventions? [97, 98]. The spectrum of ALD is extreme: on the one hand, there are individuals with alcohol use disorder (AUD) who drink regularly harmful doses and have steatosis with minimal or no liver disease; and, on the other hand, many individuals drinking the same daily doses will develop severe alcoholic hepatitis (SAH), progressive ALD, cirrhosis, AD/ACLF, hepatocellular carcinoma (HCC), and are transplanted or die [87]. The one special entity, SAH, can develop on the top of almost any stage of ALD (albeit most of patients have cirrhosis), has no durably effective therapy and up to 50% 90-day mortality [93, 99].

In the landmark study from the Perlemuter group, researchers were able to determine the specific dysbiosis which was associated with the severity of ALD and to transmit ALD by transplanting this microbiome to animals [100]. This was the proof-of-concept that alcohol drives liver disease by hijacking microbiome, its metabolites (PAMPs, beta-glucan, bile acids, low indoles, and SCFA), and gut barrier/tight junctions, as recently reviewed elsewhere [94, 101]. Alcohol-associated dysbiosis concerns all the main domains—bacteria, fungi, and viruses. As for the bacterial dysbiosis, it has been shown that, patients with AUD and AH have dysbiosis with gradually decreasing beta diversity and Shannon alpha-diversity as compared to healthy non-alcohol-drinking controls [97, 102]. However, severity of AH was not predicted by microbiome analysis [103]. There were several taxa which were associated with the severity of SAH, prognosis, and response to therapy, e.g., increased *Veillonella* and decreased *Prevotella*. However, the most striking feature of AH-associated dysbiosis was orders-of-magnitude higher abundance of *Enterococcus faecalis* in AH as compared to both AUD and healthy controls; surprisingly enough, this feature did not correlate with the clinical outcome until the subjects with *E. faecalis* were further analyzed for strains producing the toxin, **cytolysin.** Then there was a gradual increase in cytolysin-positive strains along the cohorts (controls—AUD—AH) and this time the presence of cytolysin–positive *E. faecalis* was strongly associated with mortality ($p<0.0001$). Absolutely fascinating example of personalized/precision approach is to target these cytolysin-producing strains with phages - as already shown with *C. crescentus and E. faecalis* phages in experiment [102].

Taking into account that the effective therapy for SAH is an unmet need, it is of little surprise that the clinical research focused on new therapies targeting microbiome [98, 104, 105]. The first study by Philips et al. has shown improved survival in patients with SAH not previously responding to standard of care, if they were administered FMT from healthy donors via the upper gastrointestinal tract for eight days ($p = 0.018$ vs. historical controls) [106]. More studies with FMT are needed and, according to the clinicaltrials.gov, several are ongoing (one of them at the institutions of the authors—NCT58806). A cautionary note is needed regarding FMT, as drug-resistant bacteria such as *E. coli* and viruses such as *Monkeypox* can be transmitted [107, 108]. Promising piece of evidence for a predictive, preventive and personalized potential of certain gut microbial taxa is the case of ***Akkermansia muciniphila*** as a marker, predictor and therapeutic agent in AH [109]. Yet another way of addressing microbiome in ALD and AH/SAH are antibiotics [98]. A recent study has shown a promising alleviation of dysbiosis after therapy with **rifaximin** [97]. Moreover, the interesting 3PM aspect of this multicentric study was that baseline microbiome signature was able to predict prognosis and response to therapy with rifaximin.

Very recent research from the Schnabl group has shed light on up to now rarely scrutinized virome and fungal microbiome in three cohorts (non-alcoholic controls, patients with AUD, and patients with AH). In the study on virome, authors have shown graded alterations along the three cohorts, with the most remarkable increases in AH patients of the Shannon diversity and of mammalian viruses such as Parvoviridae, Circoviridae, and Herpesviridae (especially EBV); moreover, results were corelated with the severity of liver disease as reflected in the model for end-stage liver disease (MELD) score [110]. In another set of three studies, they provided evidence of a graded fungal overgrowth in patients with AUD and AH as compared to non-drinking controls [111–113]. The most significant overgrown fungus was candida albicans. As to the fungal diversities, beta diversity was not able to discriminate between AUD and AH, but was clearly distinctive of healthy controls; Shannon alpha-diversity was highest in AH patients and lowest in controls (similar to viral-, and at a difference with bacterial diversity). One of the conclusions was that fungal overgrowth is more dependent on the alcohol intake than on the stage of ALD.

As the crucial determinants of pathogenesis and mortality in ALD are microbiome and long-term abstinence, respectively, it is logical to attempt to address them simultaneously. This has been done by Bajaj et al. in their landmark phase 1 randomized study on patients with AUD addressing craving and AUD outcomes by single-dose FMT [114]. The FMT enema was selected in the OpenBiome for enrichment with *Lachnospiraceae* and *Ruminococcaceae*. Patients in active arm post-FMT had increased Shannon diversity, increased abundance of SCFA-producing *Roseburia, Alistipes,* and *Odoribacter*—usually decreased in ALD and cirrhosis, and reduced craving and AUD-related events.

6.3 Non-Alcoholic Fatty Liver Disease (NAFLD)

With the global prevalence of 25–30%, NAFLD (currently in the process of renaming to metabolic-associated fatty liver disease—MAFLD and, in 2023 to steatotic liver disease - MASLD) is the most common etiology of CLD and, as a consequence of a pandemic of diabesity, it is the fastest growing indication for liver transplantation [76, 115, 116]. Similar to ALD, NAFLD encompasses a spectrum with only 10–20% of patients progressing to cirrhosis via non-alcoholic steatohepatitis with fibrosis over at least 10 years—the interval open for 3PM intervention [117, 118]. And, also similar to ALD, microbiome is one of the prime suspects modulating the phenotype toward benign or progressive disease or HCC [101, 119, 120]. As NAFLD is considered the liver manifestation of metabolic syndrome, transfer of obesity by FMT in animals has been taken as a proof-of-concept that NAFLD pathophysiology may be driven by dysbiosis [121, 122].

Obesity plus inactivity with sarcopenia, and insulin resistance-mediated delivery of free fatty acids from adipose tissue to the liver are the main factors leading to the first hit in **the multiple-hit hypothesis of NAFLD**. In the meantime, obesity is - according to some - associated with certain enterotypes, and certain microbiome signatures are associated with metabolic endotoxemia, low-grade inflammation, oxidative stress, endogenous alcohol production and various other "second and further hits," to the already steatotic liver; this cascade of events leads to a progression of NAFLD to NASH, cirrhosis, liver failure, and/or HCC [120, 123–125]. **NAFLD-associated dysbiosis** is characterized by reduced SCFA producing *Firmicutes, Ruminococcaceae, Prevotella, and Faecalibacterium* and over-abundance of *Bacteroides, Ruminococcus, Proteobacteria*, and *Enterobacteriaceae*—the latter linked with the production of alcohol, the pathophysiological step toward NAFLD known as **autobrewery** [120, 126, 127].

However, microbial and metabolical signatures typical for NAFLD and its progression are less well characterized and more controversial than in ALD[59, 101]. Apart from autobrewery mechanism of liver injury, over-abundant gram-negative bacteria increase levels of LPS which inflames the gut and makes it leaky, activates inflammasome in the liver and, recruit macrophages to the adipose tissue; at the same time, depleted taxa produce less SCFA with their positive functions left lacking, which closes the vicious circle of a leaky gut, translocation, inflammation, metabolic derangement, and liver injury [128, 129]. Crucial in development and progression of NAFLD and NASH is the interplay between bile acids, FXR, FGF 19, and microbiome; dysbiosis leads to a skewed bile acid signaling with downstream effect on fibrogenesis [130–132].

Outlier between the usual microbiome-based pathophysiological concepts is the relationship between SCFA-producing bacteria and progression of NAFLD [101]. While SCFA are in general, as well as in other liver diseases, considered beneficial molecules and their producers a beneficial members of microbiome—usually associated with less inflammation, better energy metabolism, satiety, better gut barrier and a good liver prognosis, in NAFLD the associations tend to differ [103, 133]: Higher stool SCFA (and their producers, such as several *Roseburia* species and *Faecalibacterium prausnitzii*) of animals and patients with NAFLD associates with a more progressive disease, more inflammation, more fibrosis, and worse prognosis [134].

The foundations of a modern predictive and personalized medicine in a wider NAFLD realm were laid by the landmark study by Zeevi et al. [135]. Authors have shown that the main determinant of a metabolic response to a defined meal (the primordial pathomechanism in NAFLD) was the microbiome. They postulated the possibility of a microbiome analysis-based **personalized nutritional intervention** in a foreseeable future. A more recent follow-ups on this line of research are personalized approach to a weight loss, tailored according to host–microbiome characteristics; and the meta-analysis showing that, *Lactobacillus* supplementation positively impacts on glycemic and lipid indices [136, 137].

Twenty-one studies (considerably heterogeneous) were scrutinized in a meta-analysis of the first-generation **probiotics** and synbiotics in NAFLD patients; improvements in liver enzymes, steatosis, and liver stiffness were found but personalized recommendations on the certain type of biotic for certain patients/phenotypes of NAFLD could not be drawn [138]. As stated above, Lactobacillus supplementation had a positive impact on glycemic and lipid indices [136, 137]. Moreover, specific strains of *Faecalibacterium prausnitzii* were found to regulate microbiome and improve NAFLD in mice [139]. Currently, there are no ongoing studies with the next-generation biotics such as phages, or engineered bacteria in NAFLD/NASH. One outstanding exception is the domain of microbiome-bile acid signaling, where the focus of recent interest has been the FXR/FGF-19 pathway; obeticholic acid and engineered FGF 19 analogue are the studied molecules, with biopsy-proven NASH the indication. Of interest in this regard is as of now unpublished finding from GwangPyo Ko group of a reduced liver steatosis by a cell-free supernatant (a postbiotic [P9]) of *Akkermansia muciniphila* via GLP-1 pathway.

FMT has been formally investigated in three studies on a metabolic syndrome and two in NAFLD; while awaiting more data, experts doubt that FMT without a causal long-term lifestyle intervention could lead to a sustained benefit [101, 140, 141].

6.4 Autoimmune Diseases and the Microbiome

Autoimmune diseases of the liver comprise three major diseases - autoimmune hepatitis (AIH) with a prevalence of 0.5–1 cases per 100,000 inhabitants [142], primary biliary cholangitis (PBC) occurring in 20–40 cases per 100,000, and primary sclerosing cholangitis (PSC) with 6–10 cases per 100,000 in the Caucasian population[143].

In general, the pathogenesis of autoimmune liver diseases is not completely understood. Recent data from the genome-wide association studies and the multi-omic (metagenomic and metabolomic) studies of the microbiome have underlined some potential mechanisms by which the microbiome could play a role in the development of autoimmunity [144, 145]: a unique pattern of genetic susceptibility to immune system recognition of antigens with various HLA haplotypes, a unique succession of changes in the microbiome during immune system maturation leading to selective immune tolerance to various antigens encountered in the environment, the state of mucosal homeostasis balancing a pro-inflammatory and gut barrier disturbing microbiota and their metabolites with anti-inflammatory and gut barrier promoting processes, a liver immune system homeostasis balancing the immune response to microbial antigens, metabolites, and signaling molecules reaching the liver from the gut by promoting either anti-inflammatory or pro-inflammatory state, a toxic effect of various food additives, industrial or household pollutants disrupting the mucosal or liver immune system homeostasis.

6.5 Autoimmune Hepatitis

Autoimmune hepatitis (AIH) is characterized by the natural history of successive bursts of varying intensity causing inflammatory destruction of hepatocytes. The actual trigger of the inflammation is unknown. The disease is not considered curable, but the established treatment is effective in the great majority of cases[146]. For patients progressing to decompensated cirrhosis liver transplantation remains the therapy of choice.

Studies of the microbiome in AIH have revealed a consistently increased abundance of *Veillonella, Streptococcus, Lactobacilli, Lachnospiraceae, Bacteroides, Roseburia, Ruminococcacae,* and *Klebsiella.* In contrast, the depletion of *Bifidobacteria* and *Clostridiales* has been reported [147]. The presence of a sufficient abundance of *Bifidobacteria* could also increase the chances of disease remission after therapy [148].

The mechanisms by which these bacteria might affect the pathogenesis of AIH are unknown. So far, there is no established cause and effect relationship. One hypothesis suggests that microbiota changes could lead to lower metabolic production of SCFA, increased intestinal permeability resulting in innate immunity (by RIP3) activation of liver macrophages. [149–151]. Moreover, the spectrum of bile acids and their metabolites has also been implicated in the regulation of T cells balancing Th17 and Treg response. Some proof-of-concept studies in animal models have confirmed these proposed mechanisms. Improvement in AIH by dietary fiber, probiotics (including Bifidobacteria and Lactobacilli), or butyrate supplementation via increase in Treg/T17 ratio, expression of tight junction proteins, decreased LPS translocation/TLR activation, and a decreased E. coli protein in the liver were displayed [150, 152, 153]. Moreover, FMT attenuated liver injury, bacterial translocation, and improved the imbalance between helper and regulatory splenic T cells [154].

6.6 Primary Biliary Cholangitis

Primary biliary cholangitis (PBC) is characterized by inflammatory destruction of the ducts transporting bile from the liver to the digestive tract. The actual trigger of the inflammation is still unknown with autoimmunity likely involved in its pathogenesis due to the frequent presence of anti-mitochondrial or specific anti-nuclear autoantibodies (anti-gp210 or anti-sp100) and the presence of lymphocytic infiltrate in the proximity of the bile ducts [155]. Without treatment, more than 50% of cases progress to cirrhosis and end-stage liver disease. Since 1987 [156], a naturally occurring secondary bile acid ursodeoxycholic acid (UDCA) has been successfully used for treatment. However, approximately 20–40% of cases do not respond to UDCA therapy [157, 158]. Second-line add-on therapy with obeticholic acid or fibrates has been used in these patients [159].

Several studies of microbiome, mainly in the Asian population, have reported an increased abundance of several species: *Haemophilus, Veillonella, Clostridiales, Lactobacilli, Streptococci, Pseudomonas, Klebsiella, Bifidobacterium*, and an unknown genus from the *Enterobacteriaceae* family [144]. In contrast, several species have been reported reduced such as Bacteroidetes, *Sutterella*, *Oscillospira*, and *Faecalibacterium*. The common ground for these changes is not completely understood but it could be associated with the decreased metabolic output of the butyric acid. In addition, the decrease in Faecalibacterium was associated with non-response to UDCA. As stated above, *Bacteroidetes* and *Faecalibacterium prausnitzi* are known butyrate-producing bacteria and a sufficient butyrate concentration in the gut is indispensable for healthy mucin production ensuring a normal function of the intestinal barrier [139].

In PBC, the autoantigen of anti-mitochondrial antibodies displays structural similarities with the human E2 component of the mitochondrial pyruvate dehydrogenase complex (PDC-E2). Since PDC-E2 is also a commonly occurring enzyme among the various bacterial species, exposition to this antigen through the disrupted intestinal barrier in a genetically susceptible individual may explain the origin of autoimmunity in PBC [160].

6.7 Primary Sclerosing Cholangitis

Primary sclerosing cholangitis (PSC) is characterized by the progressive fibrosing damage of the intrahepatic and extrahepatic bile ducts leading to impairment of bile flow and eventually biliary cirrhosis.

Natural history is marked by variable progression rate toward end-stage liver disease and less frequently to cholangiocarcinoma [155]. The trigger of the inflammation is not known, but autoimmunity is suspected due to its association with inflammatory bowel disease in 60–80% of cases, and frequent detection of autoantibodies against the cytoplasm of neutrophils.

Currently, there is no established treatment with liver transplantation remaining the only curative option. UDCA therapy is recommended by some authorities for its proven effect in lowering the markers of cholestasis and improving the quality of life. The studies have explored the mechanisms linking the genetic predisposition with the immune system and the microbiome. The microbial composition can influence the balance of the immune system directly when microbes or their fragments cross the dysfunctional intestinal barrier. Moreover, products of bacterial metabolism also influence the host immune system, as some are being absorbed into the bloodstream.

Current understanding of the pathogenesis of PSC highlights the **central role of the microbiome in the maintenance of chronic inflammation** by shifting the mucosal homeostasis toward intestinal barrier dysfunction, activation of several lineages of the immune system, and homing of gut-tropic lymphocytes in the liver endothelium [161]. Studies have reported compositional changes of the gut microbiome in PSC compared with healthy controls and newer studies are emerging with data on the functional differences.

Microbiome studies in patients with PSC have revealed consistent enrichment in various taxa including *Clostridiales, Streptococcus salivarius, Veillonella dispar, Ruminococcus gnavus, Bacteroides fragilis, Enterobacteriaceae, Lactobacilli, Blautia, Enterococcus, Rothia.* A shotgun metagenomic sequencing of the fecal microbiome also showed a markedly reduced gene richness compared to healthy controls [144]. Authors have concluded that *Veillonella* species were more prevalent, with decreased abundance after UDCA therapy; however, the mechanisms by which *Veillonella* is more abundant and how it may affect the natural history of the disease have not yet been deciphered [144].

Interestingly, patients with associated inflammatory bowel disease have a distinct profile of the microbiome compared to patients with pure PSC or healthy controls [162, 163]. A recent study of the fungal microbiota in PSC patients reported increased diversity with increased abundance of *Exophiala* genus and *Sordariomycetes* class and a decrease in *Sacharomycetacae* [164]. Bile microbiota has also been studied in PSC patients, but the results are not consistently different from healthy controls [144].

In contrast, **oral microbiome changes** copied those of the fecal microbiota displaying an increased abundance of *Streptococcus salivarius, Veillonella parvula, Actinomyces, and Bifidobacterium* in PSC patients compared to healthy controls [165].

Functional studies have revealed lowered content of the butyrate, a different metabolite content, and a decreased total bile acid pool with a lower conversion from primary to secondary bile acids [166]. Increased concentration of secondary bile acids in the liver bile has been linked to inflammation, cholestasis, gallstone formation, and carcinogenesis, as well as to modulation of FXR or TGR5 receptors on the natural killer cells, liver or intestinal macrophages, or intestinal dendritic cells. Bile acids acting on both receptors modulate the immune response against inflammation by suppressing the nuclear factor NF-kB signaling pathways and modulating the balance between the Treg and Th17 cells in the gut-liver axis.

Data from the studies with vancomycin have suggested that the observed increased conversion of primary to secondary bile acids can be reversed. Treatment with vancomycin resulted in depletion of the Gram-positive *Firmicutes* including the *Clostridium* species, which are known for their dehydroxylation activity. Indeed, vancomycin decreased fecal secondary bile acids and their postprandial plasma concentration [167, 168]. This concept has been clinically tested in small trials of patients with refractory PSC receiving oral vancomycin demonstrating a positive effect while larger randomized trials are warranted [169, 170]. Other antibiotics or fecal microbial transplantation [171] have so far reported less promising results in comparison with vancomycin alone [161, 172].

6.8 Liver Cirrhosis, Acute Decompensation and Acute-On Chronic Liver Failure

Cirrhosis is the final stage of the sufficiently long-lasting chronic liver diseases of various etiologies, characterized by an increased collagen deposition, distorted architecture and, gradually decreasing volume of hepatocytes despite their intensive regeneration [70, 173]. Being the increasing cause of morbidity and mortality globally, the prevalence of cirrhosis in Slovakia is highest in the world and, liver-related mortality is the number-one cause of death in 25–45 years old [7, 174].

Recently, dysbiosis has been proposed as the key factor associated with the transition from a pre-cirrhotic stage of CLD to cirrhosis, and from compensated to decompensated cirrhosis with the time-to-decompensation of 10 years, time-to-ACLF 2 years, and time-to-death 2 months [80, 86, 175]. Gut microbiome signatures could thus become the biomarkers discriminating asymptomatic-stage cirrhosis in population for prevention, for prediction of decompensation in diagnosed yet stable/asymptomatic cirrhosis, as well as for prediction of prognosis after decompensation.

After first defining the metagenomic signature for non-invasive detection of **advanced fibrosis** (pre-cirrhotic stage of CLD), Loomba et al. have also detected a 19–microbes-containing signature, distinguishing **cirrhosis**—with an unprecedented area under receiver operating characteristic (AUROC) of 0.91 and validated it against various geographical regions and degrees of fibrosis [32, 176]. Moreover, with the 7% of adults (not aware of any liver disease) having fibrosis, this direction of research is absolutely crucial for a modern 3PM hepatology for several other reasons [177]: First, cirrhosis fulfills all the WHO criteria for screening except one—the widely available, affordable, and patient-acceptable diagnostic marker of pre-clinical stage of disease, malleable by the recall policy (median time-to decompensation 10 years); second, current two sets of non-invasive diagnostic modalities (serological and imaging) are either not universally available, or not affordable; third, to collect a stool sample and store/transport it for examination is conceivable in a mass context akin to a colorectal cancer screening; and, fourth, the only impediment (cost) is falling exponentially over the last 15 years. Our SIRIUS Microbiome Study has been designed to detect fibrosis in community and to try to find a link with a region-relevant microbiome signature (NCT05486767).

In a more advanced stage of cirrhosis, i.e., after a decompensating event has materialized (**decompensated cirrhosis,** median time-to-ACLF 2 years), microbiome and gut microbial metabolome can serve as a predictive biomarkers and therapeutic targets [63, 83].

Cirrhosis is among diseases with the most profound dysbiosis (as compared to AUROCs in obesity, colorectal cancer, inflammatory bowel diseases, type 2 diabetes mellitus) [178].

Dysbiosis in cirrhosis is characterized by a reduction in *Bacteroidetes, Lachnospiraceae, Ruminococcaceae,* and *Clostridium incertae sedis XIV*; and increase in *Proteobacteria, Fusobacteria, Clostridium cluster XI, Streptococcaceae, Streptecoccus spp., Veilonella spp., Enterobacteriaceae, Enterococcaceae, Lactobacillaceae, Alcaligenaceae,* etc., which were derived from a stool samples, mucosal biopsies, salivary samples, etc. [14, 23, 59, 71, 80, 179–181].

Based on deviations of cirrhotic microbiome, the cirrhosis dysbiosis ratio (CDR) was developed by Bajaj et al. and has become the prime example of how to utilize a complex microbiome output in a user-friendly way to personalize risk of patients with cirrhosis and to predict outcome—especially hepatic encephalopathy, and rehospitalizations; however, CDR requires wider external validation. Taxa selected in abovementioned studies are being scrutinized as signature predictors of a response to therapy or outcome, with the **European Microb-PREDICT** being the eponymous example-endeavor in the field, whose results are expected shortly. An absolute 3PM match is the sum of a microbiome-based tools to (1) predict the risk of ACLF; (2) predict therapeutic benefit and personalize it; 3) monitor effect of therapy, with the cautionary note concerning the effect size and drug treatment confounders [80].

7 Microbiome as a Therapeutic Target in Cirrhosis and AD/ACLF

Of the three next-generation therapeutic domains defined by Schnabl and described below, most are being scrutinized against liver syndromes at the right side of CLD spectrum—i.e., in cirrhosis, AD, and ACLF. **Diets** have been shown to modulate microbiome and outcome in cirrhotics differently if of Turkish (vegetables, fermented milk) and American (typical Western diet) type [57]. **Probiotics** clearly need a more precision and personalization in cirrhosis but have already shown a potential in encephalopathy and hospitalization-rate [182, 183] . The so-called next-generation probiotics are being awaited by the community with much hope. Of quite a few antibiotics studied in cirrhosis, rifaximin has received the most focused attention with a clear effect in hepatic encephalopathy but with, as of now, contradictory performances in other indications [80]. **Fecal microbial transplantation** has been shown to be safe and improve encephalopathy, rehospitalizations, and ACLF, with a proven safety even over the long-term follow-up [114, 184–186]. Less odious/more acceptable capsule formulations of FMT have been introduced by a Bajaj's group and at least six more studies, registered in ClinicalTrials.gov are underway [187].

8 Hepatocellular Carcinoma and Microbiome

Ever since the landmark antibiotic study by Schwabe's group confirmed the role of microbiome in the evolution of liver cancer (HCC, hepatocellular carcinoma), the field has been the focus of much interest in hepatology [188, 189]). The microbiome-HCC pathogenetic pathways have been summarized recently and are the next-step evolution of the same mechanisms which lead to CLDs and cirrhosis [190–192]. At present, however, rough-level microbiome analyses based on diversity and phyla have not found a differences between cirrhosis with- and without HCC; and, although the deeper-level granularity analyses revealed small differences, predicting HCC in cirrhosis based on gut microbiome analysis remains an unmet need [193–196].

One promising direction of investigation in the predictive arm of 3PM is the intratumoral (and liver parenchymal) microbiome analysis, but the field is in its *statu nascendi* and more studies are needed [197, 198]. As for the other areas of 3PM, a microbiome-targeted prevention (primary and secondary) of HCC is scrutinized widely via all the above-mentioned pathways but, the real-life output is still to be awaited from more than forty NCT-registered studies with rifaximin, nine with norfloxacin, and one with probiotic; no HCC preventive studies with FXR agonists are underway as of 2021. As stated above, an absolutely new 3PM direction touching indirectly the HCC arena is the prediction of a microbiome-dependent effectivity of the new anti-tumor therapies such as PD-1-based immunotherapy [199–201].

9 Predictive Potential of Microbiome Analysis in Liver Diseases

Currently, there is ample evidence to suggest a predictive potential of a microbiome analysis in many liver diseases. Akin to a FOBT for colorectal cancer screening, microbiome signature can pick up cirrhosis in a general population with AUROC of

0.91. The above-mentioned associations of CLDs with microbiome / metabolome signatures notwithstanding, predicting early stage CLDs is as of now an unmet need, however. In a more advanced stages of CLD, such as in compensated cirrhosis, microbiome analysis can predict deterioration (decompensation) and, in decompensated cirrhosis, it can predict outcome.

10 Microbiome as a Target for Preventive and Personalized Medicine in Liver Diseases

Naturally, the most efficient primary prevention in this regard in hepatology is to aim at a healthy microbiome. As to ascertain healthy microbiome by daily living is often beyond the reach of the common people of the Western and westernized world, 3PM-aware medicine can step in with the region- and/or person-appropriate selection of measures from the three domains of Bugs as drugs, Drug the bug, and Drugs from bugs. The spectrum of modalities is wide, spanning from the dietary intervention to FMT and engineered phage therapy for cytolysin-positive Enterococcus faecalis. Of course, ideal prevention is as far left in this spectrum as possible but, thanks to the research done it is now clear that to claim diet and probiotics effective, it must be personalized and precise. There is accumulating evidence to suggest that the personalized diet designed according to the microbiome pattern of an individual, as well as the effectivity of probiotics predicted according to the microbiome of the recipient are the directions to be taken. As hepatology—for its inherent tight junction of liver with gut - is the area of research contributing vastly to the microbiome movement, we can expect a real-life prediction, prevention, and personalization shortly.

11 Technological Challenges of Microbiome Analysis

> *Once the diversity of the microbial world is catalogued, it will make astronomy look like a pitiful science*—(Julian Davies)

As to MS being the biggest data challenge ever (bigger than astrophysics), a teaspoon of a stool contains the data filling the memory of a ton of DVD's [16]. Conceiving of the handling these data with respect to an evolution of patient's microbiome over time or its comparisons between individuals, diseases, populations and of modeling the outcomes, a hundreds-to-thousands of years of computing time would be necessary. Not to speak of a microbiome metabolomics combined with a foodomics—the next steps of MS and 3PM. With the groundbreaking accrual of the NIH's **Human Microbiome Project** (HMP) 4.5 trillion bases freely available for analysis, MS got the necessary first impetus [10]. Then the QIIME produced an unprecedented half a million of catalogued sequences for a reasonable computing time and money (**QIIME**—Quantitative Insight into Microbial Ecology, pronounced *chime*) [202, 203]. This fascinating translation of teradata to the point on a graph—the distance metric of an evolutionary history - was described by Lozupone of Knight's then Colorado lab under the name UniFrac [56, 204] (Fig. 1).

These endeavors have enabled opening the current chapter of MS which gave birth to such projects as The American Gut, The Microsetta Initiative, The Earth Microbiome Project, The FoodOmics, The Microb-Predict and our SIRIUS Microbiome Project (NCT05486767) [205, 206]. However, to really understand a microbiome means to understand its function rather than the composition. And, if a dynamic mapping of a microbiome with a GPS navigation can be considered a reality around the corner, understanding and leveraging the host–microbiome interactions is as of yet an unmet need. **The metabolomic pathway** of microbiome → protein sequence → protein structure → protein function → molecular interactions → therapies, is just being scrutinized against the computing capacity of today's machines and community grids [20]. Over the last decade, the size of a dataset of a sequenced proteins has grown exponentially (from <10M to 175M by UniProt.org), and the size of the database of protein structures started to move (from 60K to 160K, by PDB) [207, 208]. However, even before the technology will have allowed us to leverage microbiome in our real-life 3PM clinical practice by the user-friendly gadgets, we could and should take the pains to understand more of the **predictive power of** this "dark matter" of our **patient's personal universes** [209, 210]. Because, it is quite safe to **assume that most of our patients suffer chronic dysbiosis.** And we can provide them with a general advice with a subsequent more and more personalized stewardship based on a lifestyle analysis and possibly repeated sequencing of a gut microbiome - as eponymously exemplified by Larry Smarr

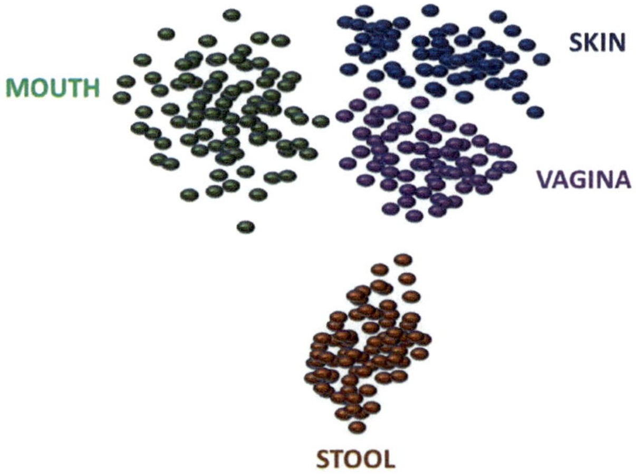

Fig. 1 The Healthy Microbiome Map. This schematic drawing has been derived from the landmark US National Institute of Health's Human Microbiome Project (HMP). By subsequently applying of certain reductive tools to the big data provided by HMP, it was possible to get output which was understandable to a non-experts, even to a lay public: Each dot represents the microbiome of one person from one body site. It can be seen that in these meticulously selected healthy people, dots tend to gravitate together to form the "continents" of the healthy microbiome map

[211–213]. Subsequently, real-life MS will translate to the lifelong endeavor of monitoring, understanding and manipulating microbiome for a better health—which is the 3PM at its best.

12 Visions and Perspectives of Microbiome Analysis in 3PM

From the teleological perspective, MS and 3PM are the perfect match. The reason for 3PM to act is the technological singularity we live on the brink of: Not much more than a decade-long revolution brought about by MS has provided a new meaning to the Heidegger‘s Question Concerning Technology, as well as to the Technological Singularity theory. Pausing over the meaning of a personalized medicine's *person*, one recalls the famous "When I think of it I know but when you ask me I do not know." If sobering before, talking the Person in the era of MS has become the experience outright humbling: Some thirty trillion human-person cells and 20,000 genes make but a 43% and 1% of the individual, respectively [47]. What are the remaining 39–100 trillion cells and 99% genes of the "human" body? Yes. They are the the human microbiota and microbiome, respectively. However, it is a holobiome's feature other than a mere quantity that makes it the prime ally for the next-generation 3PM. After the last major hurdles of price and computing time will have been overcame shortly a lay, user-friendly output will become one of the most if not The Most personal and predictive tools for an unprecedently dynamic and targeted disease prevention and therapy ever. Because, at a variance with the human genome, microbiome is malleable.

What Elon Musk said to world leaders at their summit about the artificial intelligence (AI) in politics, Rob Kight conveyed to the medical community about AI in MS: "*Do not think of it as of a science fiction. Think of it as of a science fact.*" Imagine it is morning. You have just flushed your smart toilet and now you are looking at your face in a smart mirror. The mirror is mass-spectrometering your exhaled oral microbiome metabolic output and displays the result in a lay language and pictures. A smart toilet has already sequenced your microbiome's terrabites and sent the result to your smart-phone app called by Rob Knight the microbiome GPS which will help you by QR to choose the right yogurt [10] (Fig. 2).

If your "GPS"- "You are here“ position has moved away from the healthy area of the map, you are informed about the ensuing health risks and advised what to do to compensate for it (e.g., "Exercise 20 minutes more," or "Try probiotic *Lactobacillus,*“ or "Consult your gastroenterologist for FMT") (Fig. 3).

The current price is prohibitive but, as a DNA sequencing is a million-times cheaper than 15 years ago, this technology is thought to be around the corner (genome.gov/ sequencing costs). Naturally, expected revolution in microbiome-based prediction, prevention, and personalization in medicine will inevitably concern all its areas, hepatology included [57, 60, 80, 101, 175]. After all, it has been in the realm of hepatology where Schnabl et al. proposed the next-generation approach summing the otherwise difficult-to-grasp plethora of **microbiome-directed therapeutics** (such as fermented foods/prebiotics, probiotics, synbiotics, postbiotics, and

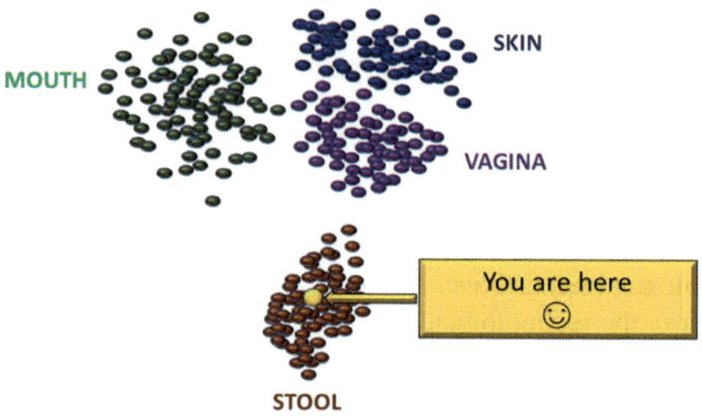

Fig. 2 The healthy microbiome map as a template against which new samples can be scrutinized. This schematic drawing has been derived from the landmark US National Institute of Health's Human Microbiome Project (HMP). Here you can see the example of a result from a stool sample (fecal microbiome) of a hypothetical healthy individual: the dot fits inside its respective healthy area (this time the "stool continent"). This reassuring result is clearly understandable to a layperson and it can be used for predictive and preventive purposes

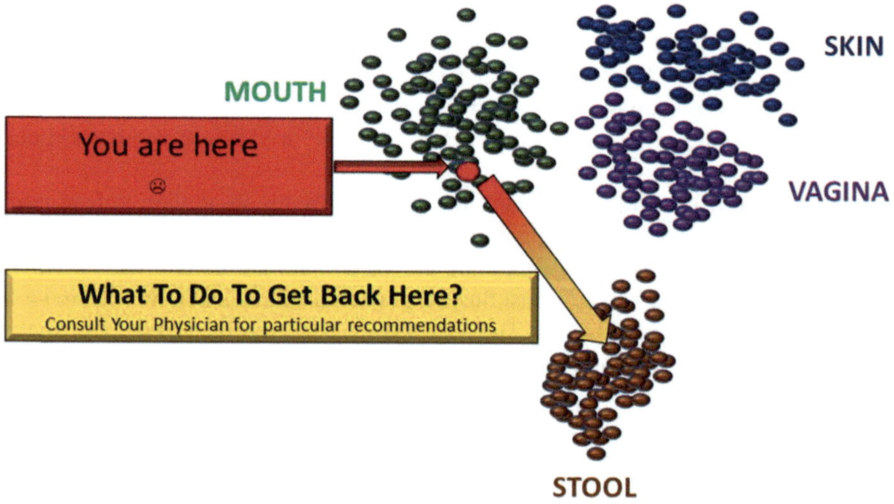

Fig. 3 The microbiome "GPS." This schematic drawing has been derived from the landmark US National Institute of Health's Human Microbiome Project (HMP). The healthy microbiome map serves as a template against which samples from individuals and patients can be scrutinized. Here is the example of result from stool sample (fecal microbiome) of a hypothetical patient with liver cirrhosis: the (red) dot is located outside the healthy area. This particular dislocation of fecal microbiome is typical for cirrhosis and is called "oralization." As it is potentially malleable, the so-called microbiome GPS can drive patient back to the healthy area ("continent") by specific measures ("What To Do To Get Back Here?") from lifestyle changes through pre–pro–post-biotics to fecal microbial transplantation. Microbiome GPS for various diseases provides the opportunity to be leveraged by predictive–preventive–personalized medicine

parabiotics) to three domains, mentioned above: "Bug as Drug," "Drug the Bug," and "Drugs from Bugs"; these next-generation microbiome-directed approaches have specific precision and 3PM as the leading principles [101, 214–218].

13 Conclusions and Recommendations

Considering the modest cumulative effect of past microbiome-based therapies in liver diseases, the next-generation approach is being launched, based on the cornerstones of prediction, prevention, and personalization as well as very specific precision, in all the three newly delineated therapeutic domains (Drugs for Bugs, Bugs as Drugs, and Drugs from Bugs). Moreover, shifts from rough-level analysis of microbiome composition to an ultimate granularity of strains are expected and, most importantly, focus on metabolic aspects will prevail. Based on a pre-emptive analysis of a functional potential of a donor stool, ideal FMT donors will be determined for particular liver diseases together with a more acceptable FMT delivery modalities.

According to the accumulated knowledge to date by the scientific research in the field of human microbiome we can undoubtedly assume that the predictive potential, potential for prevention and potential for personalization in liver diseases is simply enormous. 3PM/PPPM must essentially get ready to use this potential for the patients as well as for those who want to avoid a health deterioration. We suggest, from the point of view of liver diseases to:

- start education activities of the population in order to increase the knowledge about liver diseases in relation to microbiome, lifestyle, and healthy diet;
- start preventive and predictive monitoring of the population willing to implement particular suggestions for supporting their health;
- include the knowledge on microbiome health into the routine processes of healthcare education in the specific context of liver diseases (prehabilitation, ERAS protocols, pain chronification prediction, suboptimal health monitoring as mentioned and discussed in the other chapters of this publication);
- extend the potential of laboratory diagnostics in order to be able to provide the patient with concrete information on his/her microbiome—patterns, of dysbiosis, nutritional status, fitness status, immunity/autoimmunity status, inflammation markers monitoring, and other related factors.

References

1. National Research Council (US) Committee on Metagenomics: Challenges and Functional Applications (2007) The new science of metagenomics: revealing the secrets of our microbial planet. In: The new science of metagenomics: revealing the secrets of our microbial planet. National Academies Press, Washington, DC, pp 1–158. https://doi.org/10.17226/11902

2. Evogeneao: The Tree of Life. http://www.evogeneao.com/en. Accessed 1 Sep 2022
3. Falkowski PG, Fenchel T, Delong EF (2008) The microbial engines that drive Earth's biogeochemical cycles. Science 320:1034–1039. https://doi.org/10.1126/SCIENCE.1153213
4. Lynch SV, Pedersen O (2016) The human intestinal microbiome in health and disease. N Engl J Med 375:2369–2379. https://doi.org/10.1056/NEJMRA1600266
5. Sonnenburg ED, Smits SA, Tikhonov M, Higginbottom SK, Wingreen NS, Sonnenburg JL (2016) Diet-induced extinctions in the gut microbiota compound over generations. Nature 529:212–215. https://doi.org/10.1038/NATURE16504
6. Yatsunenko T, Rey FE, Manary MJ, Trehan I, Dominguez-Bello MG, Contreras M et al (2012) Human gut microbiome viewed across age and geography. Nature 486:222–227. https://doi.org/10.1038/NATURE11053
7. Sepanlou SG, Safiri S, Bisignano C, Ikuta KS, Merat S, Saberifiroozi M et al (2020) The global, regional, and national burden of cirrhosis by cause in 195 countries and territories, 1990-2017: a systematic analysis for the Global Burden of Disease Study 2017. Lancet Gastroenterol Hepatol 5:245–266. https://doi.org/10.1016/S2468-1253(19)30349-8
8. Zhu Q, Mai U, Pfeiffer W, Janssen S, Asnicar F, Sanders JG et al (2019) Phylogenomics of 10,575 genomes reveals evolutionary proximity between domains Bacteria and Archaea. Nat Commun 10:5477. https://doi.org/10.1038/S41467-019-13443-4
9. Woese CR, Fox GE (1977) Phylogenetic structure of the prokaryotic domain: the primary kingdoms. Proc Natl Acad Sci U S A 74:5088–5090. https://doi.org/10.1073/PNAS.74.11.5088
10. Turnbaugh PJ, Ley RE, Hamady M, Fraser-Liggett CM, Knight R, Gordon JI (2007) The human microbiome project. Nature 449:7164. https://doi.org/10.1038/nature06244
11. de Vos WM, Tilg H, van Hul M, Cani PD (2022) Gut microbiome and health: mechanistic insights. Gut 71:1020–1032. https://doi.org/10.1136/GUTJNL-2021-326789
12. Fülling C, Dinan TG, Cryan JF (2019) Gut microbe to brain signaling: what happens in Vagus…. Neuron 101:998–1002. https://doi.org/10.1016/J.NEURON.2019.02.008
13. Albillos A, de Gottardi A, Rescigno M (2020) The gut-liver axis in liver disease: pathophysiological basis for therapy. J Hepatol 72:558–577. https://doi.org/10.1016/J.JHEP.2019.10.003
14. Qin N, Yang F, Li A, Prifti E, Chen Y, Shao L et al (2014) Alterations of the human gut microbiome in liver cirrhosis. Nature 513:59–64. https://doi.org/10.1038/NATURE13568
15. Rinninella E, Raoul P, Cintoni M, Franceschi F, Miggiano GAD, Gasbarrini A et al (2019) What is the healthy gut microbiota composition? A changing ecosystem across age, environment, diet, and diseases. Microorganisms 7:14. https://doi.org/10.3390/MICROORGANISMS7010014
16. Allaband C, McDonald D, Vázquez-Baeza Y, Minich JJ, Tripathi A, Brenner DA et al (2019) Microbiome 101: studying, analyzing, and interpreting gut microbiome data for clinicians. Clin Gastroenterol Hepatol 17:218–230. https://doi.org/10.1016/J.CGH.2018.09.017
17. Belzer C, de Vos WM (2012) Microbes inside—from diversity to function: the case of Akkermansia. ISME J 6:1449–1458. https://doi.org/10.1038/ISMEJ.2012.6
18. Thursby E, Juge N (2017) Introduction to the human gut microbiota. Biochem J 474:1823–1836. https://doi.org/10.1042/BCJ20160510
19. Korpela K, de Vos WM (2018) Early life colonization of the human gut: microbes matter everywhere. Curr Opin Microbiol 44:70–78. https://doi.org/10.1016/J.MIB.2018.06.003
20. Muller EEL, Faust K, Widder S, Herold M, Martínez Arbas S, Wilmes P (2018) Using metabolic networks to resolve ecological properties of microbiomes. Curr Opin Syst Biol 8:73–80. https://doi.org/10.1016/J.COISB.2017.12.004
21. Knights D, et al. (2014) Rethinking "enterotypes". Cell Host Microbe. 8;16(4):433–7. https://doi.org/10.1016/j.chom.2014.09.013.
22. Arumugam M, Raes J, Pelletier E, Paslier D, Yamada T, Mende DR et al (2011) Enterotypes of the human gut microbiome. Nature 473:174–180. https://doi.org/10.1038/NATURE09944
23. Bajaj JS, Heuman DM, Hylemon PB, Sanyal AJ, White MB, Monteith P et al (2014) Altered profile of human gut microbiome is associated with cirrhosis and its complications. J Hepatol 60:940–947. https://doi.org/10.1016/J.JHEP.2013.12.019

24. Hsu CL, Duan Y, Fouts DE, Schnabl B (2021) Intestinal virome and therapeutic potential of bacteriophages in liver disease. J Hepatol 75:1465–1475. https://doi.org/10.1016/J.JHEP.2021.08.003
25. Rinella ME (2015) Nonalcoholic fatty liver disease: a systematic review. JAMA 313:2263–2273. https://doi.org/10.1001/JAMA.2015.5370
26. Kundu P, Blacher E, Elinav E, Pettersson S (2017) Our gut microbiome: the evolving inner self. Cell 171:1481–1493. https://doi.org/10.1016/J.CELL.2017.11.024
27. Ni JJ, Xu Q, Yan SS, Han BX, Zhang H, Wei XT et al (2022) Gut microbiota and psychiatric disorders: a two-sample Mendelian Randomization Study. Front Microbiol 12:737197. https://doi.org/10.3389/FMICB.2021.737197
28. Earle KA, Billings G, Sigal M, Lichtman JS, Hansson GC, Elias JE et al (2015) Quantitative imaging of gut microbiota spatial organization. Cell Host Microbe 18:478–488. https://doi.org/10.1016/J.CHOM.2015.09.002
29. Bäckhed F, Fraser CM, Ringel Y, Sanders ME, Sartor RB, Sherman PM et al (2012) Defining a healthy human gut microbiome: current concepts, future directions, and clinical applications. Cell Host Microbe 12:611–622. https://doi.org/10.1016/J.CHOM.2012.10.012
30. Cho I, Blaser MJ (2012) The human microbiome: at the interface of health and disease. Nat Rev Genet 13:260–270. https://doi.org/10.1038/NRG3182
31. Ridlon JM, Kang DJ, Hylemon PB, Bajaj JS (2014) Bile acids and the gut microbiome. Curr Opin Gastroenterol 30:332–338. https://doi.org/10.1097/MOG.0000000000000057
32. Loomba R, Seguritan V, Li W, Long T, Klitgord N, Bhatt A et al (2017) Gut microbiome-based metagenomic signature for non-invasive detection of advanced fibrosis in human nonalcoholic fatty liver disease. Cell Metab 25:1054–1062.e5. https://doi.org/10.1016/J.CMET.2017.04.001
33. Cryan JF, O'riordan KJ, Cowan CSM, Sandhu KV, Bastiaanssen TFS, Boehme M et al (2019) The microbiota-gut-brain axis. Physiol Rev 99:1877–2013. https://doi.org/10.1152/PHYSREV.00018.2018
34. Chambers ES, Preston T, Frost G, Morrison DJ (2018) Role of gut microbiota-generated short-chain fatty acids in metabolic and cardiovascular health. Curr Nutr Rep 7:198–206. https://doi.org/10.1007/S13668-018-0248-8
35. Muccioli GG, Naslain D, Bäckhed F, Reigstad CS, Lambert DM, Delzenne NM et al (2010) The endocannabinoid system links gut microbiota to adipogenesis. Mol Syst Biol 6:392. https://doi.org/10.1038/MSB.2010.46
36. Dong F, Hao F, Murray IA, Smith PB, Koo I, Tindall AM et al (2020) Intestinal microbiota-derived tryptophan metabolites are predictive of Ah receptor activity. Gut Microb 12:1–24. https://doi.org/10.1080/19490976.2020.1788899
37. Knauf C, Abot A, Wemelle E, Cani PD (2020) Targeting the enteric nervous system to treat metabolic disorders? "Enterosynes" as therapeutic gut factors. Neuroendocrinology 110:139–146. https://doi.org/10.1159/000500602
38. Zhang X, Han Y, Huang W, Jin M, Gao Z (2021) The influence of the gut microbiota on the bioavailability of oral drugs. Acta Pharm Sin B 11:1789–1812. https://doi.org/10.1016/J.APSB.2020.09.013
39. Kumar K, Jaiswal SK, Dhoke GV, Srivastava GN, Sharma AK, Sharma VK (2018) Mechanistic and structural insight into promiscuity based metabolism of cardiac drug digoxin by gut microbial enzyme. J Cell Biochem 119:5287–5296. https://doi.org/10.1002/JCB.26638
40. Bertani B, Ruiz N (2018) Function and biogenesis of lipopolysaccharides. EcoSal Plus 8. https://doi.org/10.1128/ECOSALPLUS.ESP-0001-2018
41. Peng Z, Cheng S, Kou Y, Wang Z, Jin R, Hu H et al (2020) The gut microbiome is associated with clinical response to anti-PD-1/PD-L1 immunotherapy in gastrointestinal cancer. Cancer Immunol Res 8:1251–1261. https://doi.org/10.1158/2326-6066.CIR-19-1014
42. Turnbaugh PJ, Ridaura VK, Faith JJ, Rey FE, Knight R, Gordon JI (2009) The effect of diet on the human gut microbiome: a metagenomic analysis in humanized gnotobiotic mice. Sci Transl Med 1:6ra14. https://doi.org/10.1126/SCITRANSLMED.3000322

43. Nagpal R, Wang S, Solberg Woods LC, Seshie O, Chung ST, Shively CA et al (2018) Comparative microbiome signatures and short-chain fatty acids in mouse, rat, non-human primate, and human feces. Front Microbiol 9:2897. https://doi.org/10.3389/FMICB.2018.02897
44. Kronsten VT, Tranah TH, Pariante C, Shawcross DL (2022) Gut-derived systemic inflammation as a driver of depression in chronic liver disease. J Hepatol 76:665–680. https://doi.org/10.1016/J.JHEP.2021.11.008
45. Kolodziejczyk AA, Federici S, Zmora N, Mohapatra G, Dori-Bachash M, Hornstein S et al (2020) Acute liver failure is regulated by MYC- and microbiome-dependent programs. Nat Med 26:1899–1911. https://doi.org/10.1038/S41591-020-1102-2
46. Davar D, Dzutsev AK, McCulloch JA, Rodrigues RR, Chauvin JM, Morrison RM et al (1979) Fecal microbiota transplant overcomes resistance to anti-PD-1 therapy in melanoma patients. Science 2021(371):595–602. https://doi.org/10.1126/science.abf3363
47. Rowan-Nash AD, Korry BJ, Mylonakis E, Belenky P (2019) Cross-domain and viral interactions in the microbiome. Microbiol Mol Biol Rev 83:e00044. https://doi.org/10.1128/MMBR.00044-18
48. Hartmann P, Lang S, Zeng S, Duan Y, Zhang X, Wang Y et al (2021) Dynamic changes of the fungal microbiome in alcohol use disorder. Front Physiol 12:699253. https://doi.org/10.3389/FPHYS.2021.699253
49. Barlow JT, Leite G, Romano AE, Sedighi R, Chang C, Celly S et al (2021) Quantitative sequencing clarifies the role of disruptor taxa, oral microbiota, and strict anaerobes in the human small-intestine microbiome. Microbiome 9:214. https://doi.org/10.1186/S40168-021-01162-2
50. Augustyn M, Grys I, Kukla M (2019) Small intestinal bacterial overgrowth and nonalcoholic fatty liver disease. Clin Exp Hepatol 5:1–10. https://doi.org/10.5114/CEH.2019.83151
51. Acharya C, Sahingur SE, Bajaj JS (2017) Microbiota, cirrhosis, and the emerging oral-gut-liver axis. JCI Insight 2:e94416. https://doi.org/10.1172/JCI.INSIGHT.94416
52. Horvath A, Rainer F, Bashir M, Leber B, Schmerboeck B, Klymiuk I et al (2019) Biomarkers for oralization during long-term proton pump inhibitor therapy predict survival in cirrhosis. Sci Rep 9:12000. https://doi.org/10.1038/S41598-019-48352-5
53. Swidsinski A, Loening-Baucke V, Verstraelen H, Osowska S, Doerffel Y (2008) Biostructure of fecal microbiota in healthy subjects and patients with chronic idiopathic diarrhea. Gastroenterology 135:568. https://doi.org/10.1053/J.GASTRO.2008.04.017
54. Tamboli CP, Neut C, Desreumaux P, Calambel JF (2004) Dysbiosis as a prerequisite for IBD. Gut 53:1057
55. Lozupone CA, Stombaugh JI, Gordon JI, Jansson JK, Knight R (2012) Diversity, stability and resilience of the human gut microbiota. Nature 489(489):220–230. https://doi.org/10.1038/nature11550
56. Huttenhower C, Gevers D, Knight R, Abubucker S, Badger JH, Chinwalla AT et al (2012) Structure, function and diversity of the healthy human microbiome. Nature 486:207–214. https://doi.org/10.1038/NATURE11234
57. Bajaj JS, Idilman R, Mabudian L, Hood M, Fagan A, Turan D et al (2018) Diet affects gut microbiota and modulates hospitalization risk differentially in an international cirrhosis cohort. Hepatology 68:234–247. https://doi.org/10.1002/HEP.29791
58. Volta U, Bonazzi C, Bianchi FB, Baldoni AM, Zoli M, Pisi E (1987) IgA antibodies to dietary antigens in liver cirrhosis. Ric Clin Lab 17:235–242. https://doi.org/10.1007/BF02912537
59. Schnabl B, Brenner DA (2014) Interactions between the intestinal microbiome and liver diseases. Gastroenterology 146:1513–1524. https://doi.org/10.1053/J.GASTRO.2014.01.020
60. Wiest R, Albillos A, Trauner M, Bajaj JS, Jalan R (2017) Targeting the gut-liver axis in liver disease. J Hepatol 67:1084–1103. https://doi.org/10.1016/J.JHEP.2017.05.007
61. Spadoni I, Zagato E, Bertocchi A, Paolinelli R, Hot E, di Sabatino A et al (2015) A gut-vascular barrier controls the systemic dissemination of bacteria. Science 350:830–834. https://doi.org/10.1126/SCIENCE.AAD0135
62. Desai MS, Seekatz AM, Koropatkin NM, Kamada N, Hickey CA, Wolter M et al (2016) A dietary fiber-deprived gut microbiota degrades the colonic mucus barrier and enhances pathogen susceptibility. Cell 167:1339–1353.e21. https://doi.org/10.1016/J.CELL.2016.10.043

63. Clària J, Stauber RE, Coenraad MJ, Moreau R, Jalan R, Pavesi M et al (2016) Systemic inflammation in decompensated cirrhosis: Characterization and role in acute-on-chronic liver failure. Hepatology 64:1249–1264. https://doi.org/10.1002/HEP.28740
64. Almeida JI, Tenreiro MF, Martinez-Santamaria L, Guerrero-Aspizua S, Gisbert JP, Alves PM et al (2022) Hallmarks of the human intestinal microbiome on liver maturation and function. J Hepatol 76:694–725. https://doi.org/10.1016/J.JHEP.2021.10.015
65. Donaldson GP, Lee SM, Mazmanian SK (2016) Gut biogeography of the bacterial microbiota. Nat Rev Microbiol 14:20–32. https://doi.org/10.1038/NRMICRO3552
66. Fukui H (2015) Gut-liver axis in liver cirrhosis: How to manage leaky gut and endotoxemia. World J Hepatol 7:425–442. https://doi.org/10.4254/WJH.V7.I3.425
67. Kinashi Y, Hase K (2021) Partners in leaky gut syndrome: intestinal dysbiosis and autoimmunity. Front Immunol 12:673708. https://doi.org/10.3389/FIMMU.2021.673708
68. Muñoz L, Borrero MJ, Úbeda M, Conde E, del Campo R, Rodríguez-Serrano M et al (2019) Intestinal immune dysregulation driven by dysbiosis promotes barrier disruption and bacterial translocation in rats with cirrhosis. Hepatology 70:925–938. https://doi.org/10.1002/HEP.30349
69. Acharya C, Bajaj JS (2021) chronic liver diseases and the microbiome-translating our knowledge of gut microbiota to management of chronic liver disease. Gastroenterology 160:556–572. https://doi.org/10.1053/J.GASTRO.2020.10.056
70. Trebicka J, Macnaughtan J, Schnabl B, Shawcross DL, Bajaj JS (2021) The microbiota in cirrhosis and its role in hepatic decompensation. J Hepatol 75(Suppl 1):S67–S81. https://doi.org/10.1016/J.JHEP.2020.11.013
71. Ponziani FR, Zocco MA, Cerrito L, Gasbarrini A, Pompili M (2018) Bacterial translocation in patients with liver cirrhosis: physiology, clinical consequences, and practical implications. Expert Rev Gastroenterol Hepatol 12:641–656. https://doi.org/10.1080/17474124.2018.1481747
72. Cani PD, Amar J, Iglesias MA, Poggi M, Knauf C, Bastelica D et al (2007) Metabolic endotoxemia initiates obesity and insulin resistance. Diabetes 56:1761–1772. https://doi.org/10.2337/DB06-1491
73. Moon AM, Singal AG, Tapper EB (2020) Contemporary epidemiology of chronic liver disease and cirrhosis. Clin Gastroenterol Hepatol 18:2650. https://doi.org/10.1016/J.CGH.2019.07.060
74. Asrani SK, Devarbhavi H, Eaton J, Kamath PS (2019) Burden of liver diseases in the world. J Hepatol 70:151–171. https://doi.org/10.1016/J.JHEP.2018.09.014
75. Asrani SK, Kouznetsova M, Ogola G, Taylor T, Masica A, Pope B et al (2018) Increasing health care burden of chronic liver disease compared with other chronic diseases, 2004-2013. Gastroenterology 155:719–729.e4. https://doi.org/10.1053/J.GASTRO.2018.05.032
76. Wong RJ, Aguilar M, Cheung R, Perumpail RB, Harrison SA, Younossi ZM et al (2015) Nonalcoholic steatohepatitis is the second leading etiology of liver disease among adults awaiting liver transplantation in the United States. Gastroenterology 148:547–555. https://doi.org/10.1053/J.GASTRO.2014.11.039
77. Pimpin L, Cortez-Pinto H, Negro F, Corbould E, Lazarus JV, Webber L et al (2018) Burden of liver disease in Europe: epidemiology and analysis of risk factors to identify prevention policies. J Hepatol 69:718–735. https://doi.org/10.1016/J.JHEP.2018.05.011
78. Moreau R, Jalan R, Gines P, Pavesi M, Angeli P, Cordoba J et al (2013) Acute-on-chronic liver failure is a distinct syndrome that develops in patients with acute decompensation of cirrhosis. Gastroenterology 144:1426. https://doi.org/10.1053/J.GASTRO.2013.02.042
79. Sarin SK, Choudhury A (2016) Acute-on-chronic liver failure: terminology, mechanisms and management. Nat Rev Gastroenterol Hepatol 13:131–149. https://doi.org/10.1038/NRGASTRO.2015.219
80. Trebicka J, Bork P, Krag A, Arumugam M (2021) Utilizing the gut microbiome in decompensated cirrhosis and acute-on-chronic liver failure. Nat Rev Gastroenterol Hepatol 18:167–180. https://doi.org/10.1038/S41575-020-00376-3

81. Bajaj JS, Khoruts A (2020) Microbiota changes and intestinal microbiota transplantation in liver diseases and cirrhosis. J Hepatol 72:1003–1027. https://doi.org/10.1016/J.JHEP.2020.01.017
82. Acharya C, Bajaj JS (2019) Altered microbiome in patients with cirrhosis and complications. Clin Gastroenterol Hepatol 17:307–321. https://doi.org/10.1016/J.CGH.2018.08.008
83. Bajaj JS, Reddy KR, O'Leary JG, Vargas HE, Lai JC, Kamath PS et al (2020) Serum levels of metabolites produced by intestinal microbes and lipid moieties independently associated with acute-on-chronic liver failure and death in patients with cirrhosis. Gastroenterology 159:1715–1730.e12. https://doi.org/10.1053/J.GASTRO.2020.07.019
84. Tripathi A, Debelius J, Brenner DA, Karin M, Loomba R, Schnabl B et al (2018) The gut-liver axis and the intersection with the microbiome. Nat Rev Gastroenterol Hepatol 15:397–411. https://doi.org/10.1038/S41575-018-0011-Z
85. Fairfield B, Schnabl B (2021) Gut dysbiosis as a driver in alcohol-induced liver injury. JHEP Rep 3:100220. https://doi.org/10.1016/J.JHEPR.2020.100220
86. Arroyo V, Moreau R, Jalan R (2020) Acute-on-chronic liver failure. N Engl J Med 382:2137–2145. https://doi.org/10.1056/NEJMRA1914900
87. Han S, Yang Z, Zhang T, Ma J, Chandler K, Liangpunsakul S (2021) Epidemiology of alcohol-associated liver disease. Clin Liver Dis 25:483–492. https://doi.org/10.1016/J.CLD.2021.03.009
88. Lee BP, Vittinghoff E, Dodge JL, Cullaro G, Terrault NA (2019) National trends and long-term outcomes of liver transplant for alcohol-associated liver disease in the United States. JAMA Intern Med 179:340–348. https://doi.org/10.1001/JAMAINTERNMED.2018.6536
89. Skladany L, Molcan P, Vnencakova J, Vrbova P, Kukla M, Laffers L et al (2021) Frailty in nonalcoholic fatty liver cirrhosis: a comparison with alcoholic cirrhosis, risk patterns, and impact on prognosis. Can J Gastroenterol Hepatol 2021:5576531
90. Skladany L, Koller T, Adamcova Selcanova S, Vnencakova J, Jancekova D, Durajova V et al (2021) Challenging management of severe chronic disorders in acute pandemic situation: chronic liver disease under COVID-19 pandemic as the proof-of-principle model to orchestrate the measures in 3PM context. EPMA J 12:1–14. https://doi.org/10.1007/s13167-021-00231-8
91. Singal AK, Bataller R, Ahn J, Kamath PS, Shah VH (2018) ACG clinical guideline: alcoholic liver disease. Am J Gastroenterol 113:175–194. https://doi.org/10.1038/AJG.2017.469
92. Dasarathy J, McCullough AJ, Dasarathy S (2017) Sarcopenia in alcoholic liver disease: clinical and molecular advances. Alcohol Clin Exp Res 41:1419–1431. https://doi.org/10.1111/acer.13425
93. Schnabl B (2016) Liver capsule: mechanisms of alcoholic hepatitis. Hepatology 64:276. https://doi.org/10.1002/HEP.28488
94. Szabo G, Thursz M, Shah VH (2022) Therapeutic advances in alcohol-associated hepatitis. J Hepatol 76:1279–1290. https://doi.org/10.1016/J.JHEP.2022.03.025
95. Habash NW, Sehrawat TS, Shah VH, Cao S (2022) Epigenetics of alcohol-related liver diseases. JHEP Rep 4:100466. https://doi.org/10.1016/j.jhepr.2022.100466
96. Mutlu EA, Gillevet PM, Rangwala H, Sikaroodi M, Naqvi A, Engen PA et al (2012) Colonic microbiome is altered in alcoholism. Am J Physiol Gastrointest Liver Physiol 302:G966. https://doi.org/10.1152/AJPGI.00380.2011
97. Kim SS, Eun JW, Cho HJ, Song DS, Kim CW, Kim YS et al (2021) Microbiome as a potential diagnostic and predictive biomarker in severe alcoholic hepatitis. Aliment Pharmacol Ther 53:540–551. https://doi.org/10.1111/APT.16200
98. German MN, Musto J, Lucey MR (2021) Novel treatments for alcoholic hepatitis. Curr Opin Gastroenterol 37:179–186. https://doi.org/10.1097/MOG.0000000000000725
99. European Association for the Study of Liver (2012) EASL clinical practical guidelines: management of alcoholic liver disease. J Hepatol 57:399–420. https://doi.org/10.1016/j.jhep.2018.03.018

100. Llopis M, Cassard AM, Wrzosek L, Boschat L, Bruneau A, Ferrere G et al (2016) Intestinal microbiota contributes to individual susceptibility to alcoholic liver disease. Gut 65:830–839. https://doi.org/10.1136/GUTJNL-2015-310585
101. Lang S, Schnabl B (2020) Microbiota and fatty liver disease-the known, the unknown, and the future. Cell Host Microbe 28:233–244. https://doi.org/10.1016/J.CHOM.2020.07.007
102. Duan Y, Llorente C, Lang S, Brandl K, Chu H, Jiang L et al (2019) Bacteriophage targeting of gut bacterium attenuates alcoholic liver disease. Nature 575:505–511. https://doi.org/10.1038/s41586-019-1742-x
103. Smirnova E, Puri P, Muthiah MD, Daitya K, Brown R, Chalasani N et al (2020) Fecal microbiome distinguishes alcohol consumption from alcoholic hepatitis but does not discriminate disease severity. Hepatology 72:271–286. https://doi.org/10.1002/HEP.31178
104. Sarin SK, Pande A, Schnabl B (2019) Microbiome as a therapeutic target in alcohol-related liver disease. J Hepatol 70:260–272. https://doi.org/10.1016/J.JHEP.2018.10.019
105. Ferrere G, Wrzosek L, Cailleux F, Turpin W, Puchois V, Spatz M et al (2017) Fecal microbiota manipulation prevents dysbiosis and alcohol-induced liver injury in mice. J Hepatol 66:806–815. https://doi.org/10.1016/J.JHEP.2016.11.008
106. Philips CA, Pande A, Shasthry SM, Jamwal KD, Khillan V, Chandel SS et al (2017) Healthy donor fecal microbiota transplantation in steroid-ineligible severe alcoholic hepatitis: a pilot study. Clin Gastroenterol Hepatol 15:600–602. https://doi.org/10.1016/J.CGH.2016.10.029
107. DeFilipp Z, Bloom PP, Torres Soto M, Mansour MK, Sater MRA, Huntley MH et al (2019) Drug-resistant E. coli bacteremia transmitted by fecal microbiota transplant. N Engl J Med 381:2043–2050. https://doi.org/10.1056/NEJMoa1910437
108. Safety Alert Regarding Use of Fecal Microbiota for Transplantation and Additional Safety Protections Pertaining to Monkeypox Virus, FDA. https://www.fda.gov/vaccines-blood-biologics/safety-availability-biologics/safety-alert-regarding-use-fecal-microbiota-transplantation-and-additional-safety-protections-0. Accessed 1 Sep 2022
109. Grander C, Adolph TE, Wieser V, Lowe P, Wrzosek L, Gyongyosi B et al (2018) Recovery of ethanol-induced Akkermansia muciniphila depletion ameliorates alcoholic liver disease. Gut 67:892–902. https://doi.org/10.1136/gutjnl-2016-313432
110. Jiang L, Lang S, Duan Y, Zhang X, Gao B, Chopyk J et al (2020) Intestinal virome in patients with alcoholic hepatitis. Hepatology 72:2182–2196. https://doi.org/10.1002/hep.31459
111. Yang AM, Inamine T, Hochrath K, Chen P, Wang L, Llorente C et al (2017) Intestinal fungi contribute to development of alcoholic liver disease. J Clin Invest 127:2829–2841. https://doi.org/10.1172/JCI90562
112. Chu H, Duan Y, Lang S, Jiang L, Wang Y, Llorente C et al (2020) The Candida albicans exotoxin Candidalysin promotes alcohol-associated liver disease. J Hepatol 72:391. https://doi.org/10.1016/j.jhep.2019.09.029
113. Lang S, Duan Y, Liu J, Torralba MG, Kuelbs C, Ventura-Cots M et al (2020) Intestinal fungal dysbiosis and systemic immune response to fungi in patients with alcoholic hepatitis. Hepatology 71:522–538. https://doi.org/10.1002/HEP.30832
114. Bajaj JS, Kassam Z, Fagan A, Gavis EA, Liu E, Cox IJ et al (2017) Fecal microbiota transplant from a rational stool donor improves hepatic encephalopathy: a randomized clinical trial. Hepatology 66:1727–1738. https://doi.org/10.1002/HEP.29306
115. Eslam M, Sanyal AJ, George J, Sanyal A, Neuschwander-Tetri B, Tiribelli C et al (2020) MAFLD: a consensus-driven proposed nomenclature for metabolic associated fatty liver disease. Gastroenterology 158:1999–2014.e1. https://doi.org/10.1053/J.GASTRO.2019.11.312
116. Byrne CD, Targher G (2015) NAFLD: a multisystem disease. J Hepatol 62:S47–S64. https://doi.org/10.1016/J.JHEP.2014.12.012
117. Loomba R, Adams LA (2019) The 20% rule of NASH progression: the natural history of advanced fibrosis and cirrhosis caused by NASH. Hepatology 70:1885–1888. https://doi.org/10.1002/HEP.30946
118. Caldwell S, Argo C (2010) The natural history of non-alcoholic fatty liver disease. Dig Dis 28:162–168. https://doi.org/10.1159/000282081

119. Boursier J, Mueller O, Barret M, Machado M, Fizanne L, Araujo-Perez F et al (2016) The severity of nonalcoholic fatty liver disease is associated with gut dysbiosis and shift in the metabolic function of the gut microbiota. Hepatology 63:764–775. https://doi.org/10.1002/HEP.28356
120. Zhu L, Baker SS, Gill C, Liu W, Alkhouri R, Baker RD et al (2013) Characterization of gut microbiomes in nonalcoholic steatohepatitis (NASH) patients: a connection between endogenous alcohol and NASH. Hepatology 57:601–609. https://doi.org/10.1002/HEP.26093
121. Bäckhed F, Ding H, Wang T, Hooper LV, Gou YK, Nagy A et al (2004) The gut microbiota as an environmental factor that regulates fat storage. Proc Natl Acad Sci U S A 101:15718–15723. https://doi.org/10.1073/PNAS.0407076101
122. Turnbaugh PJ, Ley RE, Mahowald MA, Magrini V, Mardis ER, Gordon JI (2006) An obesity-associated gut microbiome with increased capacity for energy harvest. Nature 444:1027–1031. https://doi.org/10.1038/NATURE05414
123. Wu GD, Chen J, Hoffmann C, Bittinger K, Chen YY, Keilbaugh SA et al (2011) Linking long-term dietary patterns with gut microbial enterotypes. Science 334:105–108. https://doi.org/10.1126/SCIENCE.1208344
124. Buzzetti E, Pinzani M, Tsochatzis EA (2016) The multiple-hit pathogenesis of non-alcoholic fatty liver disease (NAFLD). Metabolism 65:1038–1048. https://doi.org/10.1016/J.METABOL.2015.12.012
125. Mehal WZ (2013) The Gordian Knot of dysbiosis, obesity and NAFLD. Nat Rev Gastroenterol Hepatol 10:637–644. https://doi.org/10.1038/NRGASTRO.2013.146
126. Aron-Wisnewsky J, Vigliotti C, Witjes J, Le P, Holleboom AG, Verheij J et al (2020) Gut microbiota and human NAFLD: disentangling microbial signatures from metabolic disorders. Nat Rev Gastroenterol Hepatol 17:279–297. https://doi.org/10.1038/s41575-020-0269-9
127. Lee G, You HJ, Bajaj JS, Joo SK, Yu J, Park S et al (2020) Distinct signatures of gut microbiome and metabolites associated with significant fibrosis in non-obese NAFLD. Nat Commun 11:1–13. https://doi.org/10.1038/s41467-020-18754-5
128. Caesar R, Reigstad CS, Bäckhed HK, Reinhardt C, Ketonen M, Lundén GÖ et al (2012) Gut-derived lipopolysaccharide augments adipose macrophage accumulation but is not essential for impaired glucose or insulin tolerance in mice. Gut 61:1701–1707. https://doi.org/10.1136/GUTJNL-2011-301689
129. Wree A, McGeough MD, Peña CA, Schlattjan M, Li H, Inzaugarat ME et al (2014) NLRP3 inflammasome activation is required for fibrosis development in NAFLD. J Mol Med (Berl) 92:1069–1082. https://doi.org/10.1007/S00109-014-1170-1
130. Mouzaki M, Wang AY, Bandsma R, Comelli EM, Arendt BM, Zhang L et al (2016) Bile acids and dysbiosis in non-alcoholic fatty liver disease. PloS One 11:e0151829. https://doi.org/10.1371/JOURNAL.PONE.0151829
131. Zhang C-X, Hu J, Hu K-W, Zhang C, Wang L, Xu J-M (2011) Noninvasive analysis of portal pressure by contrast-enhanced sonography in patients with cirrhosis. J Ultrasound Med 30:205–211
132. Jiao N, Baker SS, Chapa-Rodriguez A, Liu W, Nugent CA, Tsompana M et al (2018) Suppressed hepatic bile acid signalling despite elevated production of primary and secondary bile acids in NAFLD. Gut 67:1881. https://doi.org/10.1136/GUTJNL-2017-314307
133. Schwenger KJP, Bolzon CM, Li C, Allard JP (2019) Non-alcoholic fatty liver disease and obesity: the role of the gut bacteria. Eur J Nutr 58:1771–1784. https://doi.org/10.1007/S00394-018-1844-5
134. Schwiertz A, Taras D, Schäfer K, Beijer S, Bos NA, Donus C et al (2010) Microbiota and SCFA in lean and overweight healthy subjects. Obesity 18:190–195. https://doi.org/10.1038/OBY.2009.167
135. Zeevi D, Korem T, Zmora N, Israeli D, Rothschild D, Weinberger A et al (2015) Personalized nutrition by prediction of glycemic responses. Cell 163:1079–1094. https://doi.org/10.1016/J.CELL.2015.11.001
136. Cuevas-Sierra A, Milagro FI, Guruceaga E, Cuervo M, Goni L, García-Granero M et al (2022) A weight-loss model based on baseline microbiota and genetic scores for selection

of dietary treatments in overweight and obese population. Clin Nutr 41:1712. https://doi.org/10.1016/J.CLNU.2022.06.008
137. Qiu X, Wu Q, Li W, Tang K, Zhang J (2022) Effects of Lactobacillus supplementation on glycemic and lipid indices in overweight or obese adults: a systematic review and meta-analysis. Clin Nutr 41:1787–1797. https://doi.org/10.1016/J.CLNU.2022.06.030
138. Sharpton SR, Maraj B, Harding-Theobald E, Vittinghoff E, Terrault NA (2019) Gut microbiome-targeted therapies in nonalcoholic fatty liver disease: a systematic review, meta-analysis, and meta-regression. Am J Clin Nutr 110:139–149. https://doi.org/10.1093/AJCN/NQZ042
139. Hu W, Gao W, Liu Z, Fang Z, Wang H, Zhao J et al (2022) Specific strains of Faecalibacterium prausnitzii Ameliorate nonalcoholic fatty liver disease in mice in association with gut microbiota regulation. Nutrients 14:2945. https://doi.org/10.3390/NU14142945
140. Craven L, Rahman A, Nair Parvathy S, Beaton M, Silverman J, Qumosani K et al (2020) Allogenic fecal microbiota transplantation in patients with nonalcoholic fatty liver disease improves abnormal small intestinal permeability: a randomized control trial. Am J Gastroenterol 115:1055–1065. https://doi.org/10.14309/AJG.0000000000000661
141. Witjes JJ, Smits LP, Pekmez CT, Prodan A, Meijnikman AS, Troelstra MA et al (2020) Donor fecal microbiota transplantation alters gut microbiota and metabolites in obese individuals with steatohepatitis. Hepatol Commun 4:1578–1590. https://doi.org/10.1002/HEP4.1601
142. Manns MP, Lohse AW, Vergani D (2015) Autoimmune hepatitis—update 2015. J Hepatol 62:S100–S111. https://doi.org/10.1016/j.jhep.2015.03.005
143. Boonstra K, Beuers U, Ponsioen CY (2012) Epidemiology of primary sclerosing cholangitis and primary biliary cirrhosis: a systematic review. J Hepatol 56:1181–1188. https://doi.org/10.1016/j.jhep.2011.10.025
144. Zheng Y, Ran Y, Zhang H, Wang B, Zhou L (2021) The microbiome in autoimmune liver diseases: metagenomic and metabolomic changes. Front Physiol 12:715852. https://doi.org/10.3389/FPHYS.2021.715852
145. Li B, Selmi C, Tang R, Gershwin ME, Ma X (2018) The microbiome and autoimmunity: a paradigm from the gut-liver axis. Cell Mol Immunol 15:595–609. https://doi.org/10.1038/CMI.2018.7
146. Volk M, Reau N (2021) Diagnosis and management of autoimmune hepatitis in adults and children: a patient-friendly summary of the 2019 AASLD guidelines. Clin Liver Dis 17:85–89. https://doi.org/10.1002/CLD.1080
147. Wei Y, Li Y, Yan L, Sun C, Miao Q, Wang Q et al (2020) Alterations of gut microbiome in autoimmune hepatitis. Gut 69:569–577. https://doi.org/10.1136/GUTJNL-2018-317836
148. Liwinski T, Casar C, Ruehlemann MC, Bang C, Sebode M, Hohenester S et al (2020) A disease-specific decline of the relative abundance of Bifidobacterium in patients with autoimmune hepatitis. Aliment Pharmacol Ther 51:1417–1428. https://doi.org/10.1111/APT.15754
149. Wu JL, Zou JY, de Hu E, Chen DZ, Chen L, Lu F et al (2017) Sodium butyrate ameliorates S100/FCA-induced autoimmune hepatitis through regulation of intestinal tight junction and toll-like receptor 4 signaling pathway. Immunol Lett 190:169–176. https://doi.org/10.1016/J.IMLET.2017.08.005
150. Zhang H, Liu M, Liu X, Zhong W, Li Y, Ran Y et al (2020) Bifidobacterium animalis ssp. Lactis 420 mitigates autoimmune hepatitis through regulating intestinal barrier and liver immune cells. Front Immunol 11:569104. https://doi.org/10.3389/fimmu.2020.569104
151. Zhang H, Liu M, Zhong W, Zheng Y, Li Y, Guo L et al (2021) Leaky gut driven by dysbiosis augments activation and accumulation of liver macrophages via RIP3 signaling pathway in autoimmune hepatitis. Front Immunol 12:624360. https://doi.org/10.3389/FIMMU.2021.624360
152. Liu Q, Tian H, Kang Y, Tian Y, Li L, Kang X et al (2021) Probiotics alleviate autoimmune hepatitis in mice through modulation of gut microbiota and intestinal permeability. J Nutr Biochem 98:108863. https://doi.org/10.1016/J.JNUTBIO.2021.108863
153. de Hu E, Chen DZ, Wu JL, Lu F, Chen L, Zheng MH et al (2018) High fiber dietary and sodium butyrate attenuate experimental autoimmune hepatitis through regulation of immune

regulatory cells and intestinal barrier. Cell Immunol 328:24–32. https://doi.org/10.1016/J.CELLIMM.2018.03.003
154. Liang M, Liwen Z, Jianguo S, Juan D, Fei D, Yin Z et al (2021) Fecal microbiota transplantation controls progression of experimental autoimmune hepatitis in mice by modulating the TFR/TFH immune imbalance and intestinal microbiota composition. Front Immunol 12:728723. https://doi.org/10.3389/FIMMU.2021.728723
155. Chapman MH, Thorburn D, Hirschfield GM, Webster GGJ, Rushbrook SM, Alexander G et al (2019) British Society of Gastroenterology and UK-PSC guidelines for the diagnosis and management of primary sclerosing cholangitis. Gut 68:1356–1378. https://doi.org/10.1136/GUTJNL-2018-317993
156. Poupon RE, Balkau B, Eschwege E, Poupon R (1991) A multicenter, controlled trial of ursodiol for the treatment of primary biliary cirrhosis. UDCA-PBC Study Group. N Engl J Med 324:1548–1554. https://doi.org/10.1056/NEJM199105303242204
157. Gazda J, Janicko M, Drazilova S, Grgurevic I, Kanizaj TF, Koller T et al (2021) External validation of UDCA response score in Slovak and Croatian patients with primary biliary cholangitis. Can J Gastroenterol Hepatol 2021:9928065. https://doi.org/10.1155/2021/9928065
158. Beuers U, Trauner M, Jansen P, Poupon R (2015) New paradigms in the treatment of hepatic cholestasis: from UDCA to FXR, PXR and beyond. J Hepatol 62:S25–S37. https://doi.org/10.1016/j.jhep.2015.02.023
159. Hirschfield GM, Chazouillères O, Cortez-Pinto H, Macedo G, de Lédinghen V, Adekunle F et al (2021) A consensus integrated care pathway for patients with primary biliary cholangitis: a guideline-based approach to clinical care of patients. Expert Rev Gastroenterol Hepatol 15:929–939. https://doi.org/10.1080/17474124.2021.1945919
160. Huang MX, Yang SY, Luo PY, Long J, Liu QZ, Wang J et al (2021) Gut microbiota contributes to sexual dimorphism in murine autoimmune cholangitis. J Leukoc Biol 110:1121–1130. https://doi.org/10.1002/JLB.3MA0321-037R
161. Shah A, MacDonald GA, Morrison M, Holtmann G (2020) Targeting the gut microbiome as a treatment for primary sclerosing cholangitis: a conceptional framework. Am J Gastroenterol 115:814–822. https://doi.org/10.14309/AJG.0000000000000604
162. Kummen M, Holm K, Anmarkrud JA, Nygård S, Vesterhus M, Høivik ML et al (2017) The gut microbial profile in patients with primary sclerosing cholangitis is distinct from patients with ulcerative colitis without biliary disease and healthy controls. Gut 66:611–619. https://doi.org/10.1136/GUTJNL-2015-310500
163. Bajer L, Kverka M, Kostovcik M, Macinga P, Dvorak J, Stehlikova Z et al (2017) Distinct gut microbiota profiles in patients with primary sclerosing cholangitis and ulcerative colitis. World J Gastroenterol 23:4548–4558. https://doi.org/10.3748/WJG.V23.I25.4548
164. Lemoinne S, Kemgang A, Ben Belkacem K, Straube M, Jegou S, Corpechot C et al (2020) Fungi participate in the dysbiosis of gut microbiota in patients with primary sclerosing cholangitis. Gut 69:92–102. https://doi.org/10.1136/GUTJNL-2018-317791
165. Lapidot Y, Amir A, Ben-Simon S, Veitsman E, Cohen-Ezra O, Davidov Y et al (2020) Alterations of the salivary and fecal microbiome in patients with primary sclerosing cholangitis. Hepatol Int 15:191–201. https://doi.org/10.1007/S12072-020-10089-Z
166. Torres J, Palmela C, Brito H, Bao X, Ruiqi H, Moura-Santos P et al (2018) The gut microbiota, bile acids and their correlation in primary sclerosing cholangitis associated with inflammatory bowel disease. United Eur Gastroenterol J 6:112–122. https://doi.org/10.1177/2050640617708953
167. Vrieze A, Out C, Fuentes S, Jonker L, Reuling I, Kootte RS et al (2014) Impact of oral vancomycin on gut microbiota, bile acid metabolism, and insulin sensitivity. J Hepatol 60:824–831. https://doi.org/10.1016/J.JHEP.2013.11.034
168. Tan LZ, Reilly CR, Steward-Harrison LC, Balouch F, Muir R, Lewindon PJ (2019) Oral vancomycin induces clinical and mucosal remission of colitis in children with primary sclerosing cholangitis-ulcerative colitis. Gut 68:1533–1535. https://doi.org/10.1136/gutjnl-2018-316599
169. Ali AH, Damman J, Shah SB, Davies Y, Hurwitz M, Stephen M et al (2020) Open-label prospective therapeutic clinical trials: oral vancomycin in children and adults with primary

sclerosing cholangitis. Scand J Gastroenterol 55:1–10. https://doi.org/10.1080/00365521.2020.1787501
170. Dao A, Abidian M, Lestrange A, Mattar M, Rangnekar A, Charabaty A (2019) Oral Vancomycin induces and maintains remission of ulcerative colitis in the subset of patients with associated primary sclerosing cholangitis. Inflamm Bowel Dis 25:E90–E91. https://doi.org/10.1093/IBD/IZZ027
171. Allegretti JR, Kassam Z, Carrellas M, Mullish BH, Marchesi JR, Pechlivanis A et al (2019) Fecal microbiota transplantation in patients with primary sclerosing cholangitis: a pilot clinical trial. Am J Gastroenterol 114:1071–1079. https://doi.org/10.14309/AJG.0000000000000115
172. Kummen M, Thingholm LB, Rühlemann MC, Holm K, Hansen SH, Moitinho-Silva L et al (2021) Altered gut microbial metabolism of essential nutrients in primary sclerosing cholangitis. Gastroenterology 160:1784–1798.e0. https://doi.org/10.1053/J.GASTRO.2020.12.058
173. Ginès P, Krag A, Abraldes JG, Solà E, Fabrellas N, Kamath PS (2021) Liver cirrhosis. Lancet 398:1359–1376. https://doi.org/10.1016/S0140-6736(21)01374-X
174. Health Statistics Yearbook of the Slovak Republic (2020) Národné centrum zdravotníckych infromácií. https://www.nczisk.sk/en/Publications/Health_Statistics_Yearbooks/Pages/default.aspx. Accessed 1 Sep 2022
175. Tilg H, Cani PD, Mayer EA (2016) Gut microbiome and liver diseases. Gut 65:2035–2044. https://doi.org/10.1136/GUTJNL-2016-312729
176. Oh TG, Kim SM, Caussy C, Fu T, Guo J, Bassirian S et al (2020) A universal gut-microbiome-derived signature predicts cirrhosis. Cell Metab 32:878–888.e6. https://doi.org/10.1016/J.CMET.2020.06.005
177. Ginès P, Graupera I, Lammert F, Angeli P, Caballeria L, Krag A et al (2016) Screening for liver fibrosis in the general population: a call for action. Lancet Gastroenterol Hepatol 1:256–260. https://doi.org/10.1016/S2468-1253(16)30081-4
178. Pasolli E, Truong DT, Malik F, Waldron L, Segata N (2016) Machine learning meta-analysis of large metagenomic datasets: tools and biological insights. PLoS Comput Biol 12:e1004977. https://doi.org/10.1371/JOURNAL.PCBI.1004977
179. Chen Y, Yang F, Lu H, Wang B, Chen Y, Lei D et al (2011) Characterization of fecal microbial communities in patients with liver cirrhosis. Hepatology 54:562–572. https://doi.org/10.1002/HEP.24423
180. Bajaj JS, Betrapally NS, Hylemon PB, Heuman DM, Daita K, White MB et al (2015) Salivary microbiota reflects changes in gut microbiota in cirrhosis with hepatic encephalopathy. Hepatology 62:1260–1271. https://doi.org/10.1002/HEP.27819
181. Bajaj JS, Hylemon PB, Ridlon JM, Heuman DM, Daita K, White MB et al (2012) Colonic mucosal microbiome differs from stool microbiome in cirrhosis and hepatic encephalopathy and is linked to cognition and inflammation. Am J Physiol Gastrointest Liver Physiol 303:G675. https://doi.org/10.1152/AJPGI.00152.2012
182. Holte K, Krag A, Gluud LL (2012) Systematic review and meta-analysis of randomized trials on probiotics for hepatic encephalopathy. Hepatol Res 42:1008–1015. https://doi.org/10.1111/J.1872-034X.2012.01015.X
183. Dhiman RK, Rana B, Agrawal S, Garg A, Chopra M, Thumburu KK et al (2014) Probiotic VSL#3 reduces liver disease severity and hospitalization in patients with cirrhosis: a randomized, controlled trial. Gastroenterology 147:1327–1337.e3. https://doi.org/10.1053/J.GASTRO.2014.08.031
184. Bajaj JS, Fagan A, Gavis EA, Kassam Z, Sikaroodi M, Gillevet PM (2019) Long-term outcomes of fecal microbiota transplantation in patients with cirrhosis. Gastroenterology 156:1921–1923.e3. https://doi.org/10.1053/J.GASTRO.2019.01.033
185. Kao D, Roach B, Park H, Hotte N, Madsen K, Bain V et al (2016) Fecal microbiota transplantation in the management of hepatic encephalopathy. Hepatology 63:339–340. https://doi.org/10.1002/HEP.28121
186. Shasthry SM (2020) Fecal microbiota transplantation in alcohol related liver diseases. Clin Mol Hepatol 26:294–301. https://doi.org/10.3350/CMH.2020.0057

187. Bajaj JS, Salzman NH, Acharya C, Sterling RK, White MB, Gavis EA et al (2019) Fecal microbial transplant capsules are safe in hepatic encephalopathy: a phase 1, randomized, placebo-controlled trial. Hepatology 70:1690–1703. https://doi.org/10.1002/HEP.30690
188. Dapito DH, Mencin A, Gwak GY, Pradere JP, Jang MK, Mederacke I et al (2012) Promotion of hepatocellular carcinoma by the intestinal microbiota and TLR4. Cancer Cell 21:504–516. https://doi.org/10.1016/J.CCR.2012.02.007
189. Yoshimoto S, Loo TM, Atarashi K, Kanda H, Sato S, Oyadomari S et al (2013) Obesity-induced gut microbial metabolite promotes liver cancer through senescence secretome. Nature 499:97–101. https://doi.org/10.1038/NATURE12347
190. Schwabe RF, Greten TF (2020) Gut microbiome in HCC—mechanisms, diagnosis and therapy. J Hepatol 72:230–238. https://doi.org/10.1016/J.JHEP.2019.08.016
191. Toffanin S, Cornella H, Harrington A, Llovet JM (2012) HCC is promoted by bacterial translocation and TLR-4 signaling: a new paradigm for chemoprevention and management. Hepatology 56:1998–2000. https://doi.org/10.1002/HEP.26080
192. Darnaud M, Faivre J, Moniaux N (2013) Targeting gut flora to prevent progression of hepatocellular carcinoma. J Hepatol 58:385–387. https://doi.org/10.1016/J.JHEP.2012.08.019
193. Ponziani FR, Bhoori S, Castelli C, Putignani L, Rivoltini L, del Chierico F et al (2019) Hepatocellular carcinoma is associated with gut microbiota profile and inflammation in non-alcoholic fatty liver disease. Hepatology 69:107–120. https://doi.org/10.1002/HEP.30036
194. Ren Z, Li A, Jiang J, Zhou L, Yu Z, Lu H et al (2019) Gut microbiome analysis as a tool towards targeted non-invasive biomarkers for early hepatocellular carcinoma. Gut 68:1014–1023. https://doi.org/10.1136/gutjnl-2017-315084
195. Liu Y, Li S, Li W, Wang P, Ding P, Li L et al (2019) RstA, a two-component response regulator, plays important roles in multiple virulence-associated processes in enterohemorrhagic Escherichia coli O157:H7. Gut Pathog 11:53
196. Behary J, Amorim N, Jiang XT, Raposo A, Gong L, McGovern E et al (2021) Gut microbiota impact on the peripheral immune response in non-alcoholic fatty liver disease related hepatocellular carcinoma. Nat Commun 12:187. https://doi.org/10.1038/S41467-020-20422-7
197. Chakladar J, Wong LM, Kuo SZ, Li WT, Yu MA, Chang EY et al (2020) The liver microbiome is implicated in cancer prognosis and modulated by alcohol and Hepatitis B. Cancers (Basel) 12:1–16. https://doi.org/10.3390/CANCERS12061642
198. Komiyama S, Yamada T, Takemura N, Kokudo N, Hase K, Kawamura YI (2021) Profiling of tumour-associated microbiota in human hepatocellular carcinoma. Sci Rep 11:10589. https://doi.org/10.1038/S41598-021-89963-1
199. Routy B, le Chatelier E, Derosa L, Duong CPM, Alou MT, Daillère R et al (2018) Gut microbiome influences efficacy of PD-1-based immunotherapy against epithelial tumors. Science 359:91–97. https://doi.org/10.1126/SCIENCE.AAN3706
200. Gopalakrishnan V, Spencer CN, Nezi L, Reuben A, Andrews MC, Karpinets TV et al (2018) Gut microbiome modulates response to anti-PD-1 immunotherapy in melanoma patients. Science 359:97–103. https://doi.org/10.1126/SCIENCE.AAN4236
201. Matson V, Fessler J, Bao R, Chongsuwat T, Zha Y, Alegre ML et al (2018) The commensal microbiome is associated with anti-PD-1 efficacy in metastatic melanoma patients. Science 359:104–108. https://doi.org/10.1126/SCIENCE.AAO3290
202. Hamady M, Walker JJ, Harris JK, Gold NJ, Knight R (2008) Error-correcting barcoded primers for pyrosequencing hundreds of samples in multiplex. Nat Methods 5:235–237. https://doi.org/10.1038/NMETH.1184
203. Navas-Molina JA, Peralta-Sánchez JM, González A, McMurdie PJ, Vázquez-Baeza Y, Xu Z et al (2013) Advancing our understanding of the human microbiome using QIIME. Methods Enzymol 531:371–444. https://doi.org/10.1016/B978-0-12-407863-5.00019-8
204. Lozupone CA, Hamady M, Kelley ST, Knight R (2007) Quantitative and qualitative beta diversity measures lead to different insights into factors that structure microbial communities. Appl Environ Microbiol 73:1576–1585. https://doi.org/10.1128/AEM.01996-06

205. Thompson SK, Hoye TR (2017) Organic chemistry: molecular structure assignment simplified. Nature 547:410–411. https://doi.org/10.1038/547410A
206. Microb-Predict - MICROB-PREDICT. https://microb-predict.eu/. Accessed 1 Sep 2022
207. Gligorijević V, Renfrew PD, Kosciolek T, Leman JK, Berenberg D, Vatanen T et al (2021) Structure-based protein function prediction using graph convolutional networks. Nat Commun 12:1–14. https://doi.org/10.1038/s41467-021-23303-9
208. Greener JG, Kandathil SM, Jones DT (2019) Deep learning extends de novo protein modelling coverage of genomes using iteratively predicted structural constraints. Nat Commun 10:1–13. https://doi.org/10.1038/s41467-019-11994-0
209. Loos RJF (2012) Genetic determinants of common obesity and their value in prediction. Best Pract Res Clin Endocrinol Metab 26:211–226. https://doi.org/10.1016/J.BEEM.2011.11.003
210. Knights D, Parfrey LW, Zaneveld J, Lozupone C, Knight R (2011) Human-associated microbial signatures: examining their predictive value. Cell Host Microbe 10:292–296. https://doi.org/10.1016/J.CHOM.2011.09.003
211. Why Professor Larry Smarr freezes his own faeces - BBC News. https://www.bbc.com/news/av/health-23621357. Accessed 1 Sep 2022
212. Huang S, Haiminen N, Carrieri A-P, Hu R, Jiang L, Parida L et al (2020) Human skin, oral, and gut microbiomes predict chronological age. mSystems 5:e00630. https://doi.org/10.1128/MSYSTEMS.00630-19
213. Oh J, Conlan S, Polley EC, Segre JA, Kong HH (2012) Shifts in human skin and nares microbiota of healthy children and adults. Genome Med 4:1–11. https://doi.org/10.1186/GM378/FIGURES/4
214. Koutnikova H, Genser B, Monteiro-Sepulveda M, Faurie JM, Rizkalla S, Schrezenmeir J et al (2019) Impact of bacterial probiotics on obesity, diabetes and non-alcoholic fatty liver disease related variables: a systematic review and meta-analysis of randomised controlled trials. BMJ Open 9:e017995. https://doi.org/10.1136/BMJOPEN-2017-017995
215. Sáez-Lara MJ, Robles-Sanchez C, Ruiz-Ojeda FJ, Plaza-Diaz J, Gil A (2016) Effects of probiotics and synbiotics on obesity, insulin resistance syndrome, type 2 diabetes and non-alcoholic fatty liver disease: a review of human clinical trials. Int J Mol Sci 17:928. https://doi.org/10.3390/IJMS17060928
216. Sharpton SR, Schnabl B, Knight R, Loomba R (2021) Current concepts, opportunities, and challenges of gut microbiome-based personalized medicine in nonalcoholic fatty liver disease. Cell Metab 33:21–32. https://doi.org/10.1016/J.CMET.2020.11.010
217. Acharya C, Bajaj JS (2020) Transmitting diet-related microbial benefit through fecal microbiota transplant in NASH: can microbiota cut through the fat? Hepatol Commun 4:1559–1561. https://doi.org/10.1002/HEP4.1596
218. Long-Smith C, O'Riordan KJ, Clarke G, Stanton C, Dinan TG, Cryan JF (2020) Microbiota-gut-brain axis: new therapeutic opportunities. Annu Rev Pharmacol Toxicol 60:477–502. https://doi.org/10.1146/ANNUREV-PHARMTOX-010919-023628

Computer-Aided Breast Cancer Classification Framework for Predictive, Preventive, and Personalized Medicine

Łukasz Jeleń and Michał Jeleń

Abbreviations

3P	Medicine 3P
BR	Bloom–Richardson
CAD	Computer-Aided Diagnosis
CNN	Convolutional Neural Network(s)
DPI	Dots per inch
F1	Performance measure of a classification model
FCM	Fuzzy c-means algorithm
FN	False negative
FNA	Fine needle aspiration biopsy
FP	False positive
HE	Hematoxylin and eosin
KNN	K-nearest neighbor classifier
NN	Neural network(s)
PPPM	Predictive, preventive, personalized medicine
ReLu	Rectified Linear function used in NN training
SVM	Support Vector Machines
TN	True negative
TP	True positive

Ł. Jeleń (✉)
Department of Computer Engineering, Wroclaw University of Science and Technology, Wrocław, Poland
e-mail: lukasz.jelen@pwr.edu.pl

M. Jeleń
Department of Immunopathology and Molecular Biology, Medical University of Wroclaw, Wrocław, Poland
e-mail: michal.jelen@umw.edu.pl

H. Podbielska, M. Kapalla (eds.), *Predictive, Preventive, and Personalised Medicine: From Bench to Bedside*, Advances in Predictive, Preventive and Personalised Medicine 17, https://doi.org/10.1007/978-3-031-34884-6_10

1 Introduction

World Health Organization reports that every year more than 11 million people are diagnosed with cancer [1]. In 2020 alone, ten million patients died from cancer, approximately 16.7% of deaths worldwide. These statistics place cancer as one of the leading causes of death. Additionally, breast cancer is the most frequently diagnosed caner, with 2.26 million new cases in 2020 [2] and is one of the leading causes of death among middle-aged women.

As mentioned by Barrett et al., to achieve better patient benefits from treatment, a paradigm change is needed [3]. A key element in prevention and personalized treatment is the precise diagnosis and estimation of predictive factors [4]. Correct treatment significantly reduces the high number of deaths caused by breast cancer and increases the probability of success in treatment. This typically means high diagnosis and stage estimation accuracy. Precise and early diagnosis has a significant influence on the survival rate, indicating how many patients will live after treatment.

Cancer treatment and diagnosis are an active field among researchers in the fields of medicine and computer science. The aim of this research is to find the approach for a precise diagnosis. Here, a precise diagnosis means finding a cancer as early as possible by developing computer-aided diagnostic tools that use computer vision and neural network algorithms to estimate the predictive factors of the chosen predictive factors of breast cancer. The choice of artificial intelligence tools differs depending on the type of cancer and the type of examination used for diagnosis. This work focuses on cytological images of breast cancer that are produced during a fine needle aspiration biopsy examination. This kind of examination allows pathologists to estimate the malignancy of the cancer with very high accuracy. Malignancy estimation is very important when evaluating the survival rate of patients and the type of treatment [5]. Artificial intelligence was originally defined to describe the computer's ability to make human-like decisions. Today, with the development of other fields such as image processing, pattern recognition, or neural networks, its definition is much more complex. In this work, we describe a computer vision framework that incorporates all of these fields to build a computerized system for automated breast cancer diagnosis. This framework is capable of analyzing image information from fine needle aspirates and classifying breast cancer malignancy into three malignancy classes based on characteristics calculated according to the Bloom–Richardson grading scheme (see Sect. 2.1) [6]. Estimation of tumor grade is closely related to cancer prognosis and is considered part of breast cancer staging. During breast cancer staging, the patomorphologist determines the extent of the cancerous tissue in the body. Both tumor grade and cancer staging, along with the mitotic activity index, are treated as prognostic factors for breast cancer. According to the literature, prognostic factors are crucial in increasing the survival rate. Furthermore, we can observe that tumors detected at an early stage and patients with identified slowly growing tumors show a much better prognosis [4]. Cancers in their early stages are vulnerable to treatment, while cancers in their most advanced stages are usually almost impossible to treat. Therefore, early cancer detection greatly increases the probability of successful treatment. In addition to a precise diagnosis, it is necessary to foresee the course of the cancer, and being able to predict how the cancer can develop is very important for further treatment. Computer-assisted diagnosis systems based on visual interpretation of biopsy slides with neural networks and machine learning algorithms are an important step toward prevention and personalized treatment in breast cancer therapy.

2 Computer-Aided Breast Cancer Diagnosis

Computer-assisted breast cancer diagnosis has been a rapidly growing area of research for several decades. Computer-aided diagnosis (CAD) systems are used to assist in the detection and diagnosis of cancerous tissue changes. These systems are designed to operate independently of the physician. They can be used to supplement or assist in the interpretation of diagnostic images, such as mammograms, sonograms, magnetic resonance images, biopsies, or histological slides [7–9]. CAD systems are designed to identify potential lesions or other abnormalities in images that may require further evaluation or treatment. In the literature, a description of several types of CAD systems can be found that vary in the way they analyze images, the types of data they use, and the types of output they generate [10, 11]. These systems typically use image processing techniques to analyze images and extract features [8, 12], a convolutional neural network (CNN), support vector machines (SVM), or a combination of all to analyze the data.

Here, we examine the potential of CAD systems that are designed to be used as a tool to aid in determining prognostic factors in the diagnosis of breast cancer. We also discuss how applying this artificial intelligence-driven approach can help achieve PPPM therapy. Studies show that early detection and better screening have enabled earlier and better identification of breast cancer. The detection mode could be considered a prognostic factor and therefore taken into account in the management of patients, as it can affect their survival [4].

Studies have shown that CAD systems can improve the accuracy of lesion detection and diagnosis, as well as reduce the time it takes to interpret the visual image [10, 13, 14]. In addition, CAD systems can be used to reduce the number of false negative diagnoses, which can lead to a reduction in missed diagnoses and delayed treatment [15–17].

Despite the potential benefits of CAD systems, the technology is still relatively new and research is still ongoing [18–21]. There are several potential issues that may arise when using CAD systems, including false positives, false negatives, and overreliance on technology. Furthermore, more research is still needed to determine the most effective and reliable ways to use CAD systems in the prevention and personalized treatment of breast cancer.

2.1 Breast Cancer in the Context of 3P Medicine

A healthy woman's breast anatomy contains lobules connected to a nipple by ducts. These structures are supported by fat tissue. Breast cancer is abnormal cell growth that originates in the ducts and lobules.

Breast cancer is not only one of the most commonly diagnosed cancers, but also one of the most common cancers in middle-aged women. It is also one of the most deadly cancers. Screening examinations are critically necessary to reduce the high mortality rate. Regular screening can significantly reduce the death rate. Early detection and effective treatment can reduce mortality by up to 30%. A screening examination consists of mammography, ultrasound, and palpatic examination. The last can be performed at home by the patient herself or by a doctor. During a mammographic examination, doctors can detect very small lesions that cannot be distinguished during self-examination. During an ultrasound examination, we can detect the same lesions as in mammography without the risk of excessive radiation, making it safer for the patient. Unfortunately, it cannot be used for regular screening due to the fact that microcalcifications are not as clearly visible as in mammography, which can lead to misclassification of lesions [22]. Both of these methods are said to have about 25% false positive diagnoses. Furthermore, its interpretation can vary depending on the radiologist [23].

To establish a precise diagnosis, a biopsy examination is required. There are different types of biopsies, but for the purpose of this study, we will focus only on the fine needle aspiration biopsy (FNA). During this examination, a part of the abnormal tissue is collected, placed on the glass slide, and stained (see Fig. 1). When the specimen is stained, a microscopic examination is performed, during which the type of cancer is recognized, as well as its malignancy grade and prognostic and predictive factors [24]. These factors allow pathologists to foresee overall survival and disease-free survival rates, while predictive factors allow them to foresee reaction to the treatment undertaken [25].

Today, we are looking for a more holistic approach to breast cancer treatment that focuses on prevention, prediction, and personalized treatment. In the context of 3P medicine, a physician looks at the breast cancer patient as a whole and focuses on creating a customized treatment plan that meets the individual needs of the

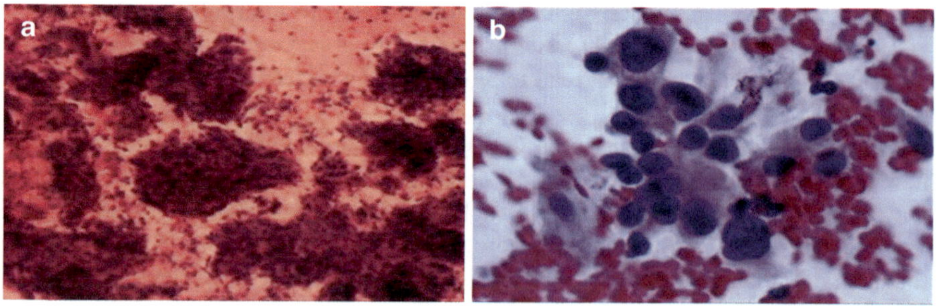

Fig. 1 Fine Needle Aspirate of a breast recorded with different magnifications. (**a**) 100×, (**b**) 400×

patient. Typically, this approach emphasizes lifestyle modifications to reduce the risk of cancer while also providing treatments to manage symptoms and improve quality of life. According to Koklesova et al., a large percentage of malignancies can be prevented with the unique properties of plant bioactive compounds [26].

When cancer is diagnosed, it is important to diagnose it quickly and accurately. As mentioned earlier, computer-aided screening and diagnosis can significantly speed up the procedure and reduce the number of false negative diagnoses, and therefore reduce missed diagnoses and delayed treatment. Here, we describe a computer-aided breast cancer classification framework that allows for the estimation of a Bloom–Richardson malignancy grade described in detail in Sect. 2.3).

Evaluation of the malignancy indicates the likelihood that the case may undergo metastasis at the time or after treatment. Personalized breast cancer treatment can include a variety of approaches depending on the type and stage of cancer and the individual's health history and preferences [27]. Surgery, radiation therapy, chemotherapy, hormone therapy, targeted therapy, and immunotherapy are some of the options offered. Target therapy is a drug specifically designed to target cancer cells. The treatment approach is typically determined by a physician based on the medical history of the individual. This path allows for the determination of the most effective and personalized treatment plan. As cancer research advances, this type of treatment is becoming increasingly popular because it can help maximize patient success [28, 29]. In the case of breast cancer, as mentioned above, the determination of cancer malignancy influences the patient's type of treatment and therefore it not only has a prognostic, but also a predictive value.

2.2 Machine Learning in Breast Cancer Diagnosis

Recent advances in imaging technology have made it possible to diagnose breast cancer more accurately. In particular, mammograms and ultrasound can be used to diagnose and identify the location, size, and shape of a tumor [9, 14]. Furthermore, magnetic resonance imaging and positron emission tomography scans can be used to identify the presence of hormone receptors in the tumor [30, 31]. Furthermore, to obtain a precise diagnosis of breast cancer, various machine learning techniques have been used to improve classification accuracy [11, 32]. In particular, supervised learning techniques, such as support vector machines (SVMs) and k-nearest neighbor (KNN), have been used to classify breast cancer tumors [12, 17, 31, 33]. These techniques have been shown to be effective in identifying the type of tumor, as well as its malignancy [8].

Here, we discuss a computerized breast cytology classification problem. It was first investigated by Wolberg et al. in 1990 [34]. The authors described an application of a multisurface pattern separation method to cancer diagnosis achieving an error rate as low as 4.1% on a fine needle aspiration biopsy database of 169 malignant cases and 201 benign. This data set was later publicly released as the Wisconsin Breast Cancer Database and is widely used by researchers to date [35]. This study was later expanded by Street et al. to describe ten nuclear features that were used for the classification and prognosis of breast cancer [36]. In 2000, Street introduced a system called XCyt, the first Remote Cytological Diagnosis and Prognosis of Breast Cancer [37]. Other approaches include more recent work of Filipczuk et al., Jeleń et al. and Kowal et al. [8, 15, 38]. All of these approaches provided different ways for image segmentation. In Jeleń et al. we can find attempts to evaluate breast cancer malignancy, while in other works a discrimination between benign and malignant cases is described. Recently, with the introduction of Le Cun's convolutional neural networks [39], we can see more studies on breast cancer classification and interpretation of visual information. Deep learning algorithms have been used for the classification and identification of subtle features in mammograms, ultrasound images, and histological slides [14, 18, 19, 40]. From the above review, it is easy to see that the use of machine learning techniques has recently improved and all the authors report high accuracy in breast cancer classification. However, there is still room for improvement, particularly in the use of deep learning techniques to identify subtle features in the imaging data. There is also a great opportunity to use the potential of artificial intelligence in the design of personalized treatment.

2.3 Bloom–Richardson Grading Scheme

In Sect. 2.1 we mentioned that prognostic and predictive factors allow pathologists to foresee the course of cancer. In the case of breast cancer, the most important prognostic factors are histological grade and mitotic count. These factors are described by the Bloom–Richardson (BR) grading scheme grading system, which is the most common malignancy grading scale used by pathologists. The system was originally introduced by Bloom and Richardson in 1957 for grading histological slides [6]. In 1989, the originally proposed scheme was modified by Scarff and is now recognized as a modified Scarff–Bloom–Richardson scheme. For the diagnosis of breast cancer, this scheme is one of the best-known prognostic factors [41]. In our studies, we use this scale to assess malignancy for cytological smears. Based on this system, three factors are considered in grading cancerous tissue, each evaluated on a three-point scale according to the following description:

1. *Degree of structural differentiation*—describes the degree of tubule formation in histological slides. In cytology, tubules are not retained, the scoring is based on the determination of cell groupings (see Fig. 2—Grade 1). For this factor, we will grant one point if cells are grouped regularly, two points are given when grouped and single cells are visible, and three points are awarded when cells are irregularly spread.
2. *Pleomorphism (P)*—This factor takes into account the differences in the size, shape, and staining of the nuclei. This scoring is fairly straightforward, since as the nuclei irregularities increase, the prognosis worsens. Here, nuclei with uniform size, shape, and staining will receive one point, while those with moderate variations will receive two points. Three points are given to the nuclei with sig-

nificant variations. These deviations are depicted in Fig. 2—Grade 2. It can be seen that G2 ductal carcinoma has more uniform nuclei and less staining variations than G3 ductal carcinoma (Fig. 2—Grade 3).

3. *Frequency of Hyperchromatic and Mitotic Figures*—this factor is used to assess the number of mitoses one can find in the image. The more mitoses are present in the image, the worse the prognosis. If occasional mitotic figures are found, then one point is awarded. Two points are given for the slides with two or three figures, and for more than three figures, we will grant three points.

The final BR grade is assigned depending on the sum of the quantitative values of the above factors. According to Bloom and Richardson, the grade distribution is as described below [6]:

$$\overbrace{\underbrace{3\,4\,5}_{\text{Grade I}}\quad\underbrace{6\,7}_{\text{Grade II}}\quad\underbrace{8\,9}_{\text{Grade III}}}^{\text{Points}}$$

where:

- Grade I—Low malignancy,
- Grade II—Intermediate malignancy,
- Grade III—High malignancy.

In the literature, other malignancy classification schemes can be found that are used for other types of cancer. The basis for all of them is similar to that of the Bloom–Richardson scheme. All assess cell pleomorphism, tubules, and mitosis. Variations usually consist of additional features that are taken into account. For histological slide grading, the most common variation of the Scraff–Bloom–Richardson scheme is the Elston and Ellis modification known as the Nottingham–Bloom–Richardson scheme. In this scoring system, the amount of gland formation or cell differentiation, nuclear features, and mitotic activity are assessed.

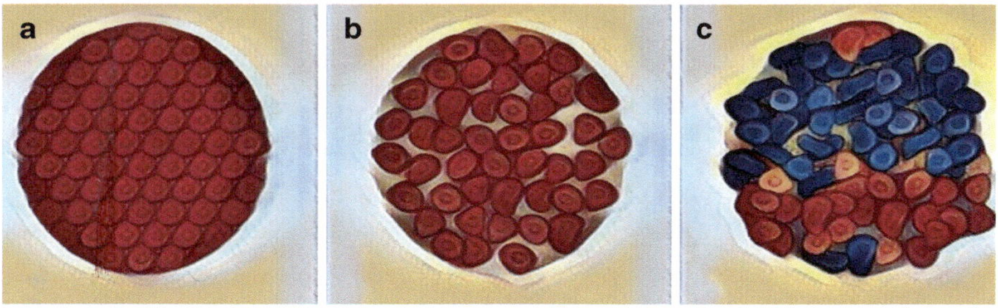

Fig. 2 Illustration of Malignancy Grades; (**a**) Grade 1, (**b**) Grade 2, (**c**) Grade 3

3 Material and Methods

In this section, a database of fine needle aspirates from breast cancer will be described, as well as the methodology of feature extraction. We will show classical features that can be calculated to resemble the Bloom–Richardson features. In addition, a set of features derived with convolutional neural networks is depicted. Based on these features, we show the classification methodology that allows for the estimation of predictive factors for breast cancer, namely the malignancy grade.

3.1 Database of Breast Cancer Slides

In our study, we have used a collection of images recorded during breast cytological examinations (see Fig. 3). Images were collected in the Department of Pathology and Clinical Cytology of the Medical University of Wrocław, Poland. The preparation of the slides includes staining with hematoxylin and eosin, known as the HE technique. The choice of staining agents allows visualization of nuclei with purple and black dyes and cytoplasm with shades of pink and red blood cells with orange and red dyes. The slides were digitized with an Olympus BX 50 microscope with CCD-IRIS camera mounted on the head of the microscope. Using MultiScan Base 08.98 software, we were able to record images with a resolution of 96 dots per inch (dpi) and a size of 764 × 572 pixels.

All images were recorded at two different magnifications of the same tissue region for each patient. On the low magnification images, we can see whether the cells are forming groups or are loosely spread in the image. These images were recorded with 100× magnification and comprise 50% of all images in the database. The low magnification images are used for the estimation of features based on the cells' tendency to form groups. Healthy and low malignant cases tend to form one or two large groups in the image, while those cases with large malignancy are loosely spread and the groups usually consist of only a few cells.

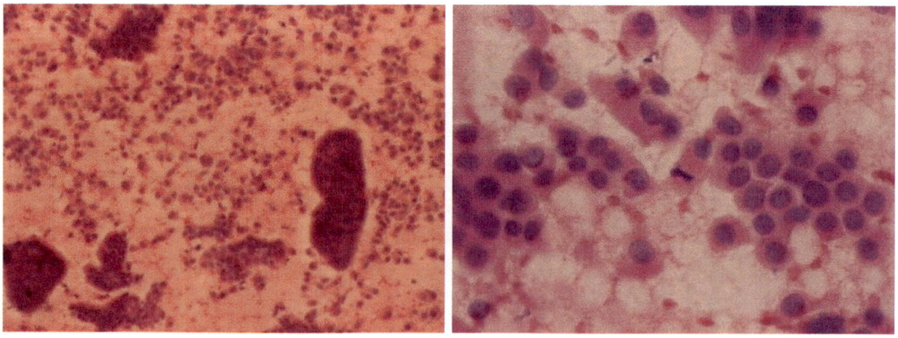

Fig. 3 Breast Cancer Fine needle aspirates. Sample Database Images: left—Low magnification, right—high magnification

The second subset of images was recorded with 400× magnification. This type of image allowed for the determination of features describing the pleomorphic cells' features. These shape-based features provide important information about cell nuclei. Here, low malignancy cases have uniform size and staining, while in more malignant cases this tendency is disturbed, and the nuclei in the image will assume nonuniform sizes and will have stronger staining variations. Currently, the database consists of 480 FNA biopsy images (both 100× and 400×) that were graded by an expert pathologist and will later be treated as the "gold standard" for malignancy classification. All images represent the three classes of cancer malignancy, namely low (G1), intermediate (G2), and high (G3) malignancy grades. There are 22 cases of low malignancy, 134 of intermediate and 84 of high malignancy. For all cases, a follow-up examination was performed. When a tissue was surgically removed, a histopathological examination was graded using the Bloom–Richardson [6] grading scale that confirmed the classification of FNA. Therefore, all the cases in our database were histopathologically confirmed.

3.2 Breast Cancer Malignancy Classification Framework

The framework described in this study uses the bright-field light microscope with an additional mirror mounted behind the objective to split the image into two visible images. The first image is visible through the eyepiece, and the second image is projected to the camera and then recorded by the camera. The data obtained in this way is then processed by machine learning algorithms, and one of the three BR grades is assigned. In Fig. 4, we show a machine learning pipeline to estimate the grade of malignancy. This scheme can be divided into several stages and will depend on the approach taken. For the classical approach, where SVM and KNN classification is performed, we need to introduce image preprocessing and segmentation (see Sect. 3.3). When deep learning is applied, we use convolutional neural networks to construct the feature vector; see Sect. 3.4 for more details.

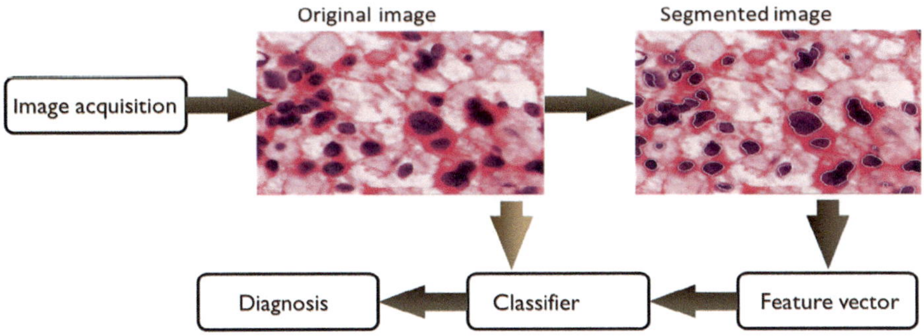

Fig. 4 Machine learning framework for malignancy classification

3.3 Preprocessing and Nuclei Segmentation

Preprocessing is a stage in which the image recorded during the acquisition step is usually modified in a way to remove unwanted noise that could have been introduced by the imaging setup. Typically, these operations would include filtering to remove noise introduced during analog-to-digital conversion. In some applications, we also try to deconvolve the image with a so-called point spread function, which should remove the aberrations of the optics of the acquisition setup. In our study, we applied a median filter that allows for the removal of random noise. When this filter is applied, the value of the pixels is replaced by a median value of the 3 × 3 neighborhood of the pixel. The main advantage of median filters is their ability to preserve edges. This allowed us to prepare the images for image segmentation by smoothing the homogeneous regions, which in fact reduces the number of colors representing these areas. For this purpose we applied a well-known segmentation technique that uses a fuzzy version of a k-means clustering, called a Fuzzy c-means segmentation.

Fuzzy c-means is an approach proposed by Klir and Yuan [42] that can be used to divide image information and extract nuclei. Generally, a set of data of $X = x_1, x_2, \ldots, x_n$ is divided into c clusters. It is assumed that $P = A_1, A_2, \ldots, A_c$ is a known pseudopartition and A_i is a vector that fits all x_k members to the i cluster. Now, using the Eq. (1), one can calculate the center of the c cluster [43].

$$v_i = \frac{\sum_{k=1}^{n} \left[A_i(x_k)\right]^m x_k}{\sum_{k=1}^{n} \left[A_i(x_k)\right]^m}, \quad i = 1, 2, \ldots, c \tag{1}$$

where $m > 1$ is a weight that controls the fuzzy membership. Memberships are defined by Eq. 2 if $\|x_k - v_i\|^2 > 0$ for all $i \in \{1, 2, \ldots, c\}$ and if $\|x_k - v_i\|^2 = 0$ for some $i \in I \subseteq \{1, 2, \ldots, c\}$ the memberships are defined as a non-negative real number that satisfies the Eq. (3) for $i \in I$.

$$A\_i(x\_k) = \left[\sum_{j=i}^{c} \left(\frac{x_k - v_i^2}{x_k - v_j^2} \right)^{\frac{1}{m-1}} \right]^{-1}, \tag{2}$$

$$\sum_{i \in I} A_i(x_k) = 1. \tag{3}$$

The clustering algorithm looks for a set P that minimizes the performance index $J_m(P)$ defined by Eq. (4).

$$J_m(P) = \sum_{k=1}^{n} \sum_{i=1}^{c} \left[A_i(x_k)\right]^m x_k - v_i^2. \tag{4}$$

In contrast to all other segmentation techniques, the fuzzy c-means algorithm (FCM) requires no additional processing and as such was applied to segment the color information in the image. In Fig. 5 an example of FCM segmentation is presented.

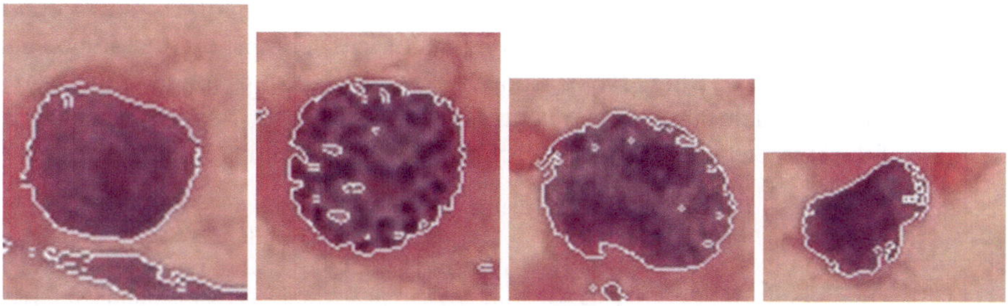

Fig. 5 Nuclei segmentation with fuzzy c-means algorithm

3.4 Feature Extraction

Feature extraction in classification is the process of selecting and extracting meaningful features from a data set to identify patterns, classify data, and make predictions. It is a crucial step in machine learning and data mining. Feature extraction involves selecting a subset of the most important, meaningful, and useful features from a larger set of raw data, which can then be used to train a machine learning model. The goal is to reduce the dimensionality of the data set while preserving important information and patterns. This helps to reduce the complexity of the model and improve its accuracy. Feature extraction can be performed manually, using domain knowledge and prior experience, or automated, using algorithms.

For the classification of the breast cancer malignancy data, two types of feature vectors were created. One used classical image processing methods and the second created with a convolutional neural network.

3.4.1 Classical Feature Extraction

The calculation of these features depended on the magnification of the image. For 100× magnification, we calculated the average area of the visible groups in the image, the number of groups, and the dispersion defined with Eq. (5).

$$\frac{1}{D} = \frac{1}{n-1}\sum_{i=1}^{n}\left(A_c - A_{100}\right)^2, \tag{5}$$

For the 400× magnification images, we calculated features that resembled nuclear features. All features were described in detail by Jeleń et al. [8] and include:

- Area that was calculated as the sum of all nuclei pixels of the nucleus [37].
- Perimeter defined as the length of the nuclear boundary of a nucleus that is approximated by a length of the polygonal approximation of the boundary.
- Convexity determined as the ratio of the nucleus area and the area of the minimal convex polygon that contains the nucleus, called a convex hull.
- Eccentricity described the circularity of the nucleus taking into account the fact that healthy nuclei will assume circular shapes, while cancerous nuclei can have arbitrary shapes. Eccentricity is calculated as a ratio of the distance between

focal points of an ellipse matched with a nucleus having the same second moments as the segmented nuclei, and its major axis length. It will assume values between 0 and 1, where 0 corresponds to a circle and 1 to a line segment.
- Centroid—For each nucleus, the centroid is a point $(\overline{x_i}, \overline{y_i})$ called a center of mass of the extracted nucleus along each row (X) and column (Y). It is calculated as follows:

$$\overline{x_i} = \frac{1}{A_i}\sum_{j=0}^{X-1}\sum_{k=0}^{Y-1} jN_{i(j,k)}; \tag{6}$$

$$\overline{y_i} = \frac{1}{A_i}\sum_{j=0}^{X-1}\sum_{k=0}^{Y-1} kN_{i(j,k)}; \tag{7}$$

where $N_i(j, k)$ equals 1 if the pixel j, k is in the nucleus N_i, and 0 otherwise.

- Orientation is also called an axis of the least second moment and contains information on the orientation of the nucleus. For the coordinate system placed at the centroid $(\overline{x_i}, \overline{y_i})$ of the nucleus, we can define the orientation as follows:

$$Or_i = \tan\left(2\theta_i\right), \tag{8}$$

where the angle θi is measured counterclockwise from the x-axis.

- Projections are calculated along rows and columns.
- Moment-based features—here we use seven normalized central moments to calculate the rotation, scaling, and translation invariant features.
- Histogram-based features are statistical features calculated based on the image histogram and included five features: mean, standard deviation, skew, energy, and width.
- Textural features—These features require a determination of the gray-level co-occurrence matrix that describes the relationships between a pair of pixels and their gray levels. Assuming that the distance between the pixels and the directions are given, we can extract energy, homogeneity, inertia, and correlation features.
- Color-based features—for these features, we treated each color component as a separate intensity image. To calculate color features, we can use the same logic as for the Textural features and applied them to each color band.

3.4.2 Convolutional Neural Networks

Convolution neural networks (CNNs) are a type of deep neural networks that are the most commonly used computer vision applications. They became a popular artificial intelligence tool because they are capable of automatic extraction of valuable information from real-world images or video streams. Unlike fully connected layers in classical neural networks, the CNN model extracts simple features from input through a single or multiple convolution layer and executes convolution operations.

Each layer is a set of nonlinear functions that combine weights in different coordinates and allow the weight to be reused from the spatial subsets of the previous layer output.

The first CNN model described by Yann LeCun in 1989 was a neural network that processed data with a known grid-like topology using at least one convolution operation instead of a matrix multiplication [39]. The convolution of two real functions can be determined with Eq. (9).

$$F_v(t) = (x - \omega)(t) \tag{9}$$

where x is an input, ω is the convolution kernel, and Fv is a feature vector. Since the images are two dimensional, the convolution kernel (Ω) should also be two dimensional. This leads to a definition of convolution with Eq. (10).

$$F_M(i,j) = (\Omega \odot \mathrm{Img})(\mathrm{I,j}) \sum_m \sum_n Img(j+m, i+n)\Omega(m,n). \tag{10}$$

To build a network capable of performing feature extraction, we build a network consisting of several convolution layers, where each layer performs several parallel convolutions that yield a set of linear activation values. Each value passes through the rectified linear function called ReLu that maintains the non-linearity of the resulting feature vector. Finally, we modify the output of the layer to reduce the output dimentionality. This is performed using a maximum output pool function (Eq. 11) and is called max-pooling.

$$O(x) = \max(O,x) \tag{11}$$

In this study, we used one of the most popular CNN architectures, called VGG-16, which was introduced by Simonyan and Zisserman in 2014 [44]. This is a CNN model that is built from 16 convolutional layers and was pretrained on the ImageNet dataset. This data set consists of more than 14 million images categorized into almost 1000 classes.

Based on the output of the VGG-16 network, we constructed a feature vector that was then used in the classification of the malignancy.

3.5 Classification Scheme

Pattern classification deals with the issue of assigning a specific class to the given pattern. There are many methods that can be used to classify data. Here, we apply the K-nearest neighbor rule, support vector machines, random forests, and neural networks to classify the data sets prepared according to the description in Sect. 3.4.

3.5.1 K-Nearest Neighbor

K-nearest neighbor (KNN) is one of the simplest classification algorithms. It is based on the distance calculation between the pattern in question and its k neighbors. The decision is made based on the closest association between the pattern and the neighbors. The pattern is classified into the closest class in terms of distance between its k neighbors.

The training procedure is very simple and is based on recording the entire training set. Testing usually uses a Euclidean distance to calculate the distances between the training samples and the tested sample. The class assigned to the sample is the one for which the distance is the smallest. To be able to calculate the Euclidean norm, it is usually necessary to normalize the data to avoid any data inconsistency. To classify our data, a KNN was calculated for five neighbors.

3.5.2 Support Vector Machines

Support vector machines are used to separate two or more classes of patterns or data points by constructing a boundary between them. An unknown point will be classified according to its orientation with respect to that boundary. To estimate the boundary between classes, we use boundary points from each class. These points are called support vectors. This procedure is an iterative approach that minimizes some error function (Eq. 12),

$$\frac{1}{2}w^T w + C\sum_{i=1}^{N}\varepsilon_i \tag{12}$$

with the following restrictions:

$$y_i\left(w^T\phi\left(x_i\right)+b\right) \geq 1-\varepsilon_i \ \text{ and } \varepsilon_i \geq 0, i = 1,\ldots,N \tag{13}$$

where C and b are constants, w is the weight vector, εi is a bias value that deals with overlapping cases, and ϕ is a kernel function that transforms the input data into the feature space. The constant C has a major influence on the error rate and has to be carefully estimated during the training process.

Depending on the error function, we can distinguish between different SVMs and different kernels. Here, we make use of the radial base function (RBF) kernel (Eq. 14).

$$\phi = \exp\left(-\gamma x_i - x_j^{\,2}\right) \tag{14}$$

The learning process uses the Adatron algorithm [45] which guarantees the convergence to the solution assuming that the solution exists.

3.5.3 Random Forests

Random forests, as their name suggests, are made up of a large number of individual decision trees that operate as a whole. Each tree in the random forest produces a class prediction and the class with the highest votes becomes our model prediction. Based on the training data, the trees are created from bootstrap data samples. During training, a random subset of attributes is drawn from which the best decision tree split is selected. The final decision is based on the majority of trees that have developed in the forest. In our case, ten trees were chosen.

3.5.4 Neural Networks

The idea of neural networks is based on the real interactions of human nerve system.

The basic element of the neural network is the neuron, sometimes also called a perceptron. It is a mathematical model of a biological neuron. Combining a few neurons together in such a way that neurons can interact with each other makes a neural network that is capable of processing input data and providing us with a certain decision.

In neural networks, each neuron accepts an input signal of the form $X = [x_1, x_2, ..., x_n]$ and each of the subsignals is assigned a weight. $F(s_i)$ is called an activation function of the neuron and, depending on the type of neuron, activates its output. In our case, the activation function used is the rectifier linear unit function—ReLu. The network architecture is based on 200 hidden layers and one input layer and one output layer. Before we can use our neural network, it is necessary to train it so that it can recognize the desired patterns. Training is based on weight adjustment depending on the output value. Our network uses the Adam optimization algorithm that iteratively updates the weights of the network [46]. Training is performed on known patterns for which the output is known. Such a set of known patterns is called a training set. Analogously, a set of unknown patterns is called a testing set.

Training of the network was carried out in a maximum of 320 iterations and for validation we used a leave-one-out technique. This technique is often used for small data sets and involves leaving one data sample for validation and the remaining samples are used for training. The procedure is repeated for all the samples in the data.

3.6 Classification Performance

To be able to say how the proposed classifiers behave and to be able to evaluate their performance, we introduce quantitative criteria. The most popular and reliable evaluation method is based on the confusion matrix that contains information on actual and predicted classifications. The fields of the matrix are filled depending on the classification result of the tested samples. Based on these responses, we can determine the number of positive classifications correctly classified as positive, called true positives (TP), the number of negative classifications correctly classified as negative, called true negatives (TN), the number of negative classifications incorrectly classified as positive, called false positives (FP), and the number of positive classifications incorrectly classified as negative, called false negatives (FN). Based on these values, we can now define additional measures such as F1, precision, and recall. Precision is the model's ability to avoid identifying irrelevant items as relevant and is calculated as a ratio of TP and the total number of predicted positives. Recall, on the other hand, measures the model's ability to identify all relevant items and is calculated as a ratio of TP to positives. F1 measure evaluates the overall performance of a classification model. It is calculated as a ratio of the sum of precision and recall and their doubled multiplication. The F1 score ranges from 0 to 1, where 1 is a perfect performance.

4 Results and Discussion

The objective of this study was to investigate the achievability of the methods described in Sect. 3.5 to computerized breast cancer malignancy and therefore for the problem of automated predictive factor estimation. The results described in this section were obtained for experimental investigations that included a comparative study of classification performance in the feature vector extracted with conventional image processing techniques called FVC23 and the feature vector created with the convolutional neural network called FVDL23 (as described in Sect. 3.4). During these tests, we made decisions only between the G2 and G3 classes, as this was the setup commonly described in the literature. Additionally, we checked how the introduction of the G1 class will influence the accuracy of the classification. These tests were performed only for the feature vector (FVDL123) extracted with the convolutional neural networks.

In Table 1 classification results for the two-class classification problem are gathered in the form of area under curve, classification accuracy, F1, precision, and recall measures. The corresponding confusion matrix is presented in Table 2. From the classification results, we can see that neural networks achieved the best classification accuracy (84.6%), which is confirmed by the high F1 measure. It can also be noticed that the Precision and Recall measures are also highest for decisions made with a neural network. Of all, kNN was the classifier with the worst performance, for which the lowest accuracy of 59.4% was observed for the feature vector created with classical image processing methods. It should be noted that accuracy and quality measures increased significantly when convolutional neural networks were used as feature extractor. These rates show that convolutional neural networks allow for the determination of more meaningful features. The accuracy obtained in this study could possibly be much higher if the fine aspirate database contained more images and the balance between classes were preserved.

The second part of the experiments was to perform a classification of breast cancer malignancies in all three malignancy classes to resemble the Bloom–Richardson grading. The results of these analyzes are presented in Table 3 as a three-class problem, and the corresponding confusion matrix is presented in Table 4. For comparison purposes, we also put the results of a two-class problem discussed earlier. Here, we can see again that the neural network is the best performing classifier achieving 78.7% accuracy with a similar 78.6% for F1 and precision measures. This means

Table 1 Classification results for the two-class problem

	FVC23					FVDL23				
Model	AUC	Acc	F1	Precision	Recall	AUC	Acc	F1	Precision	Recall
kNN	0.651	0.594	0.594	0.595	0.594	0.866	0.782	0.779	0.779	0.782
SVM	0.785	0.752	0.752	0.751	0.752	0.884	0.796	0.797	0.799	0.795
Rand. Forest	0.847	0.792	0.790	0.792	0.792	0.829	0.756	0.748	0.754	0.756
NN	0.821	0.792	0.791	0.791	0.792	0.919	0.846	0.846	0.846	0.846

Table 2 Confusion matrices for the two-class problem

	Predicted			
	FVC23		FVD23	
Actual	G2	G3	G2	G3
G2	81.0%	23.3%	87.9%	20.5%
G3	19.0%	76.7%	12.1%	79.5%

Table 3 Classification results for the three-class vs. two-class problem

	3-Class					2-Class				
Model	AUC	Acc	F1	Precision	Recall	AUC	Acc	F1	Precision	Recall
kNN	0.833	0.717	0.706	0.709	0.717	0.866	0.782	0.779	0.779	0.782
SVM	0.866	0.723	0.688	0.656	0.723	0.884	0.796	0.797	0.799	0.795
Rand. Forest	0.837	0.721	0.705	0.711	0.720	0.829	0.756	0.748	0.754	0.756
NN	0.897	0.787	0.786	0.786	0.787	0.919	0.846	0.846	0.846	0.846

Table 4 Confusion matrix for the three-class problem

	Predicted		
Actual	G1	G2	G3
G1	81.0%	18.2%	40.5%
G2	11.7%	81.2%	4.8%
G3	7.3%	0.6%	54.8%

that the introduction of an additional class did not significantly alter the results. As expected, the accuracy of the classification dropped, but for the size of the database, we can still treat it as a very good result. These additional experiments confirm that convolutional neural networks are a good choice for feature extraction. They provide accurate features that lead to good classification performance. The disadvantage of the method is the time it takes to perform the calculations. For our setup, it took roughly 1.5 times longer to evaluate one image. CNNs also require databases at least ten times larger than those used in our study, and therefore the training process tends to be time consuming. The results of this study suggest that the use of neural networks increases the precision of the classification of malignancy grade and therefore a better estimation of prognostic factors. Furthermore, the study showed that classical feature extraction methods based solely on image processing methods, such as filtering, segmentation, and geometric moments, resulted in less accurate classification.

5 Conclusions

In this chapter, a computerized framework for the estimation of breast cancer predictive factors was described. As mentioned in Sect. 2.1 Bloom–Richardson grade is one of the best prognostic and predictive factors for breast cancer [24, 25]. In this context, our research on computer-aided malignancy grading shows that machine learning algorithms have a very large potential to estimate these factors. The results presented in Sect. 4 clearly show that it is possible to create a computer vision algorithm that is capable of classifying fine needle aspiration biopsy slides and assigning one of the three malignancy grades with high accuracy and precision. Additionally, we can also conclude that.

- Computer-aided diagnosis (CAD) is an important tool for the analysis of breast imaging data. They can not only detect breast cancer by analyzing digital cytological slides, but also provide prognostic and predictive factors. It could also be used to help assess personalized treatment plans. This needs further evaluation and research. It can be pointed out as an open problem.
- Artificial intelligence can be used to analyze fine needle aspiration biopsy slides, which can then be used to detect and classify breast cancer malignancy grade.
- Deep learning (DL) algorithms have been used to extract features from biopsy images and estimate predictive factors for breast cancer. These algorithms can be used to analyze this type of data with high precision.
- Image processing techniques can also be used to analyze biopsy images to classify breast cancer. These algorithms did not show as good accuracy as the DL algorithms, but can still be treated as a good alternative if the database is small.
- The fine needle aspirate database was collected and prepared for malignancy grade classification and is maintained continuously. To the best of our knowledge, no other similar database is publicly available. To obtain better classification rates, the database needs to be enlarged, which can also be pointed out as an open problem.
- 3P medicine can benefit from artificial intelligence that provides machine learning tools for personalized predictive and preventive treatment of breast cancer.
- CAD PPPM system can be created based on machine learning algorithms that are not only capable of estimating prognostic factors but also of analyzing medical history and other personalized profiles to create an individualized risk profile.

In breast cancer, 3P medicine can be used to identify and treat patients at risk of developing breast cancer, predict the likelihood of developing certain types of breast cancer, and prevent recurrence. In this study, we focus on predictive and prognostic factors for breast cancer. Other examples of 3P approaches to breast cancer would include genetic testing to identify high-risk patients, mammogram screening to detect early stage tumors, and personalized treatments such as targeted drugs and immunotherapies. Furthermore, lifestyle modifications, such as exercise, diet, and stress management, can be incorporated into 3P approaches to reduce the risk of developing breast cancer or reduce the risk of recurrence. All these areas can be addressed for artificial intelligence-driven systems. AI can be used to detect and diagnose the disease in its early stages, allowing for the estimation of fast personalized therapy. In addition, it could also be used to analyze biopsy results to determine the best treatment options for each patient. Machine learning algorithms could also be used to analyze medical history, genetic profile, lifestyle, and environmental factors to create an individualized risk profile. This profile can be used to identify individuals who are at an increased risk of developing breast cancer and to recommend preventive measures to reduce their risk. In general, the results of this study demonstrate that the computerized malignancy grading framework will allow repeatability in the decision-making process, which is of great concern among the pathological community. The computerized scheme described in this investigation complies with this requirement, and the classification results obtained are very good. In our opinion, such a proposed solution could significantly affect physicians' day-to-day work and help in the estimation of a personalized therapy and prediction of the disease depending on the treatment undertaken. Preventing breast cancer and estimating individual risk factors could also be possible when additional patient information would be available to train machine learning algorithms. In such a case, we would be able to build a CAD PPPM system that can fulfill the requirements of the 3P paradigm change of the future.

References

1. Sung H, Ferlay J, Siegel RL, Laversanne M, Soerjomataram I, Jemal A et al (2021) Global cancer statistics 2020: Globocan estimates of incidence and mortality worldwide for 36 cancers in 185 countries. CA Cancer J Clin 71(3):209–249
2. Ferlay J, Colombet M, Soerjomataram I, Parkin DM, Pineros M, Znaor A et al (2021) Cancer statistics for the year 2020: an overview. Int J Cancer 149(4):778–789
3. Barrett M, Boyne J, Brandts J, Rocca HPB-L, Maesschalck LD, Wit KD et al (2019) Artificial intelligence supported patient self-care in chronic heart failure: a paradigm shift from reactive to predictive, preventive and personalised care. EPMA J 10:445–464. https://doi.org/10.1007/S13167-019-00188-9
4. Soerjomataram I, Louwman MWJ, Ribot JG, Roukema JA, Coebergh JWW (2008) An overview of prognostic factors for long-term survivors of breast cancer. Breast Cancer Res Treat 107:309–330
5. Jeleń Ł (2009) Computerized cancer malignancy grading of fine needle aspirates. PhD thesis, Concordia University
6. Bloom HJ, Richardson WW (1957) Histological grading and prognosis in breast cancer: a study of 1409 cases of which 359 have been followed for 15 years. Br J Cancer 11:359. https://doi.org/10.1038/bjc.1957.43
7. Eltrass AS, Salama MS (2020) Fully automated scheme for computer-aided detection and breast cancer diagnosis using digitised mammograms. IET Image Process 14:495–505. https://doi.org/10.1049/IET-IPR.2018.5953
8. Jeleń L, Krzyżak A, Fevens T, Jeleń M (2016) Influence of feature set reduction on breast cancer malignancy classification of fine needle aspiration biopsies. Comput Biol Med 79:80
9. Drukker K, Pesce L, Giger M (2010) Repeatability in computer-aided diagnosis: application to breast cancer diagnosis on sonography. Med Phys 37:2659–2669. https://doi.org/10.1118/1.3427409
10. Yassin NIR, Omran S, Houby EMFE, Allam H (2018) Machine learning techniques for breast cancer computer aided diagnosis using different image modalities: a systematic review. Comput Methods Programs Biomed 156:25–45. https://doi.org/10.1016/J.CMPB.2017.12.012
11. ElOuassif B, Idri A, Hosni M, Abran A (2021) Classification techniques in breast cancer diagnosis: a systematic literature review. Comput Methods Biomech Biomed Engin 9:50–77. https://doi.org/10.1080/21681163.2020.1811159

12. Jeleń Ł (2020) Texture description for classification of fine needle aspirates. In: Korbicz J, Maniewski R, Patan K, Kowal M (eds) Current trends in biomedical engineering and bioimages analysis. Springer, Cham, pp 107–116
13. Liu Q, Liu Z, Yong S, Jia K, Razmjooy N (2020) Computer-aided breast cancer diagnosis based on image segmentation and interval analysis. Automatika 61:496–506. https://doi.org/10.1080/00051144.2020.1785784
14. Rybiałek A, Jeleń Ł (2020) Application of densenets for classification of breast cancer mammograms. In: Saeed K, Dvorsky J (eds) Computer information systems and industrial management. Springer, Cham, pp 266–277
15. Filipczuk P, Fevens T, Krzyżak A, Monczak R (2013) Computer-aided breast cancer diagnosis based on the analysis of cytological images of fine needle biopsies. IEEE Trans Med Imaging 32:2169–2178. https://doi.org/10.1109/TMI.2013.2275151
16. Krawczyk B, Jeleń Ł, Krzyżak A, Fevens T (2012) Oversampling methods for classification of imbalanced breast cancer malignancy data. In: Computer vision and graphics, vol 7594 LNCS, pp 483–490. https://doi.org/10.1007/978-3-642-33564-8-58
17. Krawczyk B, Jeleń Ł, Krzyżak A, Fevens T (2014) One-class classification decomposition for imbalanced classification of breast cancer malignancy data. In: Artificial intelligence and soft computing, vol 8467LNAI, pp 539–550. https://doi.org/10.1007/978-3-319-07173-2-46
18. Hameed Z, Garcia-Zapirain B, Aguirre JJ, Isaza-Ruget MA (2022) Multiclass classification of breast cancer histopathology images using multilevel features of deep convolutional neural network. Sci Rep 12:1–21. https://doi.org/10.1038/s41598-022-19278-2
19. Eroglu Y, Yildirim M, Cinar A (2021) Convolutional neural networks based classification of breast ultrasonography images by hybrid method with respect to benign, malignant, and normal using MR-MR. Comput Biol Med 133:104407. https://doi.org/10.1016/j.compbiomed.2021.104407
20. Ranjbarzadeh R, Dorosti S, Ghoushchi SJ, Caputo A, Tirkolaee EB, Ali SS et al (2023) Breast tumor localization and segmentation using machine learning techniques: overview of datasets, findings, and methods. Comput Biol Med 152:106443. https://doi.org/10.1016/J.COMPBIOMED.2022.106443
21. Raaj RS (2023) Breast cancer detection and diagnosis using hybrid deep learning architecture. Biomed Signal Process Control 82:104558. https://doi.org/10.1016/J.BSPC.2022.104558
22. Kolb TM, Lichy J, Newhouse JH (1998) Occult cancer in women with dense breasts: detection with screening US–diagnostic yield and tumor characteristics. Radiology 207:191–199
23. Beam CA, Layder PM, Sullivan DC (1996) Variability in the interpretation of screening mammograms by US radiologists. Arch Intern Med 156:209–213
24. Agrawal AK, Jeleń M, Grzebieniak Z, Zukrowski P, Rudnicki J, Nienartowicz E (2008) Androgen receptors as a prognostic and predictive factor in breast cancer. Folia Histochem Cytobiol 46(3):269–276
25. Stankov A, Bargallo-Rocha JE, Silvio N-S, Ramirez MT, StankovaNinova K, Meneses-Garcia A (2012) Clinical study prognostic factors and recurrence in breast cancer: experience at the National Cancer Institute of Mexico. ISRN Oncol 2012:825258. https://doi.org/10.5402/2012/825258
26. Koklesova L, Liskova A, Samec M, Qaradakhi T, Zulli A, Smejkal K et al (2020) Genoprotective activities of plant natural substances in cancer and chemopreventive strategies in the context of 3p medicine. EPMA J 11:261–287. https://doi.org/10.1007/S13167-020-00210-5
27. Harbeck N, Salem M, Nitz U, Gluz O, Liedtke C (2010) Personalized treatment of early-stage breast cancer: present concepts and future directions. Cancer Treat Rev 36:584–594. https://doi.org/10.1016/j.ctrv.2010.04.007
28. Marcom PK, Anders CK, Ginsburg GS, Potti A, Nevins JR (2020) Utilization of genomic signatures for personalized treatment of breast cancer. In: Pharmacogenetics of breast cancer, pp 107–122. https://doi.org/10.1201/9780429137723-8
29. Kern R, Correa SC, Scandolara TB, da Silva JC, Pires BR, Panis C (2020) Current advances in the diagnosis and personalized treatment of breast cancer: lessons from tumor biology. Pers Med 17:399–420. https://doi.org/10.2217/pme-2020-0070

30. Satoh Y, Imokawa T, Fujioka T, Mori M, Yamaga E, Takahashi K et al (2022) Deep learning for image classification in dedicated breast positron emission tomography (dbPET). Ann Nucl Med 36:401–410. https://doi.org/10.1007/s12149-022-01719-7
31. Vidic I, Egnell L, Jerome NP, Teruel JR, Sjøbakk TE, Østlie A et al (2018) Support vector machine for breast cancer classification using diffusion-weighted MRI histogram features: preliminary study. J Magn Reson Imaging 47:1205–1216. https://doi.org/10.1002/jmri.25873
32. Fondon I, Sarmiento A, Garcia AI, Silvestre M, Eloy C, Polonia A et al (2018) Automatic classification of tissue malignancy for breast carcinoma diagnosis. Comput Biol Med 96:41–51. https://doi.org/10.1016/J.COMPBIOMED.2018.03.003
33. Rajyalakshmi U, Rao SK, Prasad KS (2017) Supervised classification of breast cancer malignancy using integrated modified marker controlled watershed approach. In: Proceedings - 7th IEEE international advanced computing conference, IACC 2017, pp 584–589. https://doi.org/10.1109/IACC.2017.0125
34. Wolberg WH, Mangasarian OL (1990) Multisurface method of pattern separation for medical diagnosis applied to breast cytology. Proc Natl Acad Sci U S A 87:9193–9196
35. Mangasarian OL, Setiono R, Wolberg WH (1990) Pattern recognition via linear programming: theory and application to medical diagnosis. Large-Scale Num. Opt. SIAM, Philadelphia, pp 22–31
36. Street WN, Wolberg WH, Mangasarian OL (1993) Nuclear feature extraction for breast tumor diagnosis. In: Imaging Science and Technology/Society of Photographic Instrumentation Engineers. International Symposium on Electronic Imaging: Science and Technology, San Jose, CA, vol 1905, pp 861–870
37. Street NW (2000) Xcyt: a system for remote cytological diagnosis and prognosis of breast cancer. In: Jain LC (ed) Soft computing techniques in breast cancer prognosis and diagnosis. World Scientific Publishing, Singapore, pp 297–322
38. Kowal M, Filipczuk P, Obuchowicz A, Korbicz J, Monczak R (2013) Computeraideddiagnosisofbreastcancerbasedonfineneedlebiopsymicroscopicimages. Comput Biol Med 43:1563–1572. https://doi.org/10.1016/j.compbiomed.2013.08.003
39. Cun YL, Jackel LD, Boser B, Denker JS, Graf HP, Guyon I et al (1989) Handwritten digit recognition: applications of neural network chips and automatic learning. IEEE Commun Mag 27:41–46. https://doi.org/10.1109/35.41400
40. Kowal M, Skobel M, Gramacki A, Korbicz J (2021) Breast cancer nuclei segmentation and classification based on a deep learning approach. Int J Appl Math Comput Sci 31:85–106. https://doi.org/10.34768/amcs-2021-0007
41. Doussal VL, Tubiana-Hulin M, Friedman S, Hacene K, Spyratos F, Brunet M (1989) Prognostic value of histologic grade nuclear components of Scarff-Bloom-Richardson (SBR). An improved score modification based on a multivariate analysis of 1262 invasive ductal breast carcinomas. Cancer 64:1914–1921. https://doi.org/10.1002/1097-0142(19891101)64:9<1914::aid-cncr2820640926>3.0.co;2-g
42. Klir GJ, Yuan B (1995) Fuzzy sets and fuzzy logic: theory and applications. Prentice Hall, Upper Saddle River, NJ
43. Theera-Umpon N (2005) Patch–based white blood cell nucleus segmentation using fuzzy clustering. ECTI EEC 3(1):15–19
44. Simonyan K, Zisserman A (2014) Very deep convolutional networks for large-scale image recognition. In: 3rd International Conference on Learning Representations, ICLR 2015—Conference Track Proceedings. https://doi.org/10.48550/arxiv.1409.1556
45. Friess TT, Cristianini N, Campbell C (1998) The kernel adatron algorithm: a fast and simple learning procedure for support vector machines. In: 15th International conference on machine learning. Morgan Kaufman Publishers, Burlington, MA
46. Kingma DP, Ba JL (2014) Adam: a method for stochastic optimization. arXiv preprint arXiv:1412.6980

Preventive and Personalized Strategies in Ambulatory and Clinical Cardiac Electrophysiology

Dariusz Jagielski, Przemysław Skoczyński, Andrzej Pawłowski, Bruno Hrymniak, Bartosz Skonieczny, Sebastian Stec, Dorota Zyśko, Waldemar Banasiak, and Halina Podbielska

Abbreviations

3PM	Predictive, preventive, and personalized medicine
AI	Artificial intelligence

D. Jagielski (✉) · D. Zyśko · W. Banasiak
Department of Cardiology, Center for Heart Diseases, 4th Military Hospital, Wrocław, Poland

Faculty of Medicine, Wrocław University of Science and Technology, Wrocław, Poland
e-mail: dariusz.jagielski@pwr.edu.pl; dorota.zysko@pwr.edu.pl; waldemar.banasiak@pwr.edu.pl

P. Skoczyński
Department of Cardiology, Center for Heart Diseases, 4th Military Hospital, Wrocław, Poland

Department of Emergency Medicine, Faculty of Medicine, Wroclaw Medical University, Wrocław, Poland
e-mail: przemyslaw.skoczynski@umw.edu.pl

A. Pawłowski
University of Science and Technology, Wrocław, Poland

Department of Mechanical and Industrial Engineering, University of Brescia, Brescia, Italy
e-mail: andrzej.pawlowski@unibs.it

B. Hrymniak · B. Skonieczny
Department of Cardiology, Center for Heart Diseases, 4th Military Hospital, Wrocław, Poland

S. Stec
ELMedica, EP-Network, SKA, Skarżysko-Kamienna, Poland
e-mail: smstec@wp.pl

H. Podbielska
Department of Biomedical Engineering, Wrocław University of Science and Technology, Wrocław, Poland
e-mail: halina.podbielska@pwr.edu.pl

H. Podbielska, M. Kapalla (eds.), *Predictive, Preventive, and Personalised Medicine: From Bench to Bedside*, Advances in Predictive, Preventive and Personalised Medicine 17, https://doi.org/10.1007/978-3-031-34884-6_11

AS	Aortic stenosis
AV node	Atrioventricular node
AVB	Atrioventricular block
BIS	Bispectral index scale
BMI	Body mass index
CAN	Cardioneuroablation
CDRIE	Device-related infective endocarditis
CIED	Cardiac implantable electronic devices
EACTS	European Association for Cardio-Thoracic Surgery
ECG	Electrocardiogram
ECVS	Extracardiac vagal nerve stimulation
EP	Electrophysiology
EPS	Electrophysiological study
ESC	European Society of Cardiology
IDE	Investigational Device Exemption
ILR	Implantable loop recorder
KCCQ	Kansas City Cardiomyopathy Questionnaire
LBBB	Left bundle branch block
LP	Leadless pacemaker
MAV	Micra AV (atrioventricular)
MPC	Model predictive control
MVR	Micra VR (one chamber/ventricular)
PM	Pacemaker
PONV	Postoperative nausea and vomiting
PPIPS	Permanent pacemaker implantation preventive strategy
PPM	Permanent pacemaker
PR, QRS	Parts of ECG decryption
PVI	Pulmonary vein isolation
RBBB	Right bundle branch block
RFA	Radiofrequency ablation
SAVR	Surgical aortic valve replacement
TAVR	Transcatheter aortic valve replacement
TIVA	Total intravenous anesthesia
TLE	Transvenous lead extraction
TV-PM	Transvenous pacemaker
VVI, VDD	Stimulation modes of pacemaker

1 Electrophysiology as a Success Story of the Intersection of Biomedicine and Engineering

Contemporary electrophysiology encompasses two main fields. One uses the electrical activity of living cells to evaluate biological signaling processes for medical diagnosis; the other exploits various types of currents for treating numerous lesions, both in destructive and non-destructive manners. Both of these two aspects of

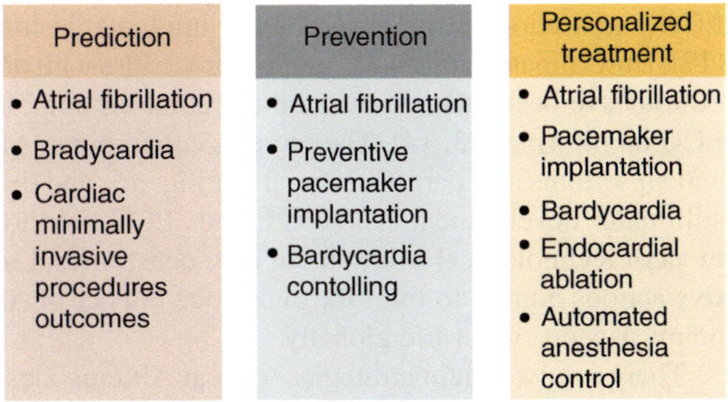

Fig. 1 3P Medicine principia in some aspects of cardiac electrophysiology

contemporary Electrophysiology require advanced technology equipment. That is why Electrophysiology is in the focus of many Biomedical Engineering education curricula worldwide (e.g. [1–4]).

Electrophysiology in medicine relates mostly to two main areas: neurology and cardiology. In neurology, it is focused on an examination of brain signals, neuroimaging and neurostimulation. There are a plethora of reports describing the diagnostic and therapeutic potential of neurologic electrophysiology [5–7].

In modern cardiology, both diagnostics and therapeutic procedures benefit from the electrophysiology approach. In this chapter, we will discuss some of them in view of 3P Medicine.

The main idea is illustrated in Fig. 1.

2 Preventive and Personalized Aspects of Atrial Fibrillation Diagnostic and Treatment Strategies

Atrial fibrillation (AF) is the most common type of heart-treated arrhythmia. It presents a completely irregular heart rate and is accompanied by an increased risk of thromboembolic and cardiovascular complications, hospitalizations, and deaths. A few percent of patients in the course of AF suffer from a stroke, apart from approx. 20% mortality rate carries complications in the form of chronic paresis, speech problems, and cognitive disorders. The above factors result in dramatic social consequences related to the costs of treatments burdening health care systems, leaving the labor market, and is a huge load for the economic systems of individual countries and societies. According to the official data, approx. 50–60 million people worldwide experience AF in its paroxysmal, persistent or permanent form [8, 9]. There are many serious scientific reasons to talk about the plague of AF, and the total number of patients is repeatedly greater [10]. The need for developing rational **predictive** and **prevention** strategies are of paramount importance. Only in the US annual treatment costs of atrial fibrillation are nearing $26 billion [11].

Several modern monitoring technologies aim to diagnose various cardiac arrhythmias as standard ECG and prolonged 24–48 h ECG Holter monitoring. Due to the fact that some episodes of AF appear relatively seldom (e.g., a few times a year), the critical issue is the recording duration. The application of a monitoring framework based on the concept of chronic registration 24 h/365 days is a gold standard of

ECG registration in the shape of the implantable loop recorder (ILR) technique [12]. Unfortunately, this is an invasive procedure with obvious limitations. Numerous efforts have been taken to develop a system for continuous non-invasive long-term ECG monitoring [13, 14]. The projects concerning a variety of hardware, software, and algorithms as a part of artificial intelligence and machine learning processes are still under development. The continuous ECG monitoring is becoming not only a modern technological solution but also constitutes a necessity to broaden **preventive** actions aiming to limit the enormous impact of AF on health, social, and economic aspects of our life globally.

There are two main strategies to treat AF episodes, i.e., rate or rhythm control therapy [15]. With growing evidence supporting early rhythm control also for asymptomatic and new-onset AF patients, we observe a change in the paradigm of AF treatment. Nevertheless, many factors influence the final decision to undertake invasive activities, such as age, comorbidities, echocardiographic parameters, potential success rate, patient's understanding of the clinical situation, etc. Because many factors influence the decision to finally undertake invasive activities like catheter ablation technologies, the effectiveness of chosen treatment method, age and category of patients, special **personalized** AF Heart Teams are established to discuss and decide about the selection decision criteria for the patients [16]. Sometimes they may range from specialist cardiologists (electrophysiologist, heart failure specialist, echocardiographist, etc.) to multidisciplinary teams (cardiologist, cardiac surgeon, endocrinologist, hematologist, nephrologist, neurologist, and others) who plan AF treatments jointly depending on individual patient needs and availability of services. Considering the significant impact of AF on a variety of aspects of our health, social and economic milieu, there is substantial space for **predictive**, **preventive,** and **personalized** actions as described previously [17].

3 Preventive Leadless Pacemaker Implantation in Patients After Tavr Procedure

Aortic stenosis (AS) is the most common valve lesion, often requiring transcatheter aortic valve replacement (TAVR) or surgical aortic valve replacement (SAVR) due to the increased risk of sudden cardiac death [18]. The AS prevalence increases with the aging of the population. Till the TAVR era, the interventional approach of the elderly and frail patients was associated with high operational risk. It changed in 2002, with the proof-of-concept first TAVR procedure performed by Cribier, which created a new treatment approach for the highest-risk patients [19]. The indisputable safety profile of the procedure mentioned above led to creating TAVR strong recommendation (IA) in ESC/EACTS Guidelines for the management of valvular heart disease from 2021 for all patients above 75 years or those with high operational risk (STS-PROM/EuroSCORE II > 8%) [18]. Since the first case, TAVR use in the elderly population has only risen. Moreover, the procedure's indications are also spreading among the younger population. It results in increase by 2.7 times the number of TAVR procedures in patients <65 years old between 2015 and 2021. That said, the TAVR procedure count reached nearly equal volume as SAVR by 2021 [20].

The safety profile in patients with severe AS presenting low operation risk was recently evaluated in the PARTNER 3 trial. In the mentioned research, study participants were randomized into groups undergoing TAVR with SAPIEN 3 system and SAVR procedure. The primary composite endpoint was death, stroke or rehospitalization at 1 year. Both 30 days and 1 year after the procedure, SAPIEN 3 system proved the safety procedure profile and was superior to SAVR in the case of the primary endpoint. Moreover, the SAVR procedure was associated with a significantly higher rate of new-onset atrial fibrillation at 30 days, a more extended index hospitalization, and a higher risk of a poor treatment outcome (death or a low KCCQ score) at 30 days compared to TAVR [21]. Developing the newer TAVR systems significantly reduced complications, which may explain the eagerness to involve younger and lower-risk patients in the TAVR procedure.

Nevertheless, new-onset or worsening conduction disturbances remain one of the most common complications after TAVR. They are found in 34.8% of patients at hospital discharge, with the Left Bundle Branch Block (LBBB) as the most common conduction disorder [22]. Randomized trials and registries show that such complications require pacemaker (PM) implantation in up to 25.9% of patients with consequent conduction disorders [23]. However, what needs to be emphasized is that AS per se increases the risk of conduction disturbances.

For example, the stenotic process of aortic valve severe calcification may involve a near-located heart conduction system. Such situation is usually observed in patients with low-flow, low-gradient AS with preserved ejection fraction. This is because the atrioventricular (AV) node is located in the triangle of Koch's apex, near the aortic valve's non-coronary cusp. Three positions of the AV node can be listed with the most common right-sided. However, the left-sided AV node, especially superficial to the endocardium, seems to be particularly vulnerable to calcification and TAVR post-procedure-related conduction disturbances.

Another heart conduction structure—the left bundle branch of the AV node—is a superficial structure positioned on the crest of the interventricular septum. It is located at the base of the interleaflet triangle, separating the aortic valve's non-coronary and right-coronary leaflets, which the TAVR procedure can easily harm. Both situations can lead to PM implantation.

3.1 Permanent Pacemaker Implantation as a Preventive Strategy

ESC Guidelines on cardiac pacing and cardiac resynchronization therapy clearly recommend: asymptomatic patients or those who do not require pacemaker implantation due to standard indications do not need a permanent pacemaker implantation preventive strategy (PPIPS) before the TAVR procedure [23].

However, due to the post-TAVR risk of further conduction disturbances advancing in the future, early PPIPS after TAVR should be considered in several cases. With pre-existing right bundle branch block, developing any other conduction disturbances during or after TAVR, even transient high-degree atrioventricular block (AVB), PR prolongation, or QRS axis change, is a clear indication of a PPIPS. Another case when PPIPS should be implemented for patients >48 h after TAVI are:

- New LBBB with QRS > 150 ms.
- Pre-existing conduction abnormality who develops prolongation of QRS or PR > 20 ms.
- PR > 240 ms.

Yet, before the PM implantation decision, one should have an electrophysiological study (EPS) that measures the His bundle -Ventricular interval. The nominal value that justifies the implantation procedure should be at least 70 ms. Those who developed bifascicular block after TAVR and did not meet above mentioned criteria, yet have had syncope after the procedure, should also be considered for PPIPS. It has been proven that in elderly patients with unexplained, recurrent syncope and bifascicular block (for example, LBBB or RBBB with left anterior fascicular block), PPIPS significantly reduces the risk of symptoms recurrence [24]. However, one in eight patients with a transvenous pacemaker (TV-PM) may experience peri- and post-procedural complications [25]. The risk of complications rises with such burdens as age, BMI, and frailty syndrome, which are all often in the characteristic spectrum for a patient after the TAVR procedure.

3.2 Leadless Pacemakers in TAVR Population

The arrival of leadless pacemakers (LPs) (Fig. 2) in 2012 became a cornerstone in the treatment of bradycardia and atrioventricular (AV) conduction disorders as an alternative to TV-PMs. Currently, the only available LPs on the market are Micra VR (MVR) and the newly developed Micra AV (MAV), which allows AV synchronous ventricle pacing (VDD mode).

However, their external construction is similar. With a low mass of 1.75 g, dimensions of 25.9 mm × 6.7 mm, and volume of 0.8 cc Micra occupies around 1% of the hearts' right ventricle volume. MVR and MAV longevity is estimated between 8 and 13 years, which depends on the pacing mode, ventricle pacing percentage, and

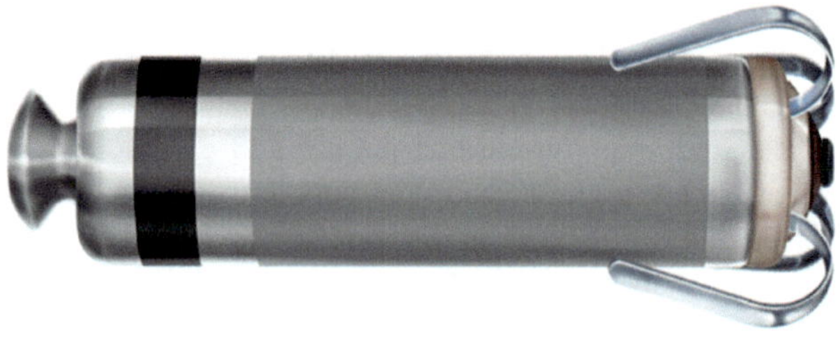

Fig. 2 Leadless Pacemaker—Micra (own picture)

implanted place's electrical parameters. Even though Micra is considered an unremovable device after a couple of months since implantation due to encapsulation [26], another implantation of Micra in the same patient is feasible and safe. However, due to the expected limited lifespan in TAVR-related, elderly and frail populations, it seems to be a relatively rare need.

The most common conduction disturbance after TAVR—the newly developed LBBB—has a relatively high long-term recovery rate to normal conductive function (26.2% at long-term follow-up [27]). Thus, such situation allows LP to work often as a backup mode extending battery life.

One of the reasons behind LP technology development was the improvement of the safety profile in cardiac pacing. The pocket and leads account for two-thirds of transvenous PM complications, and their lack in LP technology is one of their most significant advantages. Reducing the risk of infective endocarditis is essential from the point of view of a person with an artificial aortic valve.

The first study exploring the MVR safety profile was Investigational Device Exemption (IDE). The IDE study showed 48% (HR 0.52; 95% CI 0.35–0.77;) fewer complications compared to TV-PMs, a high implant success rate (99.2%), and stable low pacing thresholds at 6 months in 98.3% of patients [28]. The second one—The Post-Approval Registry—proved a low rate of major complications throughout 12 months (2.7% CI:2.0–3.6%) with no device-related infections. Major complications were mainly reduced by a 47% relative risk reduction in hospitalizations and an 82% relative risk reduction in system revisions. The all-cause mortality does not differ at 2-year follow-up in groups of LPs and TV-PMs, even though patients obtaining LP are usually burdened with more comorbidities [29]. Micra's implantation safety, performance, and post-procedural complications were also evaluated in patients who underwent MAV implantation after the TAVR procedure between November 2020 and June 2021. The short-term safety and performance of the LP were once again proved with a 1-month follow-up [30]. Most of LP's indications are similar to the TAVR population. Thus, LP should be considered for patients with frailty syndrome and chronic kidney disease, especially those on dialysis, with less than 10 years of life span, hindered access to the TV-PM, but also with a history of cardiac device-related infective endocarditis (CDRIE). The MAV should be preferred over MVR in patients with AV block but without bradycardia or persistent supraventricular arrhythmia, due to the VDD pacing mode.

This demonstrates how important is a **personalized** approach before taking a decision about the procedure to be employed.

4 Prediction, Prevention, and Personalization: A Strategy for Managing Patients with Symptomatic Bradycardia

Management of sinus node dysfunction or atrioventricular conduction disorders leading to symptomatic bradycardia remains a diagnostic and therapeutic challenge. According to the guidelines of the European and American cardiological societies ESC/EHRA/ACC/AHA/HRS, if these disorders are of internal origin and are irreversible, the treatment of choice is PM implantation [23, 31]. The method has been proven and improved for many years. However, it is burdened with significant limitations and not without the risk of complications. The recent rapid development of technology has significantly increased diagnostic possibilities and expanded the number of therapeutic options, from optimizing the stimulation itself to techniques to avoid it. Such a variety of options create a possibility to **personalize** the therapy to reduce complication risk and improve the quality of life. Saving lives, although still a priority, is no longer the only goal, and a specific therapeutic option may be an optimal solution for one patient but a difficult or unacceptable compromise for others.

It becomes possible to:

- consider the patient's individual preferences, plans, and professional and private activities.
- anticipate what limitations of potential solutions will be relevant in individual cases.
- **prevent** or minimize cumulative risk throughout chronic therapy.

Developing an optimal therapeutic strategy often requires a multidisciplinary approach and the inclusion of the patient in the decision-making process [32]. Both to know their preferences and share responsibility for decisions made.

Until recently, the only therapeutic option for a patient with symptomatic bradycardia, if it was not reversible, was PM implantation, a prosthesis of the heart's physiological pacemaker/conduction system. This method has been successfully used for many years. Subsequent PM generations are becoming more reliable and their capabilities more excellent. With new implantation technics, cardiac pacing became more physiological, i.e., His-bundle pacing or its left branch [33, 34]. However, the main limitations of this method remain the same. The generator must be replaced every few years and systematically checked by professional medical personnel.

Moreover, one should remember the possible infectious complications of implanted PMs due to periprocedural and blood–borne origin or lead damage. The risk increases with the duration of therapy. No less crucial, the PM—by itself—limits the quality of everyday life and physical activity and sometimes can force one to change a professional life. The risk of complications from PPM significantly increases in young patients with a long-life expectancy. On the other hand, often, it is the only available therapy form. Implantation procedures last shorter and shorter, and consequently, the periprocedural risk is significantly reduced. New pacing options, such as resynchronization with a left ventricle electrode, physiological pacing in the region of the His-bundle or its left branch, or the recently introduced implantation of LP, enable an individualized approach to each patient.

Cardioneuroablation (CNA)—a new therapeutic option for patients with symptomatic bradycardia—has been available for several years [35, 36]. A procedure involves modifying the heart's parasympathetic part of the autonomic nervous system of the heart's physiological pacemaker/conducting system. The vagus nerve, which belongs to the parasympathetic nervous system, has an inhibitory effect on the sinus node responsible for generating the heart rhythm and the atrioventricular junction responsible for conduction. CNA is an invasive procedure involving damage through radiofrequency electric energy to the ends of the vagal nerve (postganglionic neurons and interneurons), located in the epicardium, in the left atrium in the vicinity of the pulmonary venous ostia, interatrial septum and the mitral annulus, also in the area of the roof of the right atrium and the coronary sinus ostium. CNA is a beneficial method of bradycardia treatment caused by excessive vagal nerve tension-functional bradycardia. The rising evidence suggests that it should be a first-choice treatment in such cases [37]. It can be used in particular cases of structural damage to the heart's physiological pacemaker/conduction system, releasing its functional reserves from the vagal nerve influence. This procedure is more complicated than the implantation of a PM and, unlike it, requires general anesthesia.

Moreover, the periprocedural risk is higher, and the qualification process for CNA is more complex and time-consuming. In the short term, it requires more significant commitment and acceptance of the risk of complications and possible failure of therapy by a patient. However, in many cases, it allows for avoiding or postponing the prosthesis of the heart's physiological pacemaker/conduction system, which is PM implantation, yet not excluding this option in the future [38, 39].

The abovementioned options allow physicians to offer a more **personalized** approach to bradycardia therapy. Knowing the advantages and limitations of individual therapeutic strategies—the patient's lifestyle and preferences, as well as the estimated lifespan—allows for risk complications **prediction** and estimation related to the considered therapies. Such awareness leads to preventing and minimizing adverse events. For example, the younger the patient, with a less incriminating medical history, the longer lifespan, which entails a significant increase in the cumulative risk of long-term complications of therapy with implantable devices. However, the increased short-term periprocedural risk is more acceptable. PM implantation at a young age presupposes more PM replacement procedures in the future. Each procedure is associated with an increased risk of infectious complications. Also, the lifetime of the electrodes in pacing systems is limited due to physical damage, which can come with patient activity. It is crucial to consider the patient's lifestyle and occupational activity, i.e., transvenous pacemaker precludes some activities, such as sports involving the shoulder girdle. It also excludes the possibility of working with an electric arc and forces the avoidance of strong electromagnetic fields. It binds the patient to the center controlling the implanted device and makes him strictly, chronically dependent on the healthcare system. For this, the acceptance of an individually increased risk associated with a more complicated and arduous CNA procedure and a more complicated procedure qualification process may be accepted. The number of variables necessary to consider in this case requires a more detailed analysis of individual therapy options, optimally with the participation of a multidisciplinary team: electrophysiologists, other specialists in the case of comorbidities, a psychologist, or a career counselor (EP Heart Team) (Fig. 3).

Most importantly—the patient needs to be actively involved in this decision-making process, understanding and accepting both the short-term risk associated with the PM implantation or CNA procedure itself and the cumulative long-term risk and possible limitations resulting from such a choice. Even within the same age group, optimal therapy strategies may vary depending on other factors. The patient

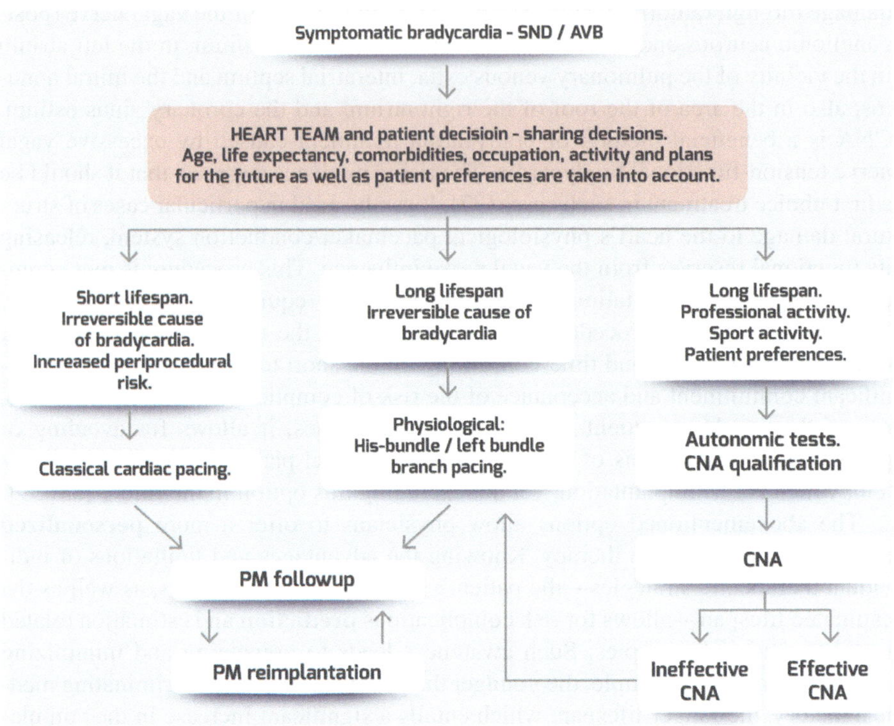

Fig. 3 The decision-making process and a strategy for personalized management of patients with symptomatic bradycardia (own scheme)

may ultimately prefer the well-established medical procedure – the PM, with all its limitations.

A more considerable challenge is the 3P Medicine approach to optimize the already implemented pacing system. An individual-**personalized** approach to each patient requires a reassessment of indications for permanent cardiac pacing. The guidelines of European and American cardiological societies ESC/EHRA/ACC/AHA/HRS [23, 31] reassures with such a procedure, requiring a reassessment of indications for continued PM therapy with PPM before each pacemaker replacement, electrode extraction and replacement and during the entire long-term follow-up.

Patients who had a conventional cardiac PM implanted a few years ago might now be qualified for physiological pacing or can avoid PPM by CNA procedure. In a study of a Danish population of patients who had a pacemaker implanted before the age of 50, it was shown that vasovagal syncope, resulting from an exaggerated reflex, the efferent arm of which is the vagus nerve, was in 5% of cases. If it is a cardioinhibitory type of reflex, i.e., when it results in bradycardia or even a pause in the heart rhythm, CNA would be a causal treatment and would avoid PM implantation. In the same population, it was shown that in 50% of patients qualified for PPM, the cause of atrioventricular node dysfunction could not be determined [40].

Continuous development of diagnostic tools, the autonomic nervous system tests improvement, or the use of implanted loop recorders undoubtedly expand the possible medical solutions for patients whose diagnostics were completed several years ago. This group would include patients who could benefit from a different therapy. Reassessment of indications for continuing PPM therapy or its possible optimization to physiological is not burdensome and should be performed in each case. However, changing the current therapy is a much more complex issue. There are various options: continuation of the current PPM, replacing it with more physiological pacing of the His-bundle or its left branch, or CNA, and discontinuation of PM therapy (Fig. 4).

Changing the current therapy, i.e., cardiac pacing to a different mode or stopping it, is not easy, even when the new method seems to be better. **Personalization** of the approach to this problem is inevitable in this case. The potential risk is no longer only due to implementing a new treatment method but also possible complications resulting from abandoning the current treatment method. Changing the pacing method to physiological or its complete cessation after a successful CNA procedure is associated with an additional risk of removal of the existing pacing system. Treatment by transvenous lead extraction (TLE) carries a 2–3% risk of severe peri-procedural complications. This risk can be minimized by performing TLE in

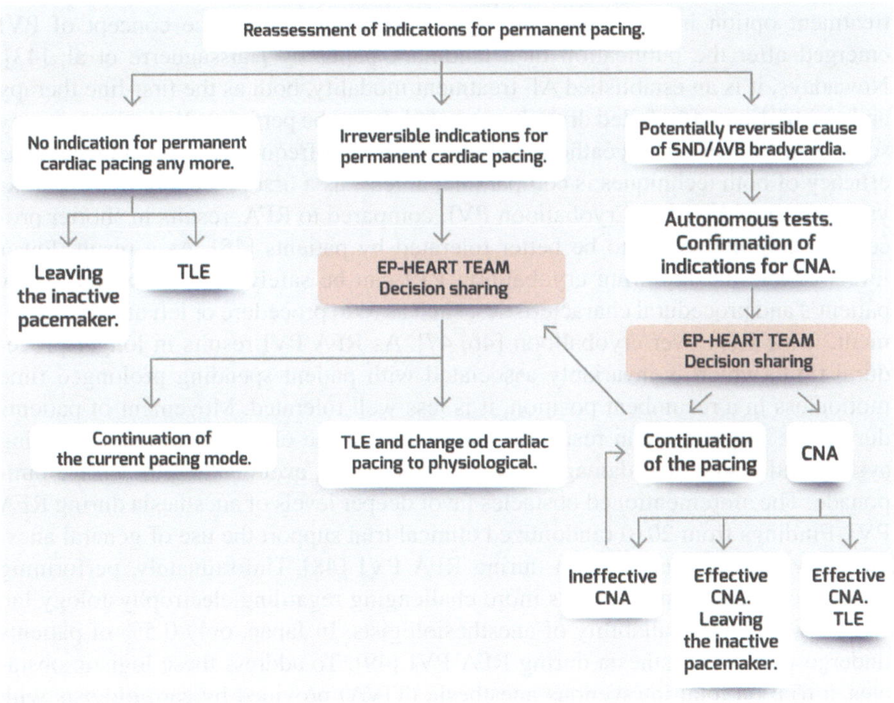

Fig. 4 Reassessment processes for permanent pacing, cardioneuroablation, and transvenous lead extraction (own scheme)

hi-volume centers [41, 42]. However, there are only a few, and they often require transporting a patient to a different center in another city for the procedure. It is an additional difficulty and stress during the treatment process. Abandonment of an inactive pacing system is not a good solution. It is associated with a long-term risk of infective endocarditis. Such a solution can be accepted only in the case of the patient's refusal to undergo the TLE procedure or a very high risk associated with this procedure.

The consideration of the potential benefits and risks of changing treatment should also be based on a multi-professional assessment by EP Heart Team and the patient. Patients who have already received PPM are more aware of its limitations and potential risks. Estimating and anticipating the risks resulting from individual options, **preventing**, and eliminating already existing limitations, such as impairment of physical activity, professional activity or social exclusion, is indispensable.

5 Automatic Control of Anesthesia for Pulmonary Vein Isolation and Cardioneuroablation Procedures

Pulmonary vein isolation (PVI) is a technique of catheter ablation of atrial fibrillation, the most often diagnosed arrhythmia worldwide and, as such, an important treatment option in modern cardiologist's armamentarium. The concept of PVI emerged after the publication of a landmark paper by Haïssaguerre et al. [43]. Nowadays, it is an established AF treatment modality, both as the first-line therapy and as a bail-out after failed drug therapy [16]. It can be performed using two energy sources: cryoballoon and catheter ablation with radiofrequency (RFA) current. The efficacy of both techniques is comparable, at least as a first procedure in the paroxysmal form of AF [44]. Cryoballoon PVI, compared to RFA, results in shorter procedure time and seems to be better tolerated by patients [45]. As a result, lower levels of anesthesia during cryoballoon PVI can be safely used. However, a few patient's and procedural characteristics, such as redo procedure or left atrial enlargement, favor RFA over cryoballoon [46, 47]. As RFA PVI results in longer procedural time, which is invariably associated with patient spending prolonged time motionless in a recumbent position, it is less well tolerated. Movement of patients during the procedure can result in disturbance of the electroanatomical mapping system and inadvertent damage of the cardiac tissue, even leading to cardiac tamponade. The aforementioned obstacles favor deeper levels of anesthesia during RFA PVI. Findings from 2010 randomized clinical trial support the use of general anesthesia over conscious sedation during RFA PVI [48]. Unfortunately, performing PVI under general anesthesia is more challenging regarding electrophysiology lab workflow and the availability of anesthesiologists. In Japan, only 0.5% of patients undergo general anesthesia during RFA PVI [49]. To address these logistic obstacles, a trial on total intravenous anesthesia (TIVA) provided by cardiologists with support from anesthesiologists was performed. TIVA using intravenous propofol and fentanyl was administered by cardiologists in the EP lab in 160 consecutive patients. Airway support was provided via i-gel, and all patients were ventilated in synchronized intermittent mandatory ventilation mode provided by a standard respirator. Doses of anesthetic were titrated to maintain a bispectral index (BIS) between 30 and 50. Only in 3% of cases the intervention of a supporting anesthesiologist was needed, and in 2%, TIVA was abandoned. There were no anesthesia-related complications [50]. This study supports the feasibility of TIVA administered by a cardiologist during RFA PVI, which is especially important in the face of an anesthesiologists' shortage.

In recent years, a novel therapy for bradyarrhythmias emerged – endocardial ablation of the vagal nerve postsynaptic neurons, i.e., CNA. During the procedure, monitoring of residual vagal innervation is essential. The monitoring can be performed by solely observing an increase in heart rate, evoking vagal reactions during high-frequency stimulation, or by direct transvenous stimulation of vagal nerve—extracardiac vagal nerve stimulation (ECVS) [51]. Due to the proximity of the accessory nerve, ECVS leads to head rotation while performed without a neuromuscular blocking agent. This unpredictable movement can result in loss of efficient vagal stimulation and even vascular damage by pacing electrode, so ECVS is generally performed after the neuromuscular blockade. However, it complicates further course of CNA, as neuromuscular blockade decreases the excitability of the diaphragm and monitoring of the phrenic nerve cannot be reliably performed so long as effect of the neuromuscular blocking agent is sustained. The remarks mentioned above makes anesthesia of patients undergoing CNA especially challenging. Method for simplified, more reliable and reproducible general anesthesia to prevent complications and ease management of patients in EP lab is sorely needed. Considering the introduced procedure, the use of the automated control system for anesthesia can be seen as the supplementary tool for support medical staff in this challenging intervention.

Recently we have witnessed an unprecedented international effort to improve the quality and availability of medical care. In this regard, researchers in clinical automation have focused on novel solutions in the field of physiological closed-loop control systems. This scientific area requires a multidisciplinary approach combining specialist knowledge to tackle the problem in a holistic manner. In this context, automated control **in personalized** therapies is one of the most promising research areas, where the application of new research techniques and cutting-edge technologies, such as artificial intelligence (AI), can expand the frontiers of this challenging field [52, 53]. Automatic control engineering has become an important enabling technology in many areas of medicine and biomedical technology. Prominent examples include the artificial pancreas, closed-loop anesthesia, and **personalized** drug-dosing strategies in neurology, oncology, endocrinology, and psychiatry [52]. It is a testament to the power of control systems that allow individualizing treatment by providing mechanisms for linking treatment goals to treatment regimens, thus achieving the desired therapeutic effect. Consequently, the arrival of control systems engineering in the clinic makes the visionary concept of "treat the patient, not the disease" technologically and economically feasible. In this regard, it is desirable to develop automated drug-dosing techniques to prevent under or overdosing issues and to provide a more personalized solution. Additionally, continuous advances in medical sensors, medical equipment and AI have created propitious conditions for incorporating closed-loop systems. For this, patient-dynamics models can be used to predict the patient's pharmacological/biological response to the drug/substance administered, which can be incorporated into the individualized control system design and tuning [52–54]. This issue is one of the open research questions that can be explored to personalize the control system in the context of model individualization.

In the setting of previously described interventions, an important aspect is related to an anesthesia process required for the proper execution of the surgery. The total intravenous anesthesia (TIVA) process generally refers to the loss of sensation. It can be described as the absence of recall and response to a noxious stimulus as the effect of the used drugs. Usually, the medications applied during intravenous anesthesia can be split into three groups: analgesic, hypnotic and those providing a neuromuscular blockade. Those drugs have a physiological effect on the loss of sensitivity to pain and loss of consciousness, interpreted as the depth of hypnosis and caused paralysis of affected skeletal muscles, respectively [52–54]. The anesthesia process is usually divided into three stages, induction, maintenance, and emergence. The simplest TIVA considers only one hypnotic drug, propofol, and its effect is measured by the depth of the hypnosis level. This scheme can be extended to a multivariable case, where more than one drug is infused, having mutual interaction between them. Nevertheless, here we will focus on the simplest case, where the potential benefits could be interpolated to even more complex control system configurations. Figure 5 shows the closed-loop control system where the main components of the analyzed scheme are indicated.

In the classical approach, the anesthesiologist observes the monitors representing patients' vital signs and manually regulates the infusion pump's rates based on their experience. While in automated control, the main idea consists of applying the control algorithm (designed software) that computes the required amount of the drug based on patient state measurements (obtained through clinical monitors equipped with specific sensors). Calculated infusion rates are applied using the computer-controlled infusion pump (actuator). Using an automated system can relieve a medical staff from continuously monitoring and modifying the drug dosage, which is a highly demanding task, especially during long interventions where

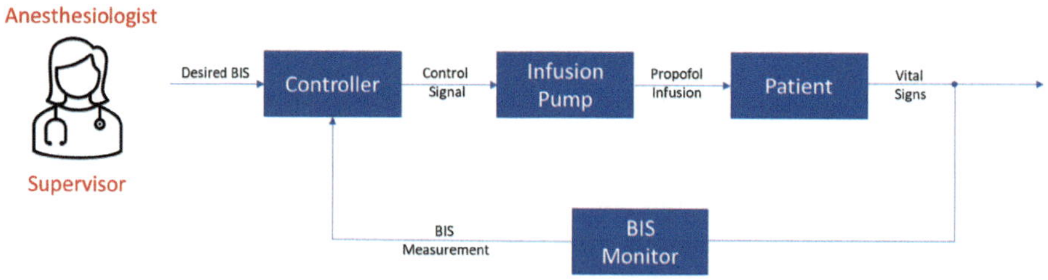

Fig. 5 Automated drug administration in anesthesia—schematic closed-control-loop for depth of hypnosis (own scheme)

it is challenging to maintain the necessary concentration for a long time. The purpose of such an automated control system is to support the anesthesiologist in this difficult process and not to replace them [53, 54]. In this way, the anesthesiologist becomes a supervisor of the process, acting only in critical situations, which permits them to focus on high-level tasks.

Nowadays, many control techniques that have been proposed for depth of hypnosis control in anesthesia process have been widely proven, e.g., A Proportional-Integrative-Derivative (PID) controllers, regulators based on fuzzy logic as well as model predictive control (MPC) techniques, to name a few [52, 55–60]. However, in the context of **personalized** medicine in anesthesia process, the MPC techniques have the greatest potential since they could use an individualized patient's model. As an example, a pharmacokinetic/pharmacodynamic (PK/PD) model for propofol could be indicated, which relates the drug infusing with its clinical effect represented by the bispectral index cale (BIS) [61]. This model is derived from the compartmental model, where some of its parameters are related to patients' physical characteristics (like; age, height, weight and gender). Finally, it should be highlighted that the **personalized** model can be exploited to predict the effect of the drug on each individual resulting in a powerful and flexible toll. When combined with an appropriate control technique, like the MPC, the resulting control action takes into account the specific patient's response to the infused drug provided by the personalized model [56–61]. The control algorithm uses this **predictive** feature to compute the optimal drug dosage, considering limitations and constraints indicated by the type of intervention and clinical practice. As a consequence, the control algorithm is able to provide the right value of the drug dosage. Simultaneously, it reduces the possibility of the drug's over/under dosage, where both could have a negative impact on the patient. The under dosage could result in the regaining consciousness and, consequently, provoking severe traumatic experiences. Whereas overdosage could result in postoperative complications such as postoperative nausea and vomiting (PONV), resulting in a longer recovery [62–65].

With these characteristics, a personalized control scheme assures the **preventive** measure to reduce postoperative complications and to limit the influence of a human factor [66–69]. Moreover, automated anesthesia is able to provide a more unified procedure due to the limited role of the subjective decision of the anesthesiologist [57–59].

6 Conclusions

Continuous ECG monitoring based on the 24 h/365 days concept could be extremely effective in clinical practice for diagnosing atrial fibrillation episodes and other arrhythmias. This might change the paradigm of recognizing not only supraventricular arrhythmias but also brain infarcts sources, syncopal episodes and influence a strategy for anticoagulation therapy.

Dedicated **personalized** AF Heart Team is of crucial importance for decisions concerning diagnostic and therapeutic options in patients with AF and numerous other arrhythmias. Such attitude will presumably influence health, social and economic policies in different countries and systems. PPM implantation **preventive** strategy after transcatheter aortic valve replacement is emphasized by cardiology guidelines and should be widely used. Not yet registered device-related infective endocarditis in patients with leadless pacemakers, a significantly lower risk of periprocedural and post-procedural complications in LPs compared to the transvenous pacemaker—also proved in a TAVR population—seems to favor the LP in frail and elderly patients. Proceeding according to the idea of **personalization**, **prediction,** and **prevention** in treating symptomatic bradycardia and its optimization should no longer be an option but a common practice. Routine application of the guidelines recommendations facilitates everyday practice but often leads to difficulty accepting and unnecessary compromises. The patient's age, occupation, plans for the future, the cumulative risk of long-term complications and difficulty in estimating other preferences cannot be easily summarized in recommendations IA or IIIA arbitrarily presented in the guidelines of cardiological societies. Each patient should be considered individually, and the decision as to the therapy method in seemingly similar cases may vary. Automatic control of anesthesia process, as described above, fits into paradigms of 3P Medicine addressing **personalized**, **predictive**, and **preventive** aspects. These properties can be of added value in the context of cardiologic surgeries, improving the overall patient state after the intervention and thus reducing their postoperative recovery time. However, it must be highlighted that significant effort must be dedicated to developing new technologies and techniques, making them reliable and widely accepted modalities that will be used in clinical practice.

Acknowledgments This work has been partially supported by EU-H2020 funds under MSCA Individual Fellowship—Grant holder: A. Pawłowski, ACTAN project ID: 837912.

References

1. University of Alabama, Department of Biomedical Engineering. https://www.uab.edu/engineering/bme/research/ce
2. University of Central Florida. https://mae.ucf.edu/research-areas/electrophysiology/
3. The University of Bologna. https://corsi.unibo.it/2cycle/BiomedicalEngineering/notice-board/advanced-training-course-bioengineer-and-the-new-technologies-in-the-electrophysiology-room
4. Albarracín AL, Farfán FD, Coletti MA, Teruya PY, Felice CJ (2016) Electrophysiology for biomedical engineering students: a practical and theoretical course in animal electrocorticography. Adv Physiol Educ 40(3):402–409. https://doi.org/10.1152/advan.00073.2015
5. Attokaren MK, Jeong N, Blanpain L, Paulson AL, Garza KM, Borron B et al (2023) BrainWAVE: a flexible method for noninvasive stimulation of brain rhythms across species. eNeuro 6:ENEURO.0257–22. Epub ahead of print. PMID: 36754625. https://doi.org/10.1523/ENEURO.0257-22.2022
6. Vial F, Merchant SHI, McGurrin P, Hallett M (2023) How to do an electrophysiological study of myoclonus. J Clin Neurophysiol 40(2):93–99. Epub 2022 Jun 30. PMID: 36735457; PMCID: PMC9898630. https://doi.org/10.1097/WNP.0000000000000885

7. Chou CY, Agin-Liebes J, Kuo SH (2023) Emerging therapies and recent advances for Tourette syndrome. Heliyon 9(1):e12874. PMID: 36691528; PMCID: PMC9860289. https://doi.org/10.1016/j.heliyon.2023.e12874
8. Kornej J, Börschel CS, Benjamin EJ, Schnabel RB (2020) Epidemiology of atrial fibrillation in the 21st century: novel methods and new insights. Circ Res 127(1):4–20. Epub 2020 Jun 18. PMID: 32716709; PMCID: PMC7577553. https://doi.org/10.1161/CIRCRESAHA.120.316340
9. Li H, Song X, Liang Y et al (2022) Global, regional, and national burden of disease study of atrial fibrillation/flutter, 1990–2019: results from a global burden of disease study, 2019. BMC Public Health 22:2015. https://doi.org/10.1186/s12889-022-14403-2
10. Khan AA, Boriani G, Lip GYH (2020) Are atrial high rate episodes (AHREs) a precursor to atrial fibrillation? Clin Res Cardiol 109:409–416. https://doi.org/10.1007/s00392-019-01545-4
11. Benjamin EJ, Virani SS, Callaway CW, Chamberlain AM, Chang AR, Cheng S et al (2018) American Heart Association Council on Epidemiology and Prevention Statistics Committee and Stroke Statistics Subcommittee. Heart Disease and Stroke Statistics-2018 update: a report from the American Heart Association. Circulation 137(12):e67–e492. Epub 2018 Jan 31. Erratum in: Circulation. 2018 Mar 20;137(12):e493. PMID: 29386200. https://doi.org/10.1161/CIR.0000000000000558
12. Kwok CS, Darlington D, Mayer J, Panchal G, Walker V, Zachariah D et al (2022) A review of the wide range of indications and uses of implantable loop recorders: a review of the literature. Heart 3:45–53. https://doi.org/10.3390/hearts3020007
13. Gautham A, Venkitaraman KR (2016) Designing of a single arm single lead ECG system for wet and dry electrode: a comparison with traditional system. Biomed Eng Appl Basis Commun 28(03):1650021. https://doi.org/10.4015/S1016237216500216
14. Nikodem J, Hrymniak B, Kluwak K, Zyśko D, Klempous R, Rozenblit J et al (2022) EUROCAST, LNCS 2023. Springer, Berlin. Chapter 60; 13789, 978-3-031-25311-9
15. Camm A, Naccarelli G, Mittal S, Crijns H, Hohnloser S, Ma C et al (2022) The increasing role of rhythm control in patients with atrial fibrillation. J Am Coll Cardiol 79(19):1932–1948. https://doi.org/10.1016/j.jacc.2022.03.337
16. Hindricks G, Potpara T, Dagres N, Arbelo E, Bax JJ, Blomström-Lundqvist C et al (2021) ESC Scientific Document Group. 2020 ESC Guidelines for the diagnosis and management of atrial fibrillation developed in collaboration with the European Association for Cardio-Thoracic Surgery (EACTS): The Task Force for the diagnosis and management of atrial fibrillation of the European Society of Cardiology (ESC) Developed with the special contribution of the European Heart Rhythm Association (EHRA) of the ESC. Eur Heart J 42(5):373–498. Erratum in: Eur Heart J. 2021 Feb 1;42(5):507. Erratum in: Eur Heart J. 2021 Feb 1;42(5):546–547. Erratum in: Eur Heart J. 2021 Oct 21;42(40):4194. PMID: 32860505. https://doi.org/10.1093/eurheartj/ehaa612
17. Golubnitschaja O, Costigliola V (2012) EPMA: general report & recommendations in predictive, preventive and personalised medicine 2012: white paper of the European association for predictive preventive and personalised medicine. EPMA J 3(1):14. https://doi.org/10.1186/1878-5085-3-14
18. Vahanian A, Beyersdorf F, Praz F, Milojevic M, Baldus S, Baucrsachs J et al (2022) 2021 ESC/EACTS guidelines for the management of valvular heart disease. Eur Heart J 43(7):561–632. https://doi.org/10.1093/eurheartj/ehab395
19. Cribier A, Eltchaninoff H, Bash A, Borenstein N, Tron C, Bauer F et al (2002) Percutaneous transcatheter implantation of an aortic valve prosthesis for calcific aortic stenosis: first human case description. Circulation 106(24):3006–3008. https://doi.org/10.1161/01.CIR.0000047200.36165.B8
20. Sharma T, Krishnan AM, Lahoud R, Polomsky M, Dauerman HL (2022) National trends in TAVR and SAVR for patients with severe isolated aortic stenosis. J Am Coll Cardiol 80(21):2054–2056. https://doi.org/10.1016/j.jacc.2022.08.787

21. Mack MJ, Leon MB, Thourani VH et al (2019) Transcatheter aortic-valve replacement with a balloon-expandable valve in low-risk patients. N Engl J Med 380(18):1695–1705. https://doi.org/10.1056/nejmoa1814052
22. Nazif TM, Williams MR, Hahn RT, Kapadia S, Babaliaros V, Rodés-Cabau J et al (2014) Clinical implications of new-onset left bundle branch block after transcatheter aortic valve replacement: analysis of the PARTNER experience. Eur Heart J 35(24):1599–1607. https://doi.org/10.1093/eurheartj/eht376
23. Glikson M, Nielsen JC, Kronborg MB, Michowitz Y, Auricchio A, Barbash I et al (2021) 2021 ESC guidelines on cardiac pacing and cardiac resynchronization therapy. Eur Heart J 42(35):3427–3520. https://doi.org/10.1093/eurheartj/ehab364
24. Palmisano P, Guerra F, Aspromonte V, Dell'Era G, Pellegrino P, Laffi M et al (2022) Management of older patients with unexplained, recurrent, traumatic syncope and bifascicular block: implantable loop recorder versus empiric pacemaker implantation—results of a propensity-matched analysis. Heart Rhythm 19(10):1696–1703. https://doi.org/10.1016/j.hrthm.2022.05.023
25. Udo EO, Zuithoff NPA, van Hemel NM, de Cock C, Hendriks T, Doevendans P et al (2012) Incidence and predictors of short- and long-term complications in pacemaker therapy: the FOLLOWPACE study. Heart Rhythm 9(5):728–735. https://doi.org/10.1016/j.hrthm.2011.12.014
26. Kypta A, Blessberger H, Lichtenauer M, Steinwender C (2016) Complete encapsulation of a leadless cardiac pacemaker. Clin Res Cardiol 105:94. https://doi.org/10.1007/s00392-015-0929-x
27. Mangieri A, Montalto C, Pagnesi M, Lanzillo G, Demir O, Testa L et al (2018) TAVI and post procedural cardiac conduction abnormalities. Front Cardiovasc Med 1:85. https://doi.org/10.3389/fcvm.2018.00085
28. El-Chami MF, Al-Samadi F, Clementy N, Garweg C, Martinez-Sande J, Piccini J et al (2018) Updated performance of the Micra transcatheter pacemaker in the real-world setting: a comparison to the investigational study and a transvenous historical control. Heart Rhythm 15(12):1800–1807. https://doi.org/10.1016/j.hrthm.2018.08.005
29. Roberts PR, Clementy N, al Samadi F, Garweg CH, Martinez-Sande J, Iacopino S et al (2017) A leadless pacemaker in the real-world setting: the Micra Transcatheter pacing system post-approval registry. Heart Rhythm 14(9):1375–1379. https://doi.org/10.1016/j.hrthm.2017.05.017
30. Mechulan A, Prevot S, Peret A, Nait-Saidi L, Miliani I, Leong-Feng L et al (2022) Micra AV leadless pacemaker implantation after transcatheter aortic valve implantation. PACE 45(11):1310–1315. https://doi.org/10.1111/pace.14545
31. Kusumoto FM, Schoenfeld MH, Barrett C, Edgerton JR, Ellenbogen KA, Gold MR et al (2019) 2018 ACC/AHA/HRS guideline on the evaluation and management of patients with bradycardia and cardiac conduction delay: executive summary: a report of the American College of Cardiology/American Heart Association task force on clinical practice guidelines, and the Heart Rhythm Society. Heart Rhythm 16(9):e227–e279. https://doi.org/10.1016/j.hrthm.2018.10.036
32. Chung MK, Fagerlin A, Wang PJ, Ajayi TB, Allen LA, Baykaner T et al (2021) Shared decision making in cardiac electrophysiology procedures and arrhythmia management. Circ Arrhythm Electrophysiol 14(12):e007958. https://doi.org/10.1161/CIRCEP.121.007958
33. Zanon F, Ellenbogen KA, Dandamudi G, Sharma PS, Huang W, Lustgarten DL et al (2018) Permanent his-bundle pacing: a systematic literature review and meta-analysis. Europace 20(11):1819–1826. https://doi.org/10.1093/europace/euy058
34. Ponnusamy SS, Arora V, Namboodiri N, Kumar V, Kapoor A, Vijayaraman P (2020) Left bundle branch pacing: a comprehensive review. J Cardiovasc Electrophysiol 31(9):2462–2473. Epub 2020 Jul 30. https://doi.org/10.1111/jce.14681
35. Pachon JC, Pachon EI, Pachon JC, Lobo TJ, Pachon MZ, Vargas RN et al (2005) "Cardioneuroablation"—new treatment for neurocardiogenic syncope, functional AV block

and sinus dysfunction using catheter RF-ablation. Europace 7:1–13. https://doi.org/10.1016/j.eupc.2004.10.003
36. Pachon JC, Pachon EI, Cunha Pachon MZ, Lobo TJ, Pachon JC, Santillana TG (2011) Catheter ablation of severe neurally mediatated reflex (neurocardiogenic or vasovagal) syncope: cardioneuroablation long-term results. Europace 13:1231–1242. https://doi.org/10.1093/europace/eur163
37. Piotrowski R, Baran J, Sikorska A, Krynski T, Kulakowski P (2022) Cardioneuroablation for reflex syncope: efficacy and effects on autonomic cardiac regulation—a prospective randomized trial. JACC Clin Electrophysiol 28:85. https://doi.org/10.1016/j.jacep.2022.08.011
38. Stec S, Jankowska-Polańska JD, Wileczek A, Josiak K, Śledź J et al (2022) Rationale and design of SAN.OK randomized clinical trial and registry: comparison of the effects of evidence-based pacemaker therapy and cardioneuroablation in sinus node dysfunction. Cardiol J 29(6):1031–1036. https://doi.org/10.5603/CJ.a2022.0103
39. Reichert A, Wileczek A, Stec S (2022) Cardioneuroablation for the effective treatment of recurrent vasovagal syncope to restore driving abilities. Kardiol Pol 80(11):1158–1160. https://doi.org/10.33963/KP.a2022.0189
40. Rudbeck-Resdal J, Christiansen MK, Johansen JB, Nielsen JC, Bundgaard H, Jensen HK (2019) Aetiologies and temporal trends of atrioventricular block in young patients: a 20-year nationwide study. Europace 21(11):1710–1716. https://doi.org/10.1093/europace/euz206
41. Tułecki Ł, Polewczyk A, Jacheć W, Nowosielecka D, Tomków K, Stefańczyk P et al (2021) A study of major and minor complications of 1500 Transvenous Lead extraction procedures performed with optimal safety at two high-volume referral centers. Int J Environ Res Public Health 18(19):10416. https://doi.org/10.3390/ijerph181910416
42. Sidhu BS, Gould J, Bunce C, Elliott M, Mehta V, Kennergren C et al (2020) ELECTRa Investigators group. The effect of Centre volume and procedure location on major complications and mortality from transvenous lead extraction: an ESC EHRA EORP European Lead extraction ConTRolled ELECTRa registry subanalysis. Europace 22(11):1718–1728. https://doi.org/10.1093/europace/euaa131
43. Haissaguerre M, Jais P, Shah DC, Takahashi A, Hocini M, Quiniou G et al (1998) Spontaneous initiation of atrial fibrillation by ectopic beats originating in the pulmonary veins. N Engl J Med 339(10):659–666. https://doi.org/10.1056/NEJM199809033391003
44. Kuck KH, Brugada J, Furnkranz A, Metzner A, Ouyang F, Chun KR et al (2016) Cryoballoon or radiofrequency ablation for paroxysmal atrial fibrillation. N Engl J Med 374:2235–2245. https://doi.org/10.1056/NEJMoa1602014
45. Defaye P, Kane A, Jacon P, Mondesert B (2010) Cryoballoon for pulmonary vein isolation: is it better tolerated than radiofrequency? Retrospective study comparing the use of analgesia and sedation in both ablation techniques. Arch Cardiovasc Dis 103(6–7):388–393. https://doi.org/10.1016/j.acvd.2010.06.004
46. Kuck KH, Albenque JP, Chun KRJ, Fürnkranz A, Busch M, Elvanet A, al. (2019) Repeat ablation for atrial fibrillation recurrence post Cryoballoon or radiofrequency ablation in the FIRE and ICE trial. Circ Arrhythm Electrophysiol 12(6):1–9. https://doi.org/10.1161/CIRCEP.119.007247
47. Ikenouchi T, Inaba O, Takamiya T, Inamura Y, Sato A, Matsumura Y et al (2021) The impact of left atrium size on selection of the pulmonary vein isolation method for atrial fibrillation: Cryoballoon or radiofrequency catheter ablation. In: Impact of LA size on selecting the PVI method, vol 231. Elsevier, Amsterdam, p 82. https://doi.org/10.1016/j.ahj.2020.10.061
48. Di Biase L, Conti S, Mohanty P, Bai R, Sanchez J, Walton D et al (2011) General anesthesia reduces the prevalence of pulmonary vein reconnection during repeat ablation when compared with conscious sedation: results from a randomized study. Heart Rhythm 8(3):368–372. https://doi.org/10.1016/j.hrthm.2010.10.043
49. Inoue K, Murakawa Y, Nogami A, Shoda M, Naito S, Kumagai K et al (2014) Current status of catheter ablation for atrial fibrillation—updated summary of the Japanese Catheter Ablation Registry of Atrial Fibrillation (J-CARAF). Circ J 78(5):1112–1120. https://doi.org/10.1253/circj.cj-13-1179

50. Yamaguchi T, Shimakawa Y, Mitsumizo S, Fukui A, Kawano Y, Otsubo T et al (2018) Feasibility of total intravenous anesthesia by cardiologists with the support of anesthesiologists during catheter ablation of atrial fibrillation. J Cardiol 72(1):19–25. https://doi.org/10.1016/j.jjcc.2017.12.008
51. Pachon MJ, Pachon ME, Santillana PT, Lobo T, Pachon C, Pachon MJ et al (2015) Simplified method for vagal effect evaluation in cardiac ablation and electrophysiological procedures. JACC Clin Electrophysiol 1(5):451–460. https://doi.org/10.1016/j.jacep.2015.06.008
52. Khodaei M, Candelino N, Mehrvarz A, Jalili N (2020) Physiological closed-loop control (PCLC) systems: review of a modern frontier in automation. IEEE Access 8:23965–24005. https://doi.org/10.1109/ACCESS.2020.2968440
53. Ghita M, Neckebroek M, Muresan C, Copot D (2020) Closed-loop control of anesthesia: survey on actual trends, challenges and perspectives. IEEE Access 8:206264–206279. https://doi.org/10.1109/ACCESS.2020.3037725
54. Ionescu C, Neckebroek M, Ghita M, Copot D (2021) An open source patient simulator for design and evaluation of computer based multiple drug dosing control for anesthetic and hemodynamic variables. IEEE Access 9:8680–8694. https://doi.org/10.1109/ACCESS.2021.3049880
55. Soltesz K, Dumont G, van Heusden K, Hägglund T, Ansermino J (2012) Simulated mid-ranging control of propofol and remifentanil using EEG measured hypnotic depth of anesthesia. In: Proceedings of 51st IEEE Conference on Decision and Control. CDC, Maui, pp 356–361. https://doi.org/10.1109/CDC.2012.6426858
56. Merigo L, Padula F, Pawlowski A, Dormido S, Guzman J, Latronico N et al (2018) A model-based control scheme for depth of hypnosis in anesthesia. Biomed Signal Process Control 42:216–229
57. Pawłowski A, Schiavo M, Latronico N, Paltenghi M, Visioli A (2023) Event-based MPC for propofol administration in anesthesia. Comput Methods Programs Biomed 229:107289. ISSN 0169-2607. https://doi.org/10.1016/j.cmpb.2022.107289
58. Pawlowski A, Schiavo M, Latronico N, Paltenghi M, Visioli A (2022) Model predictive control using MISO approach for drug co-administration in anesthesia. J Process Control 117:98–111. https://doi.org/10.1016/j.jprocont.2022.07.007
59. Pawlowski A, Merigo L, Guzmán J, Dormido S, Visioli A (2018) Two-degree-of-freedom control scheme for depth of hypnosis in anesthesia. IFAC Pap Online 51(4):72–77. https://doi.org/10.1016/j.ifacol.2018.06.034
60. Pawlowski A, Schiavo M, Latronico N, Paltenghi M, Visioli A (2022) Linear MPC for anesthesia process with external predictor. Comput Chem Eng 161:1–13. https://doi.org/10.1016/j.compchemeng.2022.107747
61. Vanluchene AL, Vereecke H, Thas O, Mortier EP, Shafer SL, Struys MM (2004) Spectral entropy as an electroencephalographic measure of anesthetic drug effect: a comparison with bispectral index and processed midlatency auditory evoked response. Anesthesiology 101(1):34–42. https://doi.org/10.1097/00000542-200407000-00008
62. Absalom A, Kenny G (2003) Closed-loop control of propofol anaesthesia using bispectral index: performance assessment in patients receiving computer controlled propofol and manually controlled remifentanil infusions for minor surgery. Br J Anaesth 90(6):737–741. https://doi.org/10.1093/bja/aeg137
63. Absalom A, Sutcliffe N, Kenny G (2002) Closed-loop control of anesthesia using bispectral index. Anesthesiology 96(1):67–73. https://doi.org/10.1097/00000542-200201000-00017
64. Liu N, Chazot T, Genty A, Landais A, Restoux A, McGee K et al (2006) Titration of propofol for anesthetic induction and maintenance guided by the bispectral index: closed-loop versus manual control. Anesthesiology 104(4):686–695. https://doi.org/10.1097/00000542-200604000-00012
65. Puri G, Kumar B, Aveek J (2007) Closed-loop anaesthesia delievery system (CLADS) using bispectral index; a performance assessment study. Anaesth Intensive Care 35(3):357–362. https://doi.org/10.1177/0310057X0703500306

66. van Heusden K, Dumont G, Soltesz K, Petersen C, Umedaly A, West N et al (2014) Design and clinical evaluation of robust PID control of propofol anesthesia in children. IEEE Trans Control Syst Technol 22(29):491–501. https://doi.org/10.1109/TCST.2013.2260543
67. Liu N, Chazot T, Hamada S, Landais A, Boichut N, Dussaussoy C et al (2011) Closed-loop coadministration of propofol and remifentanil guided by bispectral index: a randomized multicenter study. Anesth Analg 112:546–557. https://doi.org/10.1213/ANE.0b013e318205680b
68. Morley A, Derrick J, Mainland P, Lee B, Short T (2000) Closed loop control of anaesthesia: an assessment of the bispectral index as the target of control. Anesthesia 55:953–959. https://doi.org/10.1046/j.1365-2044.2000.01527.x
69. Struys M, Smet T, Versichelen L, Velde S, Broecke R, Mortier E (2001) Comparison of closed-loop controlled administration of propofol using bispectral index as the controlled variable versus standard practice controlled administration. Anesthesiology 95:6–1. https://doi.org/10.1097/00000542-200107000-00007

Wound Healing from Bench to Bedside: A PPPM Bridge Between Physical Therapies and Chronic Inflammation

Yuanhua Liu, Yongying Liang, Xiaoyuan Zhou, Jennifer E. Dent, Lucia di Nardo, Ting Jiang, Ding Qin, Youtao Lu, Dongyi He, and Christine Nardini

Yuanhua Liu, Yongying Liang, Xiaoyuan Zhou, Jennifer E. Dent contributed equally to this work.

Y. Liu
Shanghai Institute of Biochemistry and Cell Biology, Chinese Academy of Sciences, Shanghai, People's Republic of China

Group of Clinical Genomic Networks, CAS-MPG Partner Institute for Computational Biology, Shanghai Institutes for Biological Sciences, Chinese Academy of Sciences, Shanghai, China

University of Chinese Academy of Sciences, Beijing, China
e-mail: liuyuanhua@sibcb.ac.cn

Y. Liang · D. Qin · D. He
Guanghua Hospital, Shanghai, People's Republic of China
e-mail: dongyihe@medmail.com.cn

X. Zhou
Group of Clinical Genomic Networks, CAS-MPG Partner Institute for Computational Biology, Shanghai Institutes for Biological Sciences, Chinese Academy of Sciences, Shanghai, China

University of Chinese Academy of Sciences, Beijing, China

Department of Neurology, University of California, San Francisco, CA, USA
e-mail: zhouxiaoyuan@picb.ac.cn

J. E. Dent
Group of Clinical Genomic Networks, CAS-MPG Partner Institute for Computational Biology, Shanghai Institutes for Biological Sciences, Chinese Academy of Sciences, Shanghai, China

University of Chinese Academy of Sciences, Beijing, China

NORSAS Consultancy Limited, Norwich, Norfolk, UK
e-mail: j.liu@norsas.co.uk

H. Podbielska, M. Kapalla (eds.), *Predictive, Preventive, and Personalised Medicine: From Bench to Bedside*, Advances in Predictive, Preventive and Personalised Medicine 17, https://doi.org/10.1007/978-3-031-34884-6_12

L. di Nardo
Dermatology, Department of Translational Medicine and Surgery, Università Cattolica del Sacro Cuore, Rome, Italy
e-mail: lucia.dinardo@unicatt.it

T. Jiang
Department of Neurology, University of California, San Francisco, CA, USA

Y. Lu
Group of Clinical Genomic Networks, CAS-MPG Partner Institute for Computational Biology, Shanghai Institutes for Biological Sciences, Chinese Academy of Sciences, Shanghai, China

University of Chinese Academy of Sciences, Beijing, China

Department of Biology, University of Pennsylvania, Philadelphia, PA, USA
e-mail: luyoutao@sas.upenn.edu

C. Nardini (✉)
Group of Clinical Genomic Networks, CAS-MPG Partner Institute for Computational Biology, Shanghai Institutes for Biological Sciences, Chinese Academy of Sciences, Shanghai, China

University of Chinese Academy of Sciences, Beijing, China

National Research Council of Italy (CNR), Institute of Applied Calculus (IAC) "Mauro Picone", Rome, Italy
e-mail: christine.nardini@cnr.it

Abbreviations

ACR	American College of Rheumatology
AP	Acupuncture
CIA	Collagen induced arthritis
DAS	Disease activity score
EMT	Epithelial-mesenchymal transition
ERAS	Early recovery after surgery
EULAR	European Alliance of Associations for Rheumatology
GI	Gut Intestinal
GIP	Greater inflammatory pathway
HAQ	Health assessment questionnaire
LLLT	Low level laser therapy
MTX	Methotrexate
NCD	Non-communicable diseases
PBMC	Peripheral blood mononuclear cells
PBMT	PhotoBioModulation therapy
PPPM	Predictive, preventive, personalized medicine
RA	Rheumatoid arthritis
RF	Rheumatoid factor
SGD	Sustainable development goal
UN	United Nations
VNS	Vagal nerve stimulation
WH	Wound healing

1 Introduction

1.1 Inflammation

Inflammation is known to correlate with the majority of maladies we are not yet able to cure, with particular emphasis on non-communicable diseases (NCDs), responsible, worldwide, for 44 million deaths per year [1], and in Europe for 80% of expenses associated with disease [2]. The societal impact of this silent pandemic is so vast that the United Nations (UN) have recognized it as one of the 17 major obstacles to our sustainable development, and have proposed the Sustainable Development Goal (SGD) 3 to be specifically concerned in target 4 with NCDs and mental health (SGD3.4: "By 2030, reduce by one third premature mortality from non-communicable diseases through prevention and treatment and promote mental health and well-being").

In the past 10–15 years, numerous discoveries have contributed to enlighten our understanding of inflammation, including the activity of the autonomous nervous system in the control of inflammation, namely the *inflammatory reflex* [3–5], the role of the gut intestinal (GI) [6, 7] and oral [8] microbiomes. PPPMs approaches have promoted the relevance of assessing chronic inflammation and wound healing gone awry [9], two accompanying phenomena to the development of NCDs, with a long prodromic phase where subclinical inflammation plays a silent yet fundamental role [10].

It descends from these considerations that a better understanding and, importantly, a better control of inflammation must consider as many factors impinging on inflammation as possible. Our theoretical pioneering effort in this direction presents the *Greater inflammatory pathway (GIP)* [11] as the *summa* of such influences, and updates the definition of the pathway(s) whose alterations should be studied to control inflammation, including namely: the autonomous nervous system, the host–microbiome interface, and wound healing. In this frame and further [12], we have already observed that, while the recent attention on the GI microbiota and the inflammatory reflex have promoted experimental therapies ranging from *fecal transplant* [13] to vagal nerve stimulation (VNS) in bioelectronic medicine [14], respectively, therapeutic *physical stimuli* (i.e., *exploiting electric, optic, magnetic or mechanic stimuli*), which directly elicit WH, remain among the most neglected research areas.

Wound Healing (WH)-also known as epithelial-mesenchymal transition (EMT) type 2- progresses from a transient inflammatory phase, through regeneration to remodeling [15]. Its known paracrine effects are also accompanied by long distance consequences, as shown by our original work [16] and few others [17, 18], but poorly, if at all, translated into medical practice.

1.2 Recollecting a Compartmentalized and Scattered Knowledge Related to Physical Stimuli on Inflammation and Wound Healing

Indeed, research on the effects of physical stimuli on inflammation is very uneven, depending mostly on the nature of the stimulus. In fact, ample disparities exist in terms of quality and quantity of the basic biological knowledge available.

Recognizing and recollecting this scattered scientific background is the first necessary step to promote additional access to anti-inflammatory therapies, and complete the *bench* step.

1.2.1 Mechanical Stimuli

Mechanical stimuli (such as, but not limited to, vibrational therapy [17], manual acupuncture [16], massage [19, 20]) are well known to elicit all stages of WH, indeed, "injuries" are mostly thought of as mechanic. Mechanosensing and mechanostransduction are the cellular phenomena at the basis of this effect, and all cell types are known to present both these features. There exists extensive knowledge on their temporal and biochemical functional activation, including the complex transcriptional and phenotypic changes supported at the cellular level [21–23], recapitulating the inflammatory, remodeling and regenerative phases of WH. Generally, however, despite good to excellent biological knowledge of EMT type2, mechanical stimuli quantification for WH therapeutic elicitation remains empirical and translation has not proceeded to the clinics, despite relevant potential application in oncology [24] and results in muscle regeneration [25] for instance, and with the exception of the exploitation of the events occurring in the regeneration and remodeling phases (regenerative medicine), but very seldom in relation to the inflammatory phase, despite few exceptions [16–18].

1.2.2 Electric Stimuli

Electric stimuli have also received ample attention, owing to different theories that imply the usage of electricity to restore a variety of physiological features. The sensitivity to electricity of neural cells is likely the best assessed, from L. Galvani [26] onwards. Recently, as briefly introduced above, this knowledge has been expanded with a novel understanding of the effects of electrical stimulations during inflammatory episodes i.e. by *bioelectronic medicine*, where the *inflammatory reflex* [3, 5] has recently been uncovered and describes the negative feedback loop that is activated by the autonomous nervous system (ANS) in case of acute [27] and chronic [28] inflammation to control cytokines production and dampen inflammation. Electricity is also important in a different context, relevant to our purposes, as it is known to interfere with superficial wound healing. This is based on the "skin battery" concept [29–31], i.e., the difference of potential that exists in healthy and integer skin, and that is disrupted in case of physical injuries, braking the skin barrier and hence compromising the organized electrical charges that exist inside, differentially from outside, this barrier. In this case, appropriate electrostimulation (i.e., direct and of the magnitude of the skin battery) is experimentally proven to restore physiological conditions, and is known to be accompanied by improved WH (skin regeneration and remodeling), with explicit usage in dermatology and orthopedics. At the cellular level electrosensing and electrotransduction are embodied by lipid rafts [32], whose mobility within the cells' surface polarizes the membrane, deforming it with consequences that are likely to mimic mechanotransduction ones.

1.2.3 Optical Stimuli

Optosensitivity and optotransduction at the molecular and cellular level, originally emerged, similarly to electrostimulation, in a specialized context, i.e., associated to the photoreceptor cells of the retina. Nevertheless, the actuator proteins, *optins*, have also been found in fibroblasts and keratinocytes, leading the way to the exploitation of optical stimuli on the largest of our organs: skin (dermal photoreception) [33, 34]. **P**hoto**bio**modulation (PBMT) is the corresponding **t**herapeutic approach, i.e., the effect of optical signals at the organ(ism) level, generally offered as low-level laser therapy (LLLT). Despite abundant work on the application of such stimuli [35, 36], there exists very limited available literature on the explicit anti-inflammatory outcome of LLLT, reported as secondary effects (i.e., secondary to the light transduction) in the form of small molecules flux changes that do overlap exactly the non-transcriptional phase of mechanostranduction [37] (but not made explicit nor recognized as such), and as tertiary effects in terms of remodeling and regeneration. Very recently the relation between the *aryl hydrocarbon receptor* and optical stimuli has been uncovered, hopefully opening to a deeper and broader understanding of the connection with inflammation [38]. Laser applications are better known for their applications in surgery, with the majority of other types of application left to unstandardized approaches, mostly in the realm of complementary alternative medicine. Overall, at all scale levels (molecules, cells, tissues, organism) rigorous effects of optical stimuli are poorly represented.

1.2.4 Magnetic Stimuli

Magnetic stimuli are by far the most neglected in biomedicine. The usage of magnetic fields in relation to biology is in fact more commonly focused on the growth of organic crystals, using high levels of energy. Robustness of the available information is weakened by the variability of the magnetic field parameters adopted. Recent detailed work refers to mechanomagnetic [39] effects, directly indicating that the cascade of events following this type of stimulation replicates WH, other less recent results clarify the effect of static magnetic field, highly cell-dependent [40], overlooking mechanical aspects and their effects on channels, membrane, as well as Ca^{2+} fluxes change, overlapping, although generally unrecognized, with the progression of WH.

All the above information is the result of the careful collection from a large variety of publications in different research areas that remain strongly compartmentalized and rarely speak to each other (from engineering to physics to biology and biomedicine). In addition to this "horizontal" compartmentalization (related mostly to the different nature of the stimulus) there exists also a striking "vertical" compartmentalization, i.e., there is limited to no connection among the findings at the cellular level and their impact on higher scale complexes like tissues, organs and finally the human body. This vertical compartmentalization holds independently of the biological background: therapeutic dose is fully empirical based solely on the *do not harm* principle and, importantly, only rarely the medical rationale builds on the biological work, despite a large variety of attempts to exploit -in a mostly unstructured manner- physical stimuli.

2 Working Hypothesis

To move beyond this fragmentation, we hypothesize that WH can be the target phenomenon and function able to recollect under one common and complex concept the effects of therapeutic physical stimulations. In particular, knowing that WH is a highly conserved function elicited by physical stimuli and that under physiological conditions the early inflammatory phase has a transient nature, we hypothesize that purposedly eliciting this inflammatory phase by controlled physical stimuli may first elicit and then force the extinction of inflammation, not only in physiologic but also in inflamed contexts. To test our hypothesis we chose rheumatoid arthritis (RA) a model NCD whose impact on health and societal expenditure is recognized as dramatic [41]. The international organisms promoting guidelines for the control of RA (American College of Rheumatology, ACR, and the European Alliance of Associations for Rheumatology, EULAR), recommend to maximally anticipate the diagnosis of the disease [42, 43], in line with the paradigm of predictive, preventive, and personalized medicine (PPPM) [44] that promotes the identification and treatment of *ALL* inflammatory symptoms as early as possible, to minimize the devastating progression of NCDs. Moreover, International recommendations envision the use of classic and biologic disease modifying anti-rheumatic drugs (*c*- and *b*DMARD, respectively) until clinical remission (i.e., stabilization of the symptoms) with the possibility of subsequent DMARDs tapering and discontinuation [43].

3 Methods

We tested this hypothesis in a multiscale context, with animal model studies [16, 45] and a human pilot clinical trial [46] (NCT01619176, https://clinicaltrials.gov/ct2/show/NCT01619176) with the aim to assess the extent of our results' translatability.

3.1 Animal Studies

Collagen induced arthritis (CIA) [47] is a known model of RA induced in animals, recapitulating the majority of immunological and phenotypic alterations of RA. Our two studies, on Wistar rats, include control and active arms, where methotrexate (MTX), the gold standard DMARD therapy, is adopted, and mechanical stimulation [48] is performed by insertion and rotation of thin needles (acupuncture -AP) alone or in combination with MTX (MTX + AP). Phenotypic assessment of the disease was done with standard approaches (paws thickness by qualitative visual scale and quantitative with a gauge). Multiple samples from different tissues (blood peripheral blood mononuclear cells -PBMCs-, stool, subcutaneous tissue and rheumatoid arthritis fibroblast like cells -RAFLs-) and at various time points (before, at 1 h, 14 days and 32 days from the beginning of the therapy) were collected and processed with omics (miRNA, mRNA for blood and subcutaneous tissue sample, 16S-rRNA-seq for GI microbiota analysis), with all details, including therapeutic release and raw data availability, being reported in [16, 45] and summarized to explore translatability in Fig. 1.

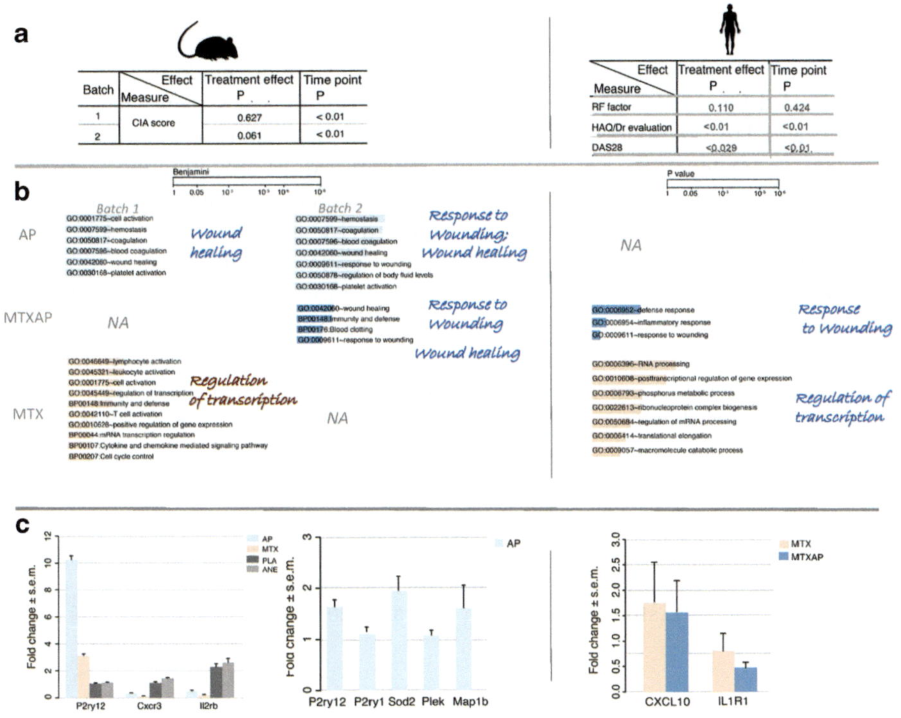

Fig. 1 Translational results, continuum between animal models (rats) and humans. Analyses were run using R version 3.6.2 or later. Panel **a**: Statistical analysis of clinical standard data, *P* indicates *p*-values based on the F-distribution. Panel **b**: blood functional results (Gene Ontology Enrichment) across batches and species including animal studies (batch1 and batch2) and the pilot human clinical trial ID: NCT01619176A, https://clinicaltrials.gov/ct2/show/NCT01619176. Blue and red bars across enriched functions indicate the associated (corrected) *p*-values for up- and down-regulated expression, respectively. Summary enriched functions are reported for enhanced clarity (handwritten style). All animal results were published in [16, 45]. Human data were aggregated to compensate for the small samples size. Namely: 18 blood samples from 9 RA patients in total, 8 before any therapy (RA), 2 AP after 2 week (AP), 5 AP + MTX after 3 months (MTXAP), 3 MTX (MTX) after 3 months. NA stands for "not available," i.e., this branch of the study was not performed. Panel C: Independent qRT-PCR analysis s.e.m. = standard error of mean. The genes studied were: Purinergic Receptor P2Y12 (P2ry12), C-X-C Motif Chemokine Receptor 3 (Cxcr3) and Interleukin 2 Receptor Subunit Beta (Il2rb) for batch 1; P2ry12, Purinergic Receptor P2Y1 (P2ry1), Superoxide Dismutase 2 (Sod2), Plekstrin (Pleck) and Microtubule Associated Protein 1B (Map1b) for batch 2; C-X-C Motif Chemokine Ligand 10 (CXCL10) and Interleukin 1 Receptor Type 1 (IL1R1) for the huma pilot trial. Rat and human icons by Freepik from www.flaticon.com

3.2 Pilot Clinical Trial

We designed a pilot study, approved by the ethical committee of Shanghai GuangHua Hospital, designed as a non-inferiority trial where 10 RA patients were enrolled, balanced by age, uniformly treated with leflunomide and non-steroidal anti-inflammatory drug and randomly assigned to MTX or AP only for the first 2 weeks and to a combination of the two (MTX-AP) or continuation of MTX alone, for 3 months in total. Details on both therapy dose and stimulation points can be found on clinicaltrials.gov, ID: NCT01619176, https://clinicaltrials.gov/ct2/show/NCT01619176. Clinical parameters for enrollment and monitoring were collected according to the American College of Rheumatology (ACR) guidelines and include Rheumatoid Factor (RF), patients and clinicians Health Assessment Questionnaire (HAQ) and DAS28 scores. Statistical phenotypic data analysis for ACR recommended parameters [49] (RF, HAQ and DAS28) was done modeling the parameters as functions of treatment and time (beginning of therapy, 3 weeks, 3 months), with fitted generalized linear models and analyzed by ANOVA (RF, DAS28) and MANOVA (HAQ). Omics were collected for assessment of the systemic effects of the therapy via blood samples (peripheral blood mononuclear cells, PBMC) processed by transcriptomics. PBMCs were analyzed via Affymetrix U133 plus 2.0 array (Gene Expression Omnibus repository, *ID* GSE59526, https://www.ncbi.nlm.nih.gov/geo/query/acc.cgi?acc=GSE59526) with the following specifics: expression intensities and calls detection filtered for the removal of probes with less than 10% of all samples, log-2 transformed and selected as differential (end of therapy samples versus all before therapy samples) with *limma* [50] for p-value <0.05 and fold-change >1.8. Further candidates for which 30% of expression intensity across all samples was absent for detection call were also removed. Functional enrichment analysis was run with DAVID functional cluster analysis [51].

For all organisms' studies, validation with an independent technology was run by qRT-PCR (Fig. 1c).

4 Results

The continuum of phenotypic and molecular data analysis results are shown in Fig. 1, where side-by-side comparison of PBMC transcriptomics highlights the translatability of the findings and the crucial involvement of WH as statistically significantly enriched function across the two organisms and the three studies, when comparing the role of the mechanical stimulation on (model) arthritis.

In particular, with respect to the human data, the phenotypic statistical analysis returned significant treatment and timepoint effects for DAS28 and qualitative results (HAQ pooled with clinicians' evaluation) – (values for MTX lower than for MTX-AP). Despite RF factor reducing over time and values for MTX being higher than for MTX-AP, due to a lack of power (missing data at multiple timepoints), the RF analyses did not return significant results (Fig. 1a). Phenotypic results are backed by the search for molecular surrogates via PBMC differential and functional analyses (Fig. 1b). The only enriched cluster (enrichment score > 1) is shown for human MTXAP2RA (MTX + AP versus baseline) comparison and all top terms (GO hierarchy) from the MTX2RA (MTX versus baseline) seven enriched clusters are shown. A similar analysis was run on animal models with detailed adaptation of the protocol and analysis reported in [16, 45]. This highlights overall the relevance of wound healing as the distinctive function elicited in the presence of the mechanical stimulation (AP), alone or in conjunction with the gold standard treatment.

5 Conclusion and Recommendations

We present, for the first time, two fundamental steps in the advancement of our knowledge on the therapeutic potential of physical stimuli. First, the introductory overview and revisitation on the shared biological functions activated by physical stimuli, independently of their nature, in an anti-inflammatory context, is to the best of our knowledge a première in this direction. Second, the continuum of systemic (PBMC) molecular effects descending from a therapeutic mechanical stimulus in a chronic inflammatory context represented by (model) arthritis, shows how this function is conserved.

The first step serves the second not only in the progression from bench (basic science) to bed (animal/clinical studies), but also from a theoretical perspective given the fact that all stimuli appear to proceed by the activation of mechanotransduction typical markers (see above, under Sect. 1.2): in this sense the loss of generality in our experiments using mechanical stimuli (i.e., manual AP) could be minimal, considering also that RA is a model NCD.

Globally, our results show that the proposed therapy progresses (also) via the elicitation of the function of *wound healing*, a transversal phenomenon, crucially impacting on the control of inflammation as we recently discussed within the transversal basic science frame of the Greater Inflammatory Pathway [52]. Such findings are relevant in the context of the ERAS ecosystem, whose evidence-based guidelines/protocols (see https://erassociety.org) are crucial for PPPM, and with particular emphasis on generally neglected clinical matters like prehabilitation, pain chronification prediction, mitochondrial health and suboptimal health, to name the major.

6 Expected PPPM Impacts

Our results, although plagued in the human study by the small sample size, represent nevertheless a fundamental starting point to explore the rationale (fundamental biology, *bench*), reproducibility (clinics, *bed*), and reimboursability (health policy, PPPM) of physical therapies. This tangible expression of the anti-inflammatory potential of the elicitation of wound healing can offer a biomedical rationale to exploit a variety of physical therapies, rapidly expanding the arsenal of approaches available to control overt and pre-clinical chronic inflammation, at the base of all

NCDs [9]. This is in line with the aforementioned ERAS initiative, which aims at promoting evidence-based best-practices for effective personalized approaches. As a consequence, conclusions for experts including all stakeholders in the rich PPPM ecosystem include **two major recommendations:**

The first is to take maximum advantage of existing basic biological (molecular and cellular) knowledge when it comes to physical stimuli transduction. Referring exclusively to previous, or historical, clinical practice may not be the only or best way to justify or take advantage of the therapeutic cascade of molecular events that descends from a savvy elicitation of wound healing [12].

Second, there is a great lack of standardization in the stimuli release, more clinical studies certainly is needed but also more basic science research is needed to guarantee robustness first, and appropriateness of dosage, i.e., effectiveness, then.

As an overall conclusion, it is to be expected that the rigorous and systematic exploration of these approaches open to a whole new area of medicine, which we call *Physicine*, with the potential to be *frugal* [53] **both for the nature of some of the stimuli (mechanical in particular) and for the opening to biomedical *devices* repurposing, along the lines of *drug* repurposing, once dosages of stimulations can be released in well informed manners.**

Acknowledgements MoST International Cooperation Program n. 2013DFA30790 "Nano-Structured Acupuncture Needle Application in Rheumatoid Arthritis ".

References

1. Saha A, Alleyne G (2018) Recognizing noncommunicable diseases as a global health security threat. Bull World Health Organ 96(11):792–793
2. Directorate-General for Health and Food Safety (2022) EU non-communicable diseases (NCDs) initiative. https://health.ec.europa.eu/publications/eu-non-communicable-diseases-ncds-initiative-guidance-document_en. Accessed 15 Sept 2022
3. Tracey KJ (2002) The inflammatory reflex. Nature 420:853–859
4. Martelli D, McKinley MJ, McAllen RM (2014) The cholinergic anti-inflammatory pathway: a critical review. Auton Neurosci 182:65–69
5. Martelli D, Farmer DG, Yao ST (2016) The splanchnic anti-inflammatory pathway: could it be the efferent arm of the inflammatory reflex? Exp Physiol 101:1245–1252
6. Bornigen D, Morgan XC, Franzosa EA, Ren B, Xavier RJ, Garrett WS et al (2013) Functional profiling of the gut microbiome in disease-associated inflammation. Genome Med 5:65
7. Honda K, Littman DR (2012) The microbiome in infectious disease and inflammation. Annu Rev Immunol 30:759–795
8. Yu JC, Khodadadi H, Baban B (2019) Innate immunity and oral microbiome: a personalized, predictive, and preventive approach to the management of oral diseases. EPMA J 10:43–50
9. Avishai E, Yeghiazaryan K, Golubnitschaja O (2017) Impaired wound healing: facts and hypotheses for multi-professional considerations in predictive, preventive and personalised medicine. EPMA J 8:23–33
10. Wang W, Yan Y, Guo Z, Hou H, Garcia M, Tan X et al (2021) All around suboptimal health—a joint position paper of the suboptimal health study consortium and European Association for predictive, preventive and personalised medicine. EPMA J 12(4):403–433

11. Maturo MG, Soligo M, Gibson G, Manni L, Nardini C (2020) The greater inflammatory pathway-high clinical potential by innovative predictive, preventive, and personalized medical approach. EPMA J 11:1–16
12. Nardini C, Candelise L, Turrini M, Addimanda O (2022) Semi-automated socio-anthropologic analysis of the medical discourse on rheumatoid arthritis: potential impact in public health. PloS One 17(12):e0279632
13. Choi HH, Cho Y-S (2016) Fecal microbiota transplantation: current applications, effectiveness, and future perspectives. Clin Endosc 49:257–265
14. Olofsson PS, Tracey KJ (2017) Bioelectronic medicine: technology targeting molecular mechanisms for therapy. J Intern Med 282:3–4
15. Kalluri R, Weinberg RA (2009) The basics of epithelial-mesenchymal transition. J Clin Invest 119:1420–1428
16. Nardini C, Devescovi V, Liu Y, Zhou X, Lu Y, Dent JE (2016) Systemic wound healing associated with local sub-cutaneous mechanical stimulation. Sci Rep 6:39043
17. Corbiere TF, Koh TJ (2020) Local low-intensity vibration improves healing of muscle injury in mice. Physiol Rep 8(2):e14356
18. Weinheimer-Haus EM, Judex S, Ennis WJ, Koh TJ (2014) Low-intensity vibration improves angiogenesis and wound healing in diabetic mice. PloS One 9:e91355
19. Crane JD, Ogborn DI, Cupido C, Melov S, Hubbard A, Bourgeois JM et al (2012) Massage therapy attenuates inflammatory signaling after exercise-induced muscle damage. Sci Transl Med 4:119ra13
20. Nelson NL, Churilla JR (2017) Massage therapy for pain and function in patients with arthritis: a systematic review of randomized controlled trials. Am J Phys Med Rehabil 96:665–672
21. Wang N (2017) Review of cellular mechanotransduction. J Phys D Appl Phys 50:233002
22. Ingber DE (2006) Cellular mechanotransduction: putting all the pieces together again. FASEB J 20:811–827
23. Martino F, Perestrelo AR, Vinarský V, Pagliari S, Forte G (2018) Cellular Mechanotransduction: from tension to function. Front Physiol 9:824
24. Northcott JM, Dean IS, Mouw JK, Weaver VM (2018) Feeling stress: the mechanics of cancer progression and aggression. Front Cell Dev Biol 6:17
25. Cezar CA, Roche ET, Vandenburgh HH, Duda GN, Walsh CJ, Mooney DJ (2016) Biologic-free mechanically induced muscle regeneration. Proc Natl Acad Sci U S A 113:1534–1539
26. Galvani L (1797) Memorie sulla elettricità animale. Stampe del Sassi. https://gutenberg.beic.it/webclient/MetadataManager?pid=12147981&descriptive_only=true. Accessed 15 Sept 2022
27. Wang D-W, Yin Y-M, Yao Y-M (2016) Vagal modulation of the inflammatory response in sepsis. Int Rev Immunol 35:415–433
28. Koopman FA, Chavan SS, Miljko S, Grazio S, Sokolovic S, Schuurman PR et al (2016) Vagus nerve stimulation inhibits cytokine production and attenuates disease severity in rheumatoid arthritis. Proc Natl Acad Sci U S A 113:8284–8289
29. Yu C, Hu Z-Q, Peng R-Y (2014) Effects and mechanisms of a microcurrent dressing on skin wound healing: a review. Mil Med Res 1:24
30. Foulds IS, Barker AT (1983) Human skin battery potentials and their possible role in wound healing. Br J Dermatol 109:515–522
31. Cheah YJ, Buyong MR, Mohd Yunus MH (2021) Wound healing with electrical stimulation technologies: a review. Polymers (Basel) 13:3790
32. Lin B-J, Tsao S-H, Chen A, Hu S-K, Chao L, Chao P-HG (2017) Lipid rafts sense and direct electric field-induced migration. Proc Natl Acad Sci U S A 114:8568–8573
33. Ahrabi B, Bahrami M, Moghadasali R, Zamanian-Azodi M, Khoramgah MS, Tabatabaei Mirakabad FS et al (2020) The effect of low-power laser therapy on the TGF/β signaling pathway in chronic kidney disease: a review. J Lasers Med Sci 11:220–225
34. Bjordal JM, Couppé C, Chow RT, Tunér J, Ljunggren EA (2003) A systematic review of low level laser therapy with location-specific doses for pain from chronic joint disorders. Aust J Physiotherapy 49:107–116

35. Baxter GD, Liu L, Petrich S, Gisselman AS, Chapple C, Anders JJ et al (2017) Low level laser therapy (Photobiomodulation therapy) for breast cancer-related lymphedema: a systematic review. BMC Cancer 17:833
36. Zarei M, Wikramanayake TC, Falto-Aizpurua L, Schachner LA, Jimenez JJ (2016) Low level laser therapy and hair regrowth: an evidence-based review. Lasers Med Sci 31:363–371
37. Hamblin MR (2017) Mechanisms and applications of the anti-inflammatory effects of photobiomodulation. AIMS Biophys 4:337–361
38. Becker A, Klapczynski A, Kuch N, Arpino F, Simon-Keller K, De La Torre C et al (2016) Gene expression profiling reveals aryl hydrocarbon receptor as a possible target for photobiomodulation when using blue light. Sci Rep 6:33847
39. Zablotskii V, Polyakova T, Lunov O, Dejneka A (2016) How a high-gradient magnetic field could affect cell life. Sci Rep 6:37407
40. Miyakoshi J (2005) Effects of static magnetic fields at the cellular level. Prog Biophys Mol Biol 87:213–223
41. Otón T, Carmona L (2019) The epidemiology of established rheumatoid arthritis. Best Pract Res Clin Rheumatol 33:101477
42. Fraenkel L, Bathon JM, England BR, St Clair EW, Arayssi T, Carandang K et al (2021) 2021 American College of Rheumatology Guideline for the treatment of rheumatoid arthritis. Arthritis Care Res (Hoboken) 73:924–939
43. Smolen JS, Landewé R, Bijlsma J, Burmester G, Chatzidionysiou K, Dougados M et al (2017) EULAR recommendations for the management of rheumatoid arthritis with synthetic and biological disease-modifying antirheumatic drugs: 2016 update. Ann Rheum Dis 76:960–977
44. Golubnitschaja O, Baban B, Boniolo G, Wang W, Bubnov R, Kapalla M et al (2016) Medicine in the early twenty-first century: paradigm and anticipation - EPMA position paper 2016. EPMA J 7:23
45. Zhou X, Devescovi V, Liu Y, Dent JE, Nardini C (2019) Host-microbiome synergistic control on sphingolipid metabolism by mechanotransduction in model arthritis. Biomolecules 9:144
46. Golubnitschaja O, Topolcan O, Kucera R, Costigliola V (2020) 10th anniversary of the European Association for Predictive, preventive and personalised (3P) medicine—EPMA world congress supplement 2020. EPMA J 11:1–133
47. Trentham D, Townes A, Kang A (1977) Autoimmunity to type II collagen: an experimental model of arthritis. J Exp Med 146:857–868
48. Langevin HM, Bouffard NA, Badger GJ, Churchill DL, Howe AK (2006) Subcutaneous tissue fibroblast cytoskeletal remodeling induced by acupuncture: evidence for a mechanotransduction-based mechanism. J Cell Physiol 207:767–774
49. Aletaha D, Neogi T, Silman AJ, Funovits J, Felson DT, Bingham CO 3rd et al (2010) 2010 rheumatoid arthritis classification criteria: an American College of Rheumatology/European League against rheumatism collaborative initiative. Ann Rheum Dis 69:1580–1588
50. Ritchie ME, Phipson B, Wu D, Hu Y, Law CW, Shi W et al (2015) Limma powers differential expression analyses for RNA-sequencing and microarray studies. Nucleic Acids Res 43:e47
51. Jiao X, Sherman BT, Huang DW, Stephens R, Baseler MW, Lane HC et al (2012) DAVID-WS: a stateful web service to facilitate gene/protein list analysis. Bioinformatics 28:1805–1806
52. Maturo MG, Soligo M, Gibson G, Manni L, Nardini C (2020) The greater inflammatory pathway—high clinical potential by innovative predictive, preventive, and personalized medical approach. EPMA J 11(1):1–16
53. Tran V-T, Ravaud P (2016) Frugal innovation in medicine for low resource settings. BMC Med 14:102

Advantages of Thermovision Imaging for PPPM Approach to Diabetic Foot

Agnieszka Dębiec-Bąk, Anna Skrzek, Agnieszka Ptak, Krzysztof Majerski, Ivana Uiberlayová, Małgorzata Stefańska, and Halina Podbielska

Abbreviations

3P Medicine, PPPM	Predictive, Preventive, Personalized Medicine
AI	Artificial Intelligence
DF	Diabetic foot
DFS	Diabetic foot syndrome
DFU	Diabetic foot ulcer
DM	Diabetes mellitus
IR camera	Infrared thermal camera
MRI	Magnetic Resonance Imaging

A. Dębiec-Bąk · A. Skrzek · M. Stefańska
Department of Physiotherapy in Dysfunctions of Organs of Movement, Faculty of Physiotherapy, Wrocław University of Health and Sport Sciences, Wrocław, Poland
e-mail: agnieszka.debiec-bak@awf.wroc.pl; anna.skrzek@awf.wroc.pl; malgorzata.stefanska@awf.wroc.pl

A. Ptak
Department of Physiotherapy in Neurology and Paediatrics, Faculty of Physiotherapy, Wrocław University of Health and Sport Sciences, Wrocław, Poland
e-mail: agnieszka.ptak@awf.wroc.pl

K. Majerski · I. Uiberlayová
Státní Léčebné Lázně Janské Lázně, státní podnik, Janské Lázně, Czech Republic
e-mail: majerskik@janskelazne.com; ivana.uiberlayova@janskelazne.com

H. Podbielska (✉)
Department of Biomedical Engineering, Wrocław University of Science and Technology, Wrocław, Poland
e-mail: halina.podbielska@pwr.edu.pl; info@halinapodbielska.pl

H. Podbielska, M. Kapalla (eds.), *Predictive, Preventive, and Personalised Medicine: From Bench to Bedside*, Advances in Predictive, Preventive and Personalised Medicine 17, https://doi.org/10.1007/978-3-031-34884-6_13

1 Diabetes Mellitus Complications in Focus of 3P Medicine

1.1 Diabetes Mellitus Complications

According to the National Diabetes Statistics Report only in the USA in 2022 more than 130 million adults were suffering from diabetes or prediabetes [1]. European chapter of the International Diabetes Federation claims that in 2021 there were 61 million adults in Europe diagnosed with diabetes, whereas the type 1 diabetes was stated in 295,000 children and adolescents [2]. DM is not more the disease of the societies living prevalently in high-income countries, but also affects poorer regions, whereas the low- and middle-income countries show the highest growth rate [3]. Moreover, there is also high incidence rate of diabetes comorbidities in low- and middle-income countries, including heart disease, kidney failure, vision impairment, and DFU [4]. DM is a global problem, affecting more and more people worldwide and resulting in several complications. DM should be treated holistically and PPPM approach seems to be the most optimal way [5].

Poorly controlled hyperglycemia affects blood vessels and peripheral nerves (Fig. 1). Recently, molecular mechanisms are studied in order to explain endothelial dysfunctions and diabetic vascular complications [6]. Genetic mechanisms are also in research focus aimed in prediction the development of vascular and neural complications [7]. Some reports also show the dependency from gender [8, 9]. Various biomarkers are examined on order to find the proper tool for predicting DM onset [10–13]. Another important aspect to be considered, is the quality of life of diabetes suffering patients, which depends often from glycaemia control and can influence also the proper treatment [14–16].

Diabetic derived neuropathies and vasculopathies result in dysfunctions of many organs of human body (Fig. 2). There is an increased risk of nephropathy, coronary heart disease and heart failure, stroke, retinopathy, glaucoma, periodontal inflammation and foot lesions and ulceration.

DM not only causes pathologic organ changes leading to dysfunctionality, but in long term also increases the risk of other pathologies such as cancer, liver diseases, cognitive and affective disorders and increases the general incidence of inflammation [17]. All these factors are a challenge for the health care system and proper care of a diabetic patient. Only an integrated approach, based on 3P Medicine, can provide a holistic method, ensuring proper therapy and preventing complications by detecting them as early as possible.

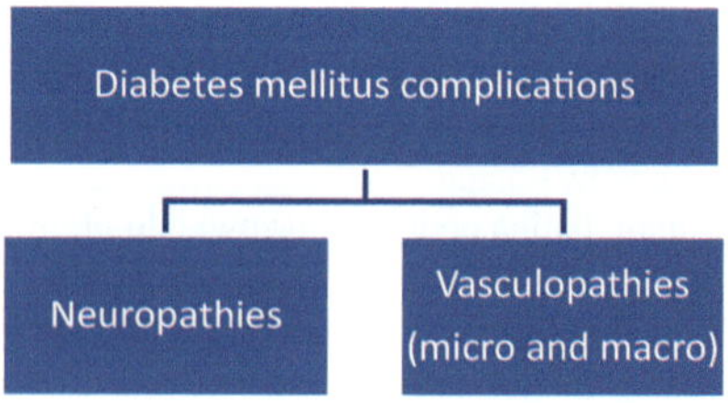

Fig. 1 Neuropathies and vasculopathies as fundamental pathologies causing DM complications

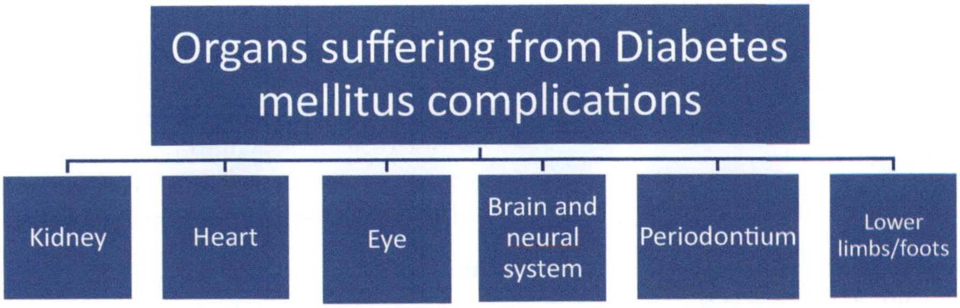

Fig. 2 Organs mostly suffering from DM complications. One has to notice that ulceration in the distal part of lower extremities and probability of amputation in diabetic patients are much higher than in non-diabetic persons

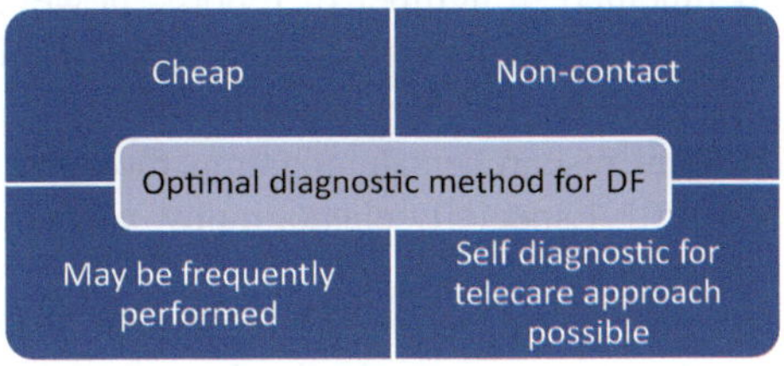

Fig. 3 Characteristics of optimal diagnostic method for prediction of diabetic foot ulcer

1.2 Diabetic Foot Syndrome

Diabetic foot ulcer (DFU) is a serious complication, resulted from many factors, as, e.g., not well controlled glycaemia, not promptly diagnosed neuropathy and vasculopathy, not proper foot care, etc. [18]. Usually, the mixture of all the abovementioned factors causes the development of ulceration on the foot. Nerves function impairment diminishes proper sensation what promotes injuries. From the other hand, vascular impairment in lower extremities causes reduced blood flow followed by hindered healing. Prediction of possible DFU leading risk factors is extremely important in view of complications prevention and introducing personalized treatment. Optimally, such diagnosis should be safe, reliable, non-contact, suitable for telecare and frequent use. This is schematically depicted by Fig. 3.

2 Imaging Technologies in Diagnosis of Diabetic Foot Syndrome

Diabetic foot syndrome may include soft-tissue infection and neuropathic osteoarthropathy, and may result even in osteomyelitis. Various imaging based diagnostic modalities are proposed for examination of DFS. Most of the reports relate to the advanced complications, including ulcerations and bones damage. There exists an extended report summarizing the criteria for use of separate imaging techniques

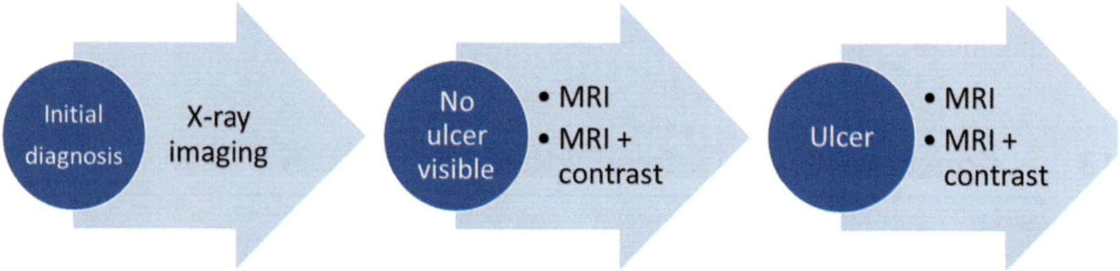

Fig. 4 Recommendations for using some of the imaging technologies in DFS diagnosis for osteomyelitis, according to [19]

[19]. The experts panel recommends to use some techniques, depending on the advancement of lesion. Here, we show this graphically on Fig. 4.

The usefulness of these techniques in advanced stages of DF complications were documented in number of reports, however, they are not suitable in prediction of DFS onset. That is why other imaging modalities should be considered for early prediction of possible complications.

Some researchers demonstrate the role of ultrasound imaging of diabetic patients' feet [20]. Especially elastography, allowing to assess mechanical tissue properties may be valuable diagnostic tool [21–23]. Mechanical properties of foot tissue may be a prognostic factor in development of DFU [24–26]. Early diagnosis of diabetic peripheral neuropathy is also important in prediction of further complications [27]. Elastography results can be a good biomarker of diabetes related peripheral neuropathy, however due to the nature of this method, non-contact measurement is not possible.

Non-contact monitoring seems to be a better option, especially in case of already existing maceration or ulceration. According to Fig. 3 imaging diagnostic should be easily adopted for telecare and telemonitoring. Some modalities were already tested as hyperspectral imaging and digital photography [28–32].

3 Thermography for Diabetic Foot Diagnosis

In recent years, thermographic recording monitoring of the diabetic foot syndrome has been examined. This method is non-invasive and non-contact, may be used multiple times, even in case of ulceration. It seems that it suits remarkably to the criteria depicted by Fig. 3. Various systems may be used for monitoring of foot temperature, including infrared thermometry, liquid crystal thermography, various temperature sensors, and thermovision [33].

The current thermovision devices became cheaper and more accurate, offering easy recording of infrared radiation emitted from leaving body. The superficial temperature distribution reflects, among others, the state of the microcirculation in the examined area. It enables to visualize and monitor, e.g., inflammation or ischemia, what is important in case of suspected DFS. One has to remember that before developing full symptoms of DFU, the first signs of damage are very rarely noticed by the patient. Occasional pain or numbness in lower extremities, is often ignored.

Some researchers noticed elevated skin temperature in DF [34], what is questioned in some other reports [35]. Yavuz et al. [34] observed higher plantar temperature in patients with the history of DFU or diabetic neuropathy. However, Stegge et al. [35] stated that the foot temperature increase before an ulcer appears, is not observed. It seems to be logic, as impairment of microcirculation and nerves functioning cause rather temperature decrease, not the opposite. From the other hand, increased local skin temperature on a callus site is regarded as precursor of diabetic foot ulcers [36]. This increase may be caused by starting inflammation process and may be deepened be by unproper footwear. Such predictor will be useful to instruct the patient how to avoid possible complications. One of the good predicting factors of foot lesion is asymmetry in superficial temperature distribution. Thermal images asymmetry may be exploited for the assessment of overall foot health in diabetic patients [37]. Anyway, more further research is required to establish proper biomarker based on temperature distribution as predictor of DHU onset.

Recently, many AI based methods are exploited for image analysis, including thermographic recordings. Machine learning methods were used for features extraction from thermal images of patients with DFU [38]. Convolutional neural networks for discrimination between non-DM and DM severity grades based plantar thermal images, were successfully exploited [39]. Such systems may be also used for automatic diagnosis of possible bacterial infection in already developed DFU [40]. Machine learning approach for classification of DFU to predict complications is prosed as well [41]. Some systems are working, using segmentation methods and prior information set [42]. Thermal imaging has the advantage that with the developing of technology and smartphone application, self-diagnostic will be possible [43].

Anyway, it does not exist a definitive biomarker based on temperature evaluation in foot region that could be exploited in prediction of DFU. In the group from the Wrocław University of Health and Sport Sciences some other approach was recently examined, namely the temperature difference between plantar and dorsal foot site [44]. This study was performed on a group of 52 patients from Provincial Specialist Healthcare Center in Wrocław, suffered from diabetes type 2 diabetes. As a control, the non-diabetes 33 persons with no feet lesions that on rehabilitation stay in SPA Center in Janské Lázně, Czech Republic. Corresponding permission from the Senate Committee on Ethics of Scientific Research at the Wrocław University of Health and Sport Sciences was obtained to perform thermographic recording in these two groups.

The thermal images were recorded from plantar and dorsal site of both feet were recorded by means of thermal imaging camera (FLIR T335) and then analyzed. Exemplary thermal images are depicted by Fig. 5. Visual inspection allows to state that there are visible differences in temperature distribution between DM patient and non-DM subject. In DM elevated temperature is observed around the toes and heels regions.

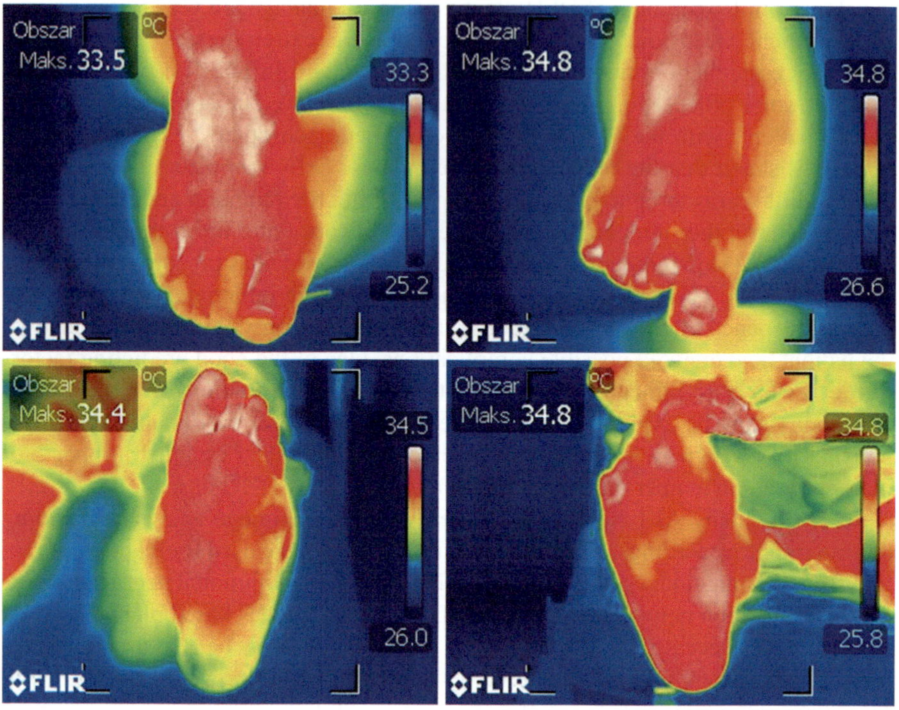

Fig. 5 Exemplary thermal images of DM patient (left) and non-diabetic persons (right). (Non-published pictures recorded by Dębiec-Bąk)

This preliminary study revealed that generally the dorsal average temperature is higher than the plantar one and the temperature differences dorsal vs. plantar were significantly greater in DM patients than in non-DM subjects. Controlling these differences may be a good predictor of developing DFU thus allowing to perform corresponding preventive and personalized curative actions.

4 Conclusion and Recommendations

As the number of DM suffering patients will be still growing, in spite of new pharmacological approaches, the health care systems may expect the growing number of DM associated complications. Regardless of the wealth of a country, health systems tend to be overburdened, understaffed, and often unable to respond quickly. Patients often receive care and treatment only when complications are advanced. This increases healthcare costs, overall social costs and can have serious consequences in the case of diabetes. Modern technologies offer the opportunity to change this paradigm and move from delayed reactive medical services to evidence-based 3P Medicine, thus fulfilling EPMA mission [45].

Table 1 PPPM recommendation to control DFU complications

PPPM steps	PPPM measures
General population	Education, screening towards DM, promotion of preventive measures
Prevention of complications in DM or prediabetes population	Education, screening In case of diagnosed DM: Thermal imaging for personal use smartphone based, telemonitoring, telecare
Prediction of DFU risk	Outpatient examination, advanced thermal imaging, AI methods for evaluation, prevention measures
Prevention of developing DFU	Thermal telemonitoring, outpatients care to prevent further complications
DFU complications prevention and personalized treatment	Thermal telemonitoring, personalized home care via dedicated specialized medical personnel

In case of developed DFU the medical care is expensive and in spite of treatment may end with an amputation, again generating huge medical and social costs [46, 47].

We propose to use thermal imaging with personal smartphone-based IR camera, followed by telemonitoring and telecare as a prevention of complications in DM or prediabetes population. If the thermal image of the feet will be remotely diagnosed as a suspicious lesion, more advanced diagnosis in medical center should be applied to predict the risk of DFU development. Further telemonitoring is advised. In case of DFU complications the measures should be undertaken towards prevention of further deterioration and personalized treatment should be introduced. These recommendations are depicted in Table 1.

References

1. Centers for Disease Control and Prevention. National Diabetes Statistics Report. https://www.cdc.gov/diabetes/data/statistics-report/index.html. Accessed 6 Feb 2023
2. IDF Diabetes Atlas 2021. https://diabetesatlas.org/atlas/tenth-edition/. Accessed 6 Feb 2023
3. Liu J, Bai R, Chai Z, Cooper ME, Zimmet PZ, Zhang L (2022) Low- and middle-income countries demonstrate rapid growth of type 2 diabetes: an analysis based on Global Burden of Disease 1990–2019 data. Diabetologia 65:1339–1352. https://doi.org/10.1007/s00125-022-05713-6
4. Lam AA, Lepe A, Wild SH, Jackson C (2021) Diabetes comorbidities in low- and middle-income countries: an umbrella review. J Glob Health 11:04040. https://doi.org/10.7189/jogh.11.04040
5. Mozaffari MS (2014) New strategies to advance pre/diabetes care: integrative approach by PPPM. EPMA J 5(Suppl 1):A14. https://doi.org/10.1186/1878-5085-5-S1-A14
6. Bhamidipati T, Kumar M, Verma SS, Mohanty SK, Kacar S, Reese D, Martinez MM, Kamocka MM, Dunn KW, Sen CK, Singh K (2022) Epigenetic basis of diabetic vasculopathy. Front Endocrinol 13:989844. https://doi.org/10.3389/fendo.2022.989844
7. Cole JB, Florez JC (2020) Genetics of diabetes mellitus and diabetes complications. Nat Rev Nephrol 16(7):377–390. https://doi.org/10.1038/s41581-020-0278-5
8. Golubnitschaja O (2014) Gender specific complications in female diabetic patients: an integrative view. EPMA J 5(Suppl 1):A78. https://doi.org/10.1186/1878-5085-5-S1-A78

9. Ciarambino T, Crispino P, Leto G, Mastrolorenzo E, Para O, Giordano M (2022) Influence of gender in diabetes mellitus and its complication. Int J Mol Sci 23(16):8850. Published 2022 Aug 9. https://doi.org/10.3390/ijms23168850
10. Meng X, Wang F, Gao X et al (2022) Association of IgG N-glycomics with prevalent and incident type 2 diabetes mellitus from the paradigm of predictive, preventive, and personalized medicine standpoint. EPMA J 14:1. https://doi.org/10.1007/s13167-022-00311-3
11. Dorcely B, Katz K, Jagannathan R, Chiang SS, Oluwadare B, Goldberg IJ, Bergman M (2017) Novel biomarkers for prediabetes, diabetes, and associated complications. Diabetes Metab Syndr Obes 10:345–361. https://doi.org/10.2147/DMSO.S100074
12. Ma Y, Xiong J, Zhang X, Qiu T, Pang H, Li X, Zhu J, Wang J, Pan C, Yang X, Chu X, Yang B, Wang C, Zhang J (2021) Potential biomarker in serum for predicting susceptibility to type 2 diabetes mellitus: free fatty acid 22:6. J Diabetes Investig 12(6):950–962. Epub 2020 Dec 4. https://doi.org/10.1111/jdi.13443
13. Dias S, Pheiffer C, Abrahams Y, Rheeder P, Adam S (2018) Molecular biomarkers for gestational diabetes mellitus. Int J Mol Sci 19(10):2926. https://doi.org/10.3390/ijms19102926
14. Rodríguez-Almagro J, García-Manzanares Á, Lucendo AJ, Hernández-Martínez A (2018) Health-related quality of life in diabetes mellitus and its social, demographic and clinical determinants: a nationwide cross-sectional survey. J Clin Nurs 27(21–22):4212–4223. Epub 2018 Jul 27. https://doi.org/10.1111/jocn.14624
15. Podbielska H, Madziarska K, Demczuk-Włodarczyk E (2014) Quality of life of people suffering from the diabetes type 2—examination of the influence of various factors to prevent complications. EPMA J 5(Suppl 1):A72. https://doi.org/10.1186/1878-5085-5-S1-A72
16. Castellano-Guerrero AM, Guerrero R, Ruiz-Aranda D et al (2020) Gender differences in quality of life in adults with long-standing type 1 diabetes mellitus. Diabetol Metab Syndr 12:64. https://doi.org/10.1186/s13098-020-00571-x
17. Tomic D, Shaw JE, Magliano DJ (2022) The burden and risks of emerging complications of diabetes mellitus. Nat Rev Endocrinol 18:525–539. https://doi.org/10.1038/s41574-022-00690-7
18. Oliver TI, Mutluoglu M (2022) Diabetic foot ulcer. In: StatPearls [internet]. StatPearls Publishing, Treasure Island, FL
19. Expert Panel on Musculoskeletal Imaging, Walker EA, Beaman FD, Wessell DE, Cassidy RC, Czuczman GJ, Demertzis JL, Lenchik L, Motamedi K, Pierce JL, Sharma A, Ying-Kou Yung E, Kransdorf MJ (2019) ACR appropriateness criteria® suspected osteomyelitis of the foot in patients with diabetes mellitus. J Am Coll Radiol 16(11S):S440–S450. https://doi.org/10.1016/j.jacr.2019.05.027
20. Pieruzzi L, Napoli V, Goretti C, Adami D, Iacopi E, Cicorelli A, Piaggesi A (2020) Ultrasound in the modern management of the diabetic foot syndrome: a multipurpose versatile toolkit. Int J Low Extrem Wounds 19(4):315–333. Epub 2020 Aug 21. https://doi.org/10.1177/1534734620948351
21. Lung CW, Wu FL, Liao F, Pu F, Fan Y, Jan YK (2020) Emerging technologies for the prevention and management of diabetic foot ulcers. J Tissue Viability 29(2):61–68. Epub 2020 Mar 17. https://doi.org/10.1016/j.jtv.2020.03.003
22. Zhang F, Wang J, Ma Y, Wang Y, Wang W, Wang Y (2022) Evaluation of Achilles tendon in patients with diabetic foot ulcer by high-frequency ultrasound combined with real-time shear-wave elastography. J Healthc Eng 28(2022):4866240. https://doi.org/10.1155/2022/4866240
23. Chen SP, Ye TT, Hong J, Zhu H (2023) Evaluation of sciatic nerve stiffness using shear wave Elastography in patients with unilateral diabetic foot ulcers. Diagnostics (Basel) 13(3):547. https://doi.org/10.3390/diagnostics13030547
24. Naemi R, Chatzistergos P, Suresh S, Sundar L, Chockalingam N, Ramachandran A (2017) Can plantar soft tissue mechanics enhance prognosis of diabetic foot ulcer? Diabetes Res Clin Pract 126:182–191. Epub 2017 Feb 10. https://doi.org/10.1016/j.diabres.2017.02.002
25. Naemi R, Romero Gutierrez SE, Allan D, Flores G, Ormaechea J, Gutierrez E, Casado-Pena J, Anyosa-Zavaleta S, Juarez M, Casado F, Castaneda AB (2022) Diabetes status is associated with plantar soft tissue stiffness measured using ultrasound reverberant shear wave

Elastography approach. J Diabetes Sci Technol 16(2):478–490. Epub 2020 Oct 23. https://doi.org/10.1177/1932296820965259
26. Patwari M, Chatzistergos P, Sundar L, Chockalingam N, Ramachandran A, Naemi R (2022) A quantitative comparison of plantar soft tissue strainability distribution and homogeneity between ulcerated and non-ulcerated patients using ultrasound strain elastography. Proc Inst Mech Eng H 236(5):722–729. Epub 2022 Feb 24. https://doi.org/10.1177/09544119221074786
27. Dong B, Lyu G, Yang X, Wang H, Chen Y (2022) Shear wave elastography as a quantitative biomarker of diabetic peripheral neuropathy: a systematic review and meta-analysis. Front Public Health 22(10):915883. https://doi.org/10.3389/fpubh.2022.915883
28. Hazenberg CEVB, Aan de Stegge WB, Van Baal SG, Moll FL, Bus SA (2020) Telehealth and telemedicine applications for the diabetic foot: a systematic review. Diabetes Metab Res Rev 36(3):e3247. Epub 2019 Dec 20. https://doi.org/10.1002/dmrr.3247
29. Hazenberg CE, van Baal JG, Manning E, Bril A, Bus SA (2010) The validity and reliability of diagnosing foot ulcers and pre-ulcerative lesions in diabetes using advanced digital photography. Diabetes Technol Ther 12:1011–1017. https://doi.org/10.1089/dia.2010.0088
30. Cabal Mirabal CA, Berlanga Acosta J, Fernández Montequín J, Oramas Díaz L, González Dalmau E, Herrera Martínez L, Sauri JE, Baldomero Hernández J, Savigne Gutiérrez W, Valdés JL, Tabio Reyes AL, Pérez Pérez SC, Valdés Pérez C, Armstrong AA, Armstrong DG (2019) Quantitative studies of diabetic foot ulcer evolution under treatment by digital stereotactic photography. J Diabetes Sci Technol 13(5):821–826. Epub 2019 Jun 13. https://doi.org/10.1177/1932296819853843
31. Rajbhandari SM, Harris ND, Sutton M, Lockett C, Eaton S, Gadour M, Tesfaye S, Ward JD (1999) Digital imaging: an accurate and easy method of measuring foot ulcers. Diabet Med 16(4):339–342. https://doi.org/10.1046/j.1464-5491.1999.00053.x
32. Kounas K, Dinh T, Riemer K, Rosenblum BI, Veves A, Giurini JM (2023) Use of hyperspectral imaging to predict healing of diabetic foot ulceration. Wound Repair Regen 31:199. Epub ahead of print. https://doi.org/10.1111/wrr.13071
33. Grech J, Mizzi S, Falzon O (2022) A technical review of foot temperature measurement systems. J Am Podiatr Med Assoc 112(2):21–065. https://doi.org/10.7547/21-065
34. Yavuz M, Ersen A, Hartos J, Lavery LA, Wukich DK, Hirschman GB, Armstrong DG, Quiben MU, Adams LS (2019) Temperature as a causative factor in diabetic foot ulcers: a call to revisit ulceration pathomechanics. J Am Podiatr Med Assoc 109(5):345–350. Epub 2018 Nov 14. https://doi.org/10.7547/17-131
35. Stegge WBA, Van Netten JJ, Bus SA (2023) Does the skin heat up before it breaks down in diabetic foot ulceration? Diabetes Metab Res Rev 8:e3621. Epub ahead of print. https://doi.org/10.1002/dmrr.3621
36. Qin Q, Oe M, Ohashi Y, Shimojima Y, Imafuku M, Dai M, Nakagami G, Yamauchi T, Yeo S, Sanada H (2022) Factors associated with the local increase of skin temperature, 'Hotspot,' of callus in diabetic foot: a cross-sectional study. J Diabetes Sci Technol 16(5):1174–1182. Epub 2021 May 20. https://doi.org/10.1177/19322968211011181
37. Evangeline NC, Srinivasan S, Suresh E (2022) Development of AI classification model for angiosome-wise interpretive substantiation of plantar feet thermal asymmetry in type 2 diabetic subjects using infrared thermograms. J Therm Biol 110:103370. Epub 2022 Oct 9. https://doi.org/10.1016/j.jtherbio.2022.103370
38. Hernandez-Guedes A, Arteaga-Marrero N, Villa E, Callico GM, Ruiz-Alzola J (2023) Feature ranking by variational dropout for classification using thermograms from diabetic foot ulcers. Sensors (Basel) 23(2):757. https://doi.org/10.3390/s23020757
39. Muralidhara S, Lucieri A, Dengel A, Ahmed S (2022) Holistic multi-class classification & grading of diabetic foot ulcerations from plantar thermal images using deep learning. Health Inf Sci Syst 10(1):21. https://doi.org/10.1007/s13755-022-00194-8
40. Yogapriya J, Chandran V, Sumithra MG, Elakkiya B, Shamila Ebenezer A, Suresh Gnana Dhas C (2022) Automated detection of infection in diabetic foot ulcer images using convolutional neural network. J Healthc Eng 2022:2349849. https://doi.org/10.1155/2022/2349849

41. Khandakar A, Chowdhury MEH, Reaz MBI, Ali SHM, Kiranyaz S, Rahman T, Chowdhury MH, Ayari MA, Alfkey R, Bakar AAA, Malik RA, Hasan A (2022) A novel machine learning approach for severity classification of diabetic foot complications using Thermogram images. Sensors (Basel) 22(11):4249. https://doi.org/10.3390/s22114249
42. Bougrine A, Harba R, Canals R, Ledee R, Jabloun M, Villeneuve A (2022) Segmentation of plantar foot thermal images using prior information. Sensors (Basel) 22(10):3835. https://doi.org/10.3390/s22103835
43. Qin Q, Nakagami G, Ohashi Y, Dai M, Sanada H, Oe M (2022) Development of a self-monitoring tool for diabetic foot prevention using smartphone-based thermography: plantar thermal pattern changes and usability in the home environment. Drug Discov Ther 16(4):169–176. Epub 2022 Aug 25. https://doi.org/10.5582/ddt.2022.01050
44. Dębiec-Bąk A, Skrzek A, Ptak A, Majerski K, Uiberlayová I, Stefańska M (2023) Evaluation of the surface temperature distribution of the feet in patients with type 2 diabetes using the thermovision method. Physiother Q 31:92
45. EPMA. https://www.epmanet.eu/mission/epma-mission, Accessed 28 Feb 2023
46. Kerr M, Barron E, Chadwick P, Evans T, Kong WM, Rayman G, Sutton-Smith M, Todd G, Young B, Jeffcoate WJ (2019) The cost of diabetic foot ulcers and amputations to the National Health Service in England. Diabet Med 36(8):995–1002. Epub 2019 Jun 5. https://doi.org/10.1111/dme.13973
47. Raghav A, Khan ZA, Labala RK, Ahmad J, Noor S, Mishra BK (2018) Financial burden of diabetic foot ulcers to world: a progressive topic to discuss always. Ther Adv Endocrinol Metab 9(1):29–31. Epub 2017 Dec 12. PMID: 29344337. https://doi.org/10.1177/2042018817744513

Predictive, Preventive, and Personalized Approach in Sleep Medicine

Kneginja Richter, Nikola Gjorgov, and Stojan Bajraktarov

Abbreviations

ADHD	Attention deficit hyperactivity disorder
ADS	Attention deficit syndrome
CBT-I	Cognitive behavioural therapy for insomnia
CPAP	Continuous positive air pressure
CVD	Cardiovascular disease
CVH	Cardiovascular health
dCBT-I	Digital cognitive behavioural therapy for insomnia
DCs	Antigen-presenting dendritic cells
IARC	International Agency for Research on Cancer
ICU	Intensive Care Unit
LSAT	Low oxyhaemoglobin desaturation
OSAS	Obstructive Sleep Apnoea

K. Richter (✉)
CuraMed Tagesklinik Nürnberg GmbH, Nuremberg, Germany

University Clinic for Psychiatry and Psychotherapy, Paracelsus Medical University Nuremberg, Nuremberg, Germany

Technical University for Applied Sciences, Nuremberg, Germany

Faculty for Medical Sciences, University Goce Delcev Stip, Skopje, North Macedonia
e-mail: kneginja.Richter@gmx.de

N. Gjorgov
Head, Heart Rhythm Management, Zan Mitrev Clinic, Skopje, North Macedonia
e-mail: nikola.gjorgov@zmc.mk

S. Bajraktarov
University Clinic for Psychiatry, University Cyril and Methodius (UKIM) Skopje, Skopje, North Macedonia

H. Podbielska, M. Kapalla (eds.), *Predictive, Preventive, and Personalised Medicine: From Bench to Bedside*, Advances in Predictive, Preventive and Personalised Medicine 17, https://doi.org/10.1007/978-3-031-34884-6_14

PCR	Polymerase chain reaction
PER	Period
PTBS	Post-traumatic stress disorder
QIDS	Quick Inventory of Depressive Symptomatology QIDS
SA	Suicide attempts
SI	Suicidal ideation
TIM	Timeless

1 Introduction to Sleep and Health

Sleep quality and quantity plays very important role for the maintaining of the physical and mental health. There is not any organ, hormone, vessel or neurotransmitter in the human body out of the influence of the sleep process. The most prominent part of the human brain that is essential for the regulation of the sleep and also sleep-wake activity is the suprachiasmatic nucleus located in the middle of hypothalamus. This nucleus is the inner pacemaker setting the rhythm of the rest-activity cycles of all cells of the body, including the regeneration, inactivity, and multiplication of the cells.

There is intrinsic rhythm not only of the body cells, but also of the proteins synthesis done by the cells. The Nobel Prize winner Jeffrey C. Hall, Michael Rosbash and Michael W. Young who won the Nobel Prize for chronobiology in Year 2017 for very important discovery, has investigated this intrinsic rhythm on the cellular level.

The story about the rest-activity cycle is much older: Jean Jaques d'Ortous de Mairan was French astronomer –he discovered that mimosa leaflets opened at day and closed at night. In addition, even when Mimosas were kept in artificial light, they were able to express the identical rest-activity rhythm. So-what was the answer? It was found in the protein PER as a product of the Gen Period which accumulate and breaks down in oscillations within the period of 24 h. PER reaches the maximal concentration at midnight. TIM (Timeless) is second identified gene that express a synchronized switch-on and switch-off activity with PER. In the following years, new genes were explored: clock and cycle. PER and TIM support the production of CLOCK and CYCLE, while CLOCK and CYCLE inhibit the production of PER and TIM.

This is very important explanation of the science of chronobiology describing the genetic and molecular origin of the circadian rhythm of the human body cells, organs, metabolism immune answer, and cognition. However, the most prominent role in the maintaining of the physical and mental health plays the sleep-wake rhythm [1–4].

1.1 Sleep and Suboptimal Health Conditions

Many non-communicable diseases as cardiovascular diseases, the type 2 diabetes mellitus, breast, lung, liver and prostate malignancies, neurological, sleep, mood, and eye disorders, are rapidly increasing in the last 20 years. Most of them become chronic character progressing from suboptimal health conditions to irreversible severe illnesses with many comorbidities and clinical complications. The period between the occurring of sleep disorders as a part of Suboptimal Health Condition and the clinical onset of the Illness should be used for prediction, prevention, and personalized approach with the aim to reduce the risk factors and the chronification, reduced work ability, and increasing costs for treatment. Suboptimal health condition is characterized by declines in vitality, reduced physiological function including sleep, but does not meet the defined criteria of diseases [5].

People with beginning sleep disturbances as a sign of suboptimal health condition suffer from the perception of health complaints, general weakness, and low energy and have predispositions to physical or mental diseases, especially non-communicable diseases. This complains can progress over many years from a reversible suboptimal health condition to irreversible pathology with corresponding complications.

1.2 Sleep and Mental Health

Prediction, prevention, and personalized approach to insomnia is important for the prevention of mood disorders because of the role of sleep disturbance in the development of depression. Data from large longitudinal studies suggest that insomnia and evening circadian preference are risk factors for depression. Patients with depression and comorbid sleep disturbances show poorer outcomes compared with patients without sleep disorder. It means that sleep disturbances are modifiable risk factors as well in the development as also in the maintenance of depression. There is some evidence suggesting that the treatment of the sleep disturbance can improve overall outcomes of depression and may prevent the future depressive episodes [6].

Newer research papers have reported insomnia symptoms as a risk factor for suicidal ideation (SI), suicide attempts (SA), and suicide death, [3] indicating that the treatment of insomnia symptoms may help to reduce the risk of suicide. The Study of Kambach et al. analyses the results of 658 Participants with insomnia in a RCT Study including insomnia treatment with digital CBT-I (dCBT-I) versus a sleep education control group. The dCBT-I was fully automated and self-paced with six sessions to be completed one-per-week. Depressive symptoms were measured with the self-rated Quick Inventory of Depressive Symptomatology (QIDS). The QIDS SI item was scored from zero to three, with a score of "3" defined as "thinks of suicide/death several times a day in depth or has made specific plans to commit or attempted suicide" and insomnia was measured with the Insomnia Severity Index. Remission of insomnia after treatment with CBT-I was associated with lower odds of incident Suicidal Ideation at post-treatment (OR = 0.18). A mediation analysis supported the role of dCBT-I as a driver of the remission of insomnia, which in turn was associated with a reduction in Suicidal Ideation [7]. Suicide death is on the 10-th place as death cause, and from the PPP View, it is important to use approved tools for *Prediction* of Insomnia (female sex, adolescence, high level of stress), *Prevention* using Sleep Education in the Companies, Schools, Universities, and *personalized Treatment* with cognitive behavioural Therapies for Insomnia (CBT-I) as face to face, or, as digital treatment [8].

Burnout syndrome, anxiety, and insomnia can affect the healthcare workers, who mostly work in shifts. The cross-sectional study including 1011 Health care workers and 679 (67.2%) of the study respondents were women, with a mean age of 35.67 ± 8.61 years. Fifty-eight percent (n = 589) of the participants were rotating shift workers. Age and on-call duty led to a significant difference in the severity of insomnia ($p = 0.028$, $p < 0.001$, respectively) and Insomnia was found to be statistically significant positively correlated with the Burnout-Score [9]. An increased awareness of the impact of sleep deprivation, burnout and anxiety among Health care Workers and *Preventing* interventions on the Topics Sleep and Mental Health are needed in every health care facility.

1.3 Sleep in Adolescents

Some previous studies have found associations between sleep disturbances and health related quality of life in children with other health disturbances as ADHD or PTBS [10, 11].

These findings implicate the importance and need for *prevention* strategy for sleep disorders in the childhood and adolescence. The strategy should consist of sleep health promotion in kindergarten and schools, as well as sleep education for the caregivers and parents. The sleep primary *prevention* should be part of the health policy similar as already known healthy food promotion or promotion of physical activity in young person's [12]. Adolescence is a critical life period associated with finally maturation of the physical and mental habitus. Life stress, insomnia, and ADS (attention deficit syndrome) in the adolescence are bidirectional related to one another, whereas insomnia was found to be a mediator of life stress and subsequent ADS in the adolescent age. These findings underline the importance of sleep and mental health assessment and intervention in adolescents following life stress [13].

There is a bidirectional relationship between daily stress and night sleep, with daily stress negatively affecting sleep, which can lead to more stress in adolescents. Insomnia in adolescence can be complex and the core clinical features (perceived sleep difficulties) and the critical factors (stress/worry) not necessarily reflected in objective sleep indicators.

The study of Menghini et al. present the results of 93 adolescents (59 girls; 16–19 years old) with ($N = 47$; 26 with clinical and 21 with sub-clinical) and without (N = 46; control) DSM-5 insomnia symptomatology, being measured by 2 months of continuous wearable tracking and daily diary ratings in free-living conditions using Fitbit Charge 3 tracked sleep, heart rate, and steps. Evening electronic diaries collected ratings of daily stress, pre sleep worry, and mood.

Participants with insomnia reported higher levels of stress and worry, being mainly related to "school." Stress and worry predicted shorter sleep duration and earlier wake up times, which, in turn, predicted higher stress the following day. Moreover, higher-than-usual stress predicted higher sleep time heart rate, with a more prominent effect in adolescents with insomnia [14].

1.4 Shift Work, Sleep, and Cancer

Night work is necessity in many sectors of the 24-h society. The exposure to light-at-night suppresses the nocturnal hormone melatonin that shows oncostatic properties and causes circadian misalignment between cells and organs, which has been examined as important pathogenetic mechanisms involved in carcinogenesis [15]. In 2007, the International Agency for Research on Cancer (IARC) classified shift work as probably carcinogenic to humans based on limited evidence from eight epidemiologic studies on breast cancer, in addition to sufficient evidence from animal experiments. The review of Hansen et al. is a critical update of the IARC evaluation, including the epidemiologic evidence on breast cancer risk after shift and night work [16, 17].

Nine new case-control studies, one case-cohort study, and eight cohort studies have been analysed: There is some evidence that high number of consecutive night shifts has impact on the extent of circadian disruption, and thereby increased breast cancer risk, but this information is missing in almost all cohort studies. The heterogeneity of the study methods and definitions of outcomes makes the overall interpretation difficult, especially the question concerning the association between night work and breast cancer, but overall there is tendency in the direction of an increased breast cancer risk, in particular after over 20 years of night shifts or after shorter periods with many consecutive shifts. Beside the need of more studies, there is a need for evidence-based preventive interventions [16]. One prevention method could be the implementation of Sleep Education and Sleep *Prevention* implementing the digital CBT-I on Companies employing Shift Worker as Hospital Facilities, Industry, Police, and many others [17, 18].

2 Sleep Quality and Immune Defence

Sleep could play very important role for the immune defence of the human body. The newest scientific research data show up that the sleep deprivation can severely impair the immune system functionality either caused by Insomnia, Circadian disruption, Shift Work or induced by sleep deprivation because people are over busy.

[Richter et al]. During the sleep there is higher activity of two subtypes of lymphocyte that play pivotal role for the immune response and general disease prevention, called CD4+ "helper" T cells and cytotoxic CD8+ "killer" T cells [12, 19–24]. Night-time sleep enables the synchronization between the pro-inflammatory hormones and cytokines and can facilitate the onset of an adaptive immune response, because increased production of pro-inflammatory cytokines and decreased activity of natural killer cells are important for the immune defence of the host against different pathogens including viral and also bacterial infections. The cytokines TNF-α and IL-12 and the antigen-presenting dendritic cells (DCs) express their highest activity during the night. Second important information is that the peak time of the circadian rhythms of cortisol, epinephrine, norepinephrine, and the cytokine IL-10 occurs in the early morning hours around the physiological; time of awakening. It indicates that we have to re-think the effect of forced awakening in the morning for the health, instead of awakening in the natural way. Cortisol and norepinephrine show peak value rhythms similar to sleep values, which Nadir values, for both, are higher under conditions of constant wakefulness, which indicates higher activity of the stress axis [20]. In sleep deprived subjects reduced activities of natural killer cell activity and T cell cytokine production have been found compared with subjects with a full undisturbed night of sleep [22, 23].

Fatigue and tiredness are common symptoms of COVID-19 infection, vaccination, and of long COVID symptoms lasting up to 6 months after infection. In some cases, disturbed sleep quality could explain at least one part of fatigue. That is the reason to indicate examination of the sleep quality in affected persons. Huang et al. examined a sample of N = 1655 participants and found that 437 individuals (26%) showed sleep problems and fatigue associated with COVID-19 [24].

Another important reason to investigate the sleep quality is the fact that sleep regulates glucose metabolism and weight gain, which are risk factors of diabetes, obesity, and sleep apnoea, and both of them are associated with a higher risk for disease on viral infections and for COVID-19 disease progression [25–27].

In a previous study, we found that insomnia symptoms persist in 36–88% of all COVID-19 patients and that this level is significantly higher compared to the prevalence in the general population, which has been estimated, with 10–40% [24].

3 Sleep and Cardiovascular Health

Despite the high prevalence of Obstructive Sleep Apnoea, which varies between 40 and 80% in patients with hypertension, heart failure, coronary artery disease, pulmonary hypertension, atrial fibrillation, stroke, OSA is often under recognized and undertreated in cardiovascular practice. The American Heart Association recommends regular screening for OSA in patients with hypertension, pulmonary hypertension, and recurrent atrial fibrillation after either cardioversion or ablation. Also, in patients with New York Heart Association class II to IV heart failure and suspicion of sleep-disordered breathing or excessive daytime sleepiness, a formal sleep assessment can be reasonable. Further recommendation for Apnoea Screening are patients with tachy-brady syndrome, ventricular tachycardia, survivors of sudden cardiac death, patients with nocturnally occurring angina, myocardial infarction, arrhythmias, and patients with appropriate shocks from implanted cardioverter-defibrillators. The early recognition of *predictive* factors as hypertension and cardiovascular symptoms can lead to early recognition of OSAS and prevention of severe cardiovascular events and complications through personalized treatment including behavioural modifications, weight loss, continuous positive airway pressure or oral appliances [28].

Although sufficient and healthy sleep is inversely associated with cardiovascular disease (CVD) and its risk factors, the American Heart Association's Life's Simple 7 (LS7), as a measure of cardiovascular health (CVH), did not include sleep. Makarem et al. evaluated in their study an expanded measure of CVH that includes sleep as an eighth metric in relation to CVD risk. The analytic sample consisted of 1920 participants (mean age: 69 ± 9 years; 54% female) of MESA (Multi-Ethnic Study of Atherosclerosis) Sleep Study who had completed overnight polysomnography, 7-day wrist actigraphy, and validated questionnaires. The Life's Simple 7 LS7 score was extended for four iterations of a new CVH score: score 1 included sleep duration, score 2 included sleep characteristics linked to CVD in the literature (sleep duration, insomnia, daytime sleepiness, and obstructive sleep apnoea), scores 3 and 4 included sleep characteristics associated with CVD in MESA (score 3: sleep duration and efficiency, daytime sleepiness, and obstructive sleep apnoea; score 4: score 3 + sleep regularity). Among there were 95 prevalent CVD events and 93 incident cases (mean follow-up, 4.4 years). Participants in the highest versus lowest tertile of CVH score 1, which included sleep duration, and CVH score 4, which included multidimensional sleep health, had 43% and 47% lower incident CVD risk (hazard ratio, 0.57 [95% CI, 0.33–0.97]; and hazard ratio, 0.53 [95% CI, 0.32–0.89]), respectively. CVH scores that include sleep health predicted CVD risk in older US adults. The authors recommend incorporation of sleep as a CVH metric, akin to other health behaviours, may enhance CVD primordial and primary prevention efforts [29].

4 Obstructive Sleep Apnoea in Patients with COVID-19

Some form of coronavirus infections has continuously been present throughout our history. The current coronavirus infection first appeared in China in 2019 and due to the high transmission rate of this disease it quickly spread worldwide [30, 31]. Based on phylogenic analysis of the virus, initially the infection was named Severe Acute Respiratory Syndrome Coronavirus 2 (SARS-CoV-2) by the International Committee on Taxonomy of Viruses. As the infection evolved and progressed into pandemic it was renamed as Coronavirus Disease of 2019 (COVID-19). This Coronavirus is highly contagious, spreads rapidly and continuously evolve and mutates in the human population.

COVID-19 infection often presents with variable symptoms, which frequently include fever cough, headache, fatigue, breathing difficulties, loss of smell, and loss of taste [32–34]. Symptoms usually appear after one and up to 14 days following exposure to the virus. A sizable proportion (up to 33%) of those exposed to the virus do not develop symptoms [35]. In majority of patients (81%) that develop symptoms, the symptoms are mild to moderate, while in 14% severe symptoms such as dyspnoea, and hypoxia develop. When imaged (CXR or CT scan) these patients with severe symptoms present with >50% lung involvement. Of these patients, 5% develop critical symptoms such as respiratory failure, shock, or multiorgan failure [36]. The clinical data has shown that older people are at a higher risk of developing these severe symptoms. As of September 19, 2022, there are reported over 617 million patients with COVID-19 with over six, five million total reported deaths [37]. Most of the patients who developed severe symptoms, with accompanying clinically significant hypoxia, were subsequently put on ventilation. Initially during the

COVID-19, pandemic most of the clinically severe patients who were unable to breathe on their own were placed on invasive ventilation with endotracheal intubation. As the pandemic progressed Non-invasive ventilation, (NIV) was used in greater amount for respiratory support. To maintain blood oxygen saturation at acceptable levels NIV is administered through a tight-fitting facemask with supplemented oxygen depending on the clinical presentation of the patient.

One group of patients considered to pose with increased risk from COVID-19 are those suffering from Sleep Apnoea. Even though this cohort of patients are not prone to a higher risk for contracting the Coronavirus, they tend to develop more severe outcomes, including a 31% higher rate of hospitalization and mortality [38]. It is not clear why these patients developed more severe outcomes even though they were using a continuous positive air pressure (CPAP) machine prior to contracting COVID-19.

4.1 Case Report of Patient with OSA Enduring COVID-19

Patients with Obstructive sleep apnoea (OSA) dread the notion of going through a respiratory illness. Reporting on a patient with obstructive sleep apnoea (OSA) with daily CPAP use who had been twice vaccinated for COVID-19 and twice boosted with Pfizer's COVID-19 vaccine but in constant contact with potential COVID-19 patients.

Initially our patient presented with low-grade fever of 37.6 °C and a headache. These were his only symptoms, and when they first appeared, three initial rapid tests (from various manufactures) were performed and all results came back negative. The next day the PCR test for SARS-CoV-2 came back positive.

The patient expressed concerns regarding the upcoming managements of COVID-19 since he is a long-time user of CPAP. Initial fears of undesirable disease outcome presented, but his knowledge of the current illness seemed to bring confidence that he could manage this upcoming event. He was reminded that he had previously endured respiratory infections with no serious consequences, and that his experience would help him get through this respiratory infection.

Following current worldwide medical recommendations, the patient was isolated in separate quarters in his household. The new area of accommodations and confinement were comfortable, and in the upcoming days, he would need to establish regular sleeping routine. The patient's greatest concern was that he would not be able to continue using his CPAP machine, due to circumstance that he only used nasal mask. His chief concern was that most of COVID-19 patients presented with nasal congestion, while stuffy and runny nose would make breathing through the nose difficult if not impossible. Reflecting on experience with nasal congestion, our patient devised a plan how to overcome the nasal congestion. Thoroughly blowing his nose and immediately starting the use of the CPAP machine can achieve drying up of the nasal cavity. In the next 10–15 min before falling asleep, he would be breathing positive air pressure, which in most instances dried up the nasal cavity and made it possible to sleep with the CPAP machine over night without any difficulty. This manoeuvre would be attempted each night, as he did not have a full-face mask at his disposal, and immediate procurement of full-face mask was not possible. In order to achieve maximal dryness of the nasal cavity at bedtime, if needed, the patient would also take over-the-counter nasal decongestant and antihistamine (either Bilastine or Pseudoephedrine + Triprolidine).

Initial night passed without any difficulty, but the COVID-19 infection was not yet in full swing. Sleeping alone did not require the need for night-time ventilation, but in the morning and much throughout the day his quarters was aired as to clean the room as much as possible from the presence of ambient coronavirus. Initially no concern was placed on cleaning the CPAP machine as the patient had previously used a cleaner and sanitizer device that automatically cleaned and dried the CPAP machine with the use of activated oxygen. The next day the patient called and informed us that he had previously discontinued the use of this cleaning device as it had destroyed the CPAP machine and had to pay a sizable repair bill to get the CPAP machine fixed. He did not want to damage his new machine while waiting for replacement of the CPAP machine. He opted to manually parts of the CPAP apparatus. With regular medical grade liquid soap, he cleaned the mask and hose each morning following instruction from established routine surgical scrubbing. A minimum of 3 min of washing would be enough for the facemask, but what about the hose? The same medical grade liquid soap was poured into the hose and repeatedly ran from one to another end in the hose for 3 min. Afterwards one end of the shower hose was hooked up to the rubbery end of the hose and lukewarm water was allowed to run and rinse the hose for 3–5 min. The distal end of the hose was elevated above the shower hose entrance point as to thoroughly rinse the hose. In order to prevent further reinfection from the Coronavirus, and prevention of new infection from either bacteria or fungi, this daily cleaning of the facemask and hose would prove acceptable. With proper care given to hygiene of the CPAP equipment, attention was shifted to managing the clinical symptoms that regularly accompany COVID-19 (Figs. 1 and 2).

Regular measurement of fever was easy to resolve with infrared thermometer. Portable pulse oximeter is sufficient to follow the all-important oxygen saturation changes. Changes in heart activity was followed with Kardia AliveCor ECG [39]. The CPAP machine provided recorded information on sleeping patterns. An open-source application was used to review data provided by the CPAP machine [40]. During nights, commercially available devices such as I Watch provided measurement of blood oxygen saturation. Although not 100% accurate it was, close enough [41]. This night-time data also provided accurate heart rate measurements throughout the night. These were simple yet powerful tools for home patient management. To our patients fortune the next 10 days were uneventful. Everyday routine involved regular cleaning of the CPAP facemask and hose, and review of symptoms obtained by the commercially available apps. We are happy to report that our patient made full recovery with no lasting complications.

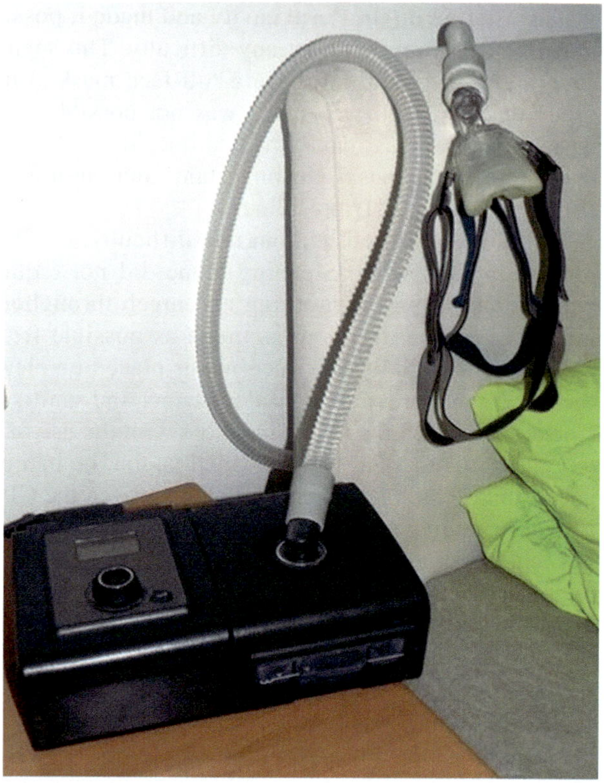

Fig. 1 Continuous positive air pressure (CPAP) machine, hose, and nasal mask

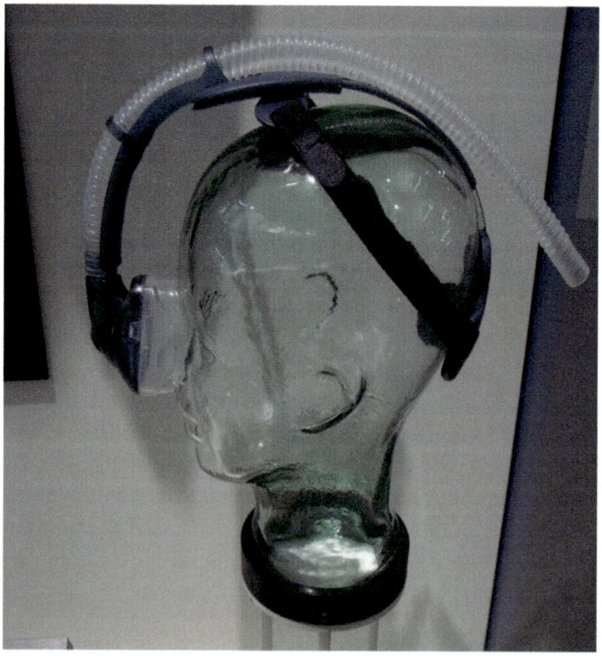

Fig. 2 Typical position of the nasal mask

5 AI and Big Data in Sleep Research

There is growing scientific evidence exploring big data in the field of sleep medicine. Big data have been collected from polysomnography and are used for stratification und subtyping of the different types of sleep apnoea. The data from wrist wearables that have been used for collection of hand movements can calculate the activity-inactivity cycles based solely on the measuring of the acceleration of the hand movement. Implementing a specific algorithm, the hand movement activity can be transformed into activity –rest cycle and can be visually presented as time periods of wake and sleep status. Sigga et al. examined how sleep duration, timing, misalignment, and variability develop with age and vary by gender and BMI collecting the data of 11.14 million nights from 69,650 adult non-shift workers aged 19–67 from 47 countries from wearable activity trackers.

The results of this study show that with growing age, the sleep duration decreases, while the frequency of awakenings at night increases, and also that sleep onset and offset advance become earlier with age. Generally, men tend to sleep less than women do across the lifespan; yet, night-time awakenings are more frequently for women, with the peak in the life stage associated with child rearing. This dataset was collected by consumer wearable devices from different companies and confirmed age-related and gender-related changes in sleep patterns. The results indicate a big potential for the implementation of the data of the wearables in the field of sleep medicine with the goal to improve the diagnosis and the treatment of sleep disorders. Still, it is too early to implement this data in the medical services because to do that, validations studied are needed for different manufacturer [42, 43]. Insomnia and the mental health status should be evaluated with wearables measuring the sleep quality, rest-activity cycle, heart rate variability, and the mood via digital questionnaires. There is a need of validation of the wearables that can be used for health tracking and medical use. In the actual market, there is a big number of wearables from different manufacturers using not approved algorithm for the measuring of the data. The reason for the lack of validated wearables for measuring of sleep-wake rhythm is that the most manufacturer do not allow the export of the raw data so that it is still not possible to prove if the used algorithm are the same algorithm used in the medical devices as actography [44].

In the future, the big sleep data from validated wearables should be collected enabling the early recognition of disturbed sleep quality. The *prediction* of prolonged sleep latency, interruption of the night sleep, early awakening, and reduced daily motor activity could be used to **predict** insomnia, to *prevent* it by sleep education and for *personalized* treatment using the digital cognitive – behavioural Therapy for Insomnia- CBT-I [8, 44].

6 Expert Recommendation in Sleep and Preventive, Predictive, and Personalized Medicine -PPP

6.1 How Much Sleep Is Healthy?

Answer on this question according to *PPP*M Strategy:
Getting the individual amount of sleep to load the own "battery" can improve the optimal physical and mental health. The individual amount of sleep can be recognized by following outcomes: 1. sleep duration- Totals Sleep time, 2. time needed to get asleep-Sleep Latency, 3. frequency of the awakening after getting asleep, 4. awakening in the early morning time (waking up too early), and the 5. Amount of deep sleep. Because these outcomes can vary according to the age, occupation, and the general health condition, every person should learn to find the own outcomes for perfect sleep.

Knowing the facts how long how deep the person should sleep, and also how long time showed it take to get asleep, can be helpful indicator to set some conditions in personal and professional life how to get enough sleep.

These five sleep outcomes can be seen as ***predictors*** for many known health conditions:

- Deficiency of deep sleep can lead immune deficiency.
- Sleep deprivation caused by insomnia can induce depression.
- Sleep deprivation in childhood and adolescence can induce emotional instability and school failure.
- Sleep deprivation in the adolescence can be associated to internet addiction.
- Fifth predictor if the third predictor does not count for two predictors.

Knowing the possible *predictors*, according *prevention measures* can be implemented:

Prevention of insomnia, sleep-wake disorders and any kind of sleep deprivation using the Sleep Education and Elements of evidence-based strategy of CBT-I (cognitive behavioural therapy for insomnia) [44, 45]. The Sleep Education should be implemented in schools, faculties, military, small and big companies, police, health sector, and other person centered activities. This can be made by online platforms [8, 17, 18].

***Personalization* of Sleep Education:**

Finding the perfect quality of sleep for every person can be achieved by acquisition of personal data using the wearables collecting the data on individual sleep habits. In the second step, the individual habits can be analysed by sleep specialist, sleep online platforms, or sleep apps. Sleep apps connected with wearables are on the public market, but most of them have not be validated. The reason is the luck of transparency considering in used algorithm and amount of "dirty data." Now, the only validated wearable for monitoring of the sleep-wake rhythm according to the measuring of the movement acceleration of the hand is actometry [43].

It means, that actualla only small number of persons has a chance (possibiliity) to recieve a sleep education which is esentialy important for the humant health.

To improve this problem in the future, the artificial intelligence methods could help to collect a big amount of sleep data collected by wearables and collected by online- sleep – platforms via digital questionnaires. Second, using the methods of machine learning, automatically generated recommendation can be developed for the different phenotypes of sleep disturbances.

Sleep omics should be further defined collected and shared in a way of open-source data [46].

6.2 Predicting, Preventing, and Personalizing Treatment of Patients with OSA

Early recognition of Risk Factors as arterial Hypertension, Obesity, Screening of Cardiovascular Health by validated digital devices and wearables could spread the possibility for health monitoring of big number of people and van also reduce the costs for the treatment of cardiovascular diseases if they are wide implemented in the health systems in many countries [47]. The importance of *predicting* and properly identifying risk factors in OSA patient will provide for appropriate management and most importantly prevent mortality. The early detection of Risk Factors will enable *preventive* measures using digital screening of digital ECG, oxygen saturation, ambulatory polygraphy, and others risk factors as glycose level control, education measures for reduction of obesity. For the *personalized* Treatment of OSAS the new Methods of Tele monitoring including CPAP Control at home will be expanding in the future.

6.3 Recommendation for Management COVID-19 Patients with OSA

Thinking of the illness in a time of COVID-19 pandemic will provide for timely diagnosis, as most patients will present with varying symptoms. The timely diagnosis provided with time to reflect on the health condition and develop a plan for management of the infection. The previous vaccinations and subsequent booster doses certainly help to keep the infection under control, but this did not happen in all COVID-19 patients with OSA. In a publication by Strausz et al., it was reported the presence of OSA is associated with COVID-19 severity in a way that OSA was associated with higher risk for hospitalization [48].

In a study by JP Ho, it was shown that the degree of OSA was not significantly associated with the rate of hospitalization, but that it was the low oxyhaemoglobin desaturation (LSAT) that was associated with COVID-19 severity. Furthermore, higher LSAT values represented lower risk for hospitalization while lower LSAT values were associated with higher ICU admission or death [49].

As the pandemic continues on, more and more patients are still being infected. Many of them are with OSA and although the severity of COVID-19 can vary among individuals, COVID-19 still has a detrimental outcome in most with OSA. To optimize patient care in these patients, physicians need to understand and quickly identify patient risk factors and threat these patients appropriately (Fig. 3).

In order to believe that we can *predict* outcome from illness, we have to understand the pathophysiology that defines Obstructive Sleep Apnoea. Although we still do not fully understand the mechanism of COVID-19 infection, we can reflect on our past actions for our future guidelines by analysing what we did and did not do correctly.

In patients with uncomplicated course of COVID-19 illness that did not need hospitalization, we can safely conclude that the outcome of OSA patients using a CPAP machine do not differ from those that do not have OSA. In patients that required hospitalization and subsequently needed ventilator support due to low oxygen saturation, the outcome was poorer for OSA patients on CPAP. Not all of the negative outcomes could be solely prescribed to the OSA. Many of these patients are diabetic, hypertensive and with other metabolic conditions that contribute to the severity of COVID-19 [38]. Data suggest that in patients with OSA who are not fully compliant with the use of their CPAP machine, the resultant sleep-related hypoxia is associated with progression of hypoxic insult and hypoxia-related injury

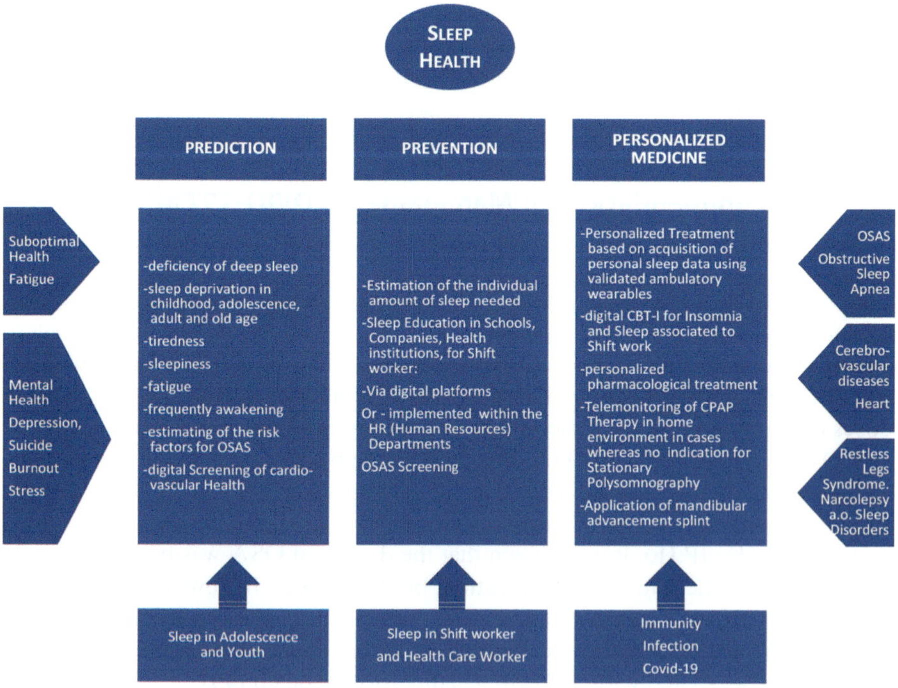

Fig. 3 Principles of PPP in Sleep Medicine

during COVID-19 infection [50]. Even though it is shown that hypoxia potentiates both viral replication [51, 52] and inflammation [53] data from research suggest that sleep-related hypoxia is not associated with increased likelihood of contracting SARS-CoV-2. However, hypoxia may play a role in worsening outcomes as the illness evolves. Hypoxia contribution in COVID-19 lung injury is likely multifactorial, including micro-infarctions, pulmonary parenchymal inflammation, hypoxic pulmonary vasoconstriction [54, 55], which in turn influence future treatment direction [56]. Many studies are consistent with the observation that hypoxemia below 90% (despite oxygen supplementation) is associated with increased mortality in critically ill patients with COVID-19 [57].

This important hypoxic event present during COVID-19 infection is most likely the principal *predicting* factor for higher mortality in countries with low awareness for use of CPAP therapy in patients with OSA. Perhaps the greatest measures that can be undertaken in reduction of mortality in OSA patients is education of medical providers for the presence of OSA, and the benefits from use of *personalized* CPAP therapy. Besides correctly diagnosing patients, various cultural beliefs will also have to be overcome which in some places might be a bigger hurdle to overcome.

References

1. Richter K, Rodenbeck A (2022) Current developments in sleep research and sleep medicine: an assessment of the chronobiology taskforce. Somnology 26(3):152–154. https://doi.org/10.1007/s11818-022-00383-3
2. Osterkamp J. https://www.spektrum.de/news/medizin-nobelpreis-fuer-die-innere-uhr/1507805. Accessed 10 Jul 2022
3. Roenneberg T (2019) Chronobiologische Aspekte der Sommerzeit. Somnologie 23:247–252
4. Begemann K, Oster H (2021) Zirkadiane Uhren und Schlaf – nachgeschaltete Funktion oder Crosstalk? Somnologie 25:126–130. https://doi.org/10.1007/s11818-020-00275-4
5. Wang W, Yan Y, Guo Z et al (2021) All around suboptimal health—a joint position paper of the Suboptimal Health Study Consortium and European Association for predictive, preventive and personalised medicine. EPMA J 12:403–433. https://doi.org/10.1007/s13167-021-00253-2
6. Mirchandaney R, Asarnow LD, Kaplan KA (2023) Recent advances in sleep and depression. Curr Opin Psychiatry 36(1):34–40. Epub 2022 Nov 16. https://doi.org/10.1097/YCO.0000000000000837
7. Kalmbach DA et al (2022) Cognitive-behavioral therapy for insomnia prevents and alleviates suicidal ideation: insomnia remission is a suicidolytic mechanism. Sleep 45:zsac251. https://doi.org/10.1093/sleep/zsac251
8. Retzer L, Feil M, Reindl R, Richter K, Lehmann R, Stemmler M, Graessel E (2021) Anonymous online cognitive behavioral therapy for sleep disorders in shift workers-a study protocol for a randomized controlled trial. Trials 22(1):539. https://doi.org/10.1186/s13063-021-05437-9
9. Aydin Guclu O, Karadag M, Akkoyunlu ME, Acican T, Sertogullarindan B, Kirbas G, Selimoglu Sen H, Lakadamyali H, Intepe YS, Arslan S, Firat Gursoy S, Kaya A (2022) Association between burnout, anxiety and insomnia in healthcare workers: a cross-sectional study. Psychol Health Med 27(5):1117–1130. Epub 2021 Jan 25. https://doi.org/10.1080/13548506.2021.1874434
10. Lewis KJS, Martin J, Gregory AM et al (2022) Sleep disturbances in ADHD: investigating the contribution of polygenic liability for ADHD and sleep-related phenotypes. Eur Child Adolesc Psychiatry 32:1253. https://doi.org/10.1007/s00787-021-01931-2

11. Agorastos Agorastos & Miranda Olff (2021) Sleep, circadian system and traumatic stress. Eur J Psychotraumatol 12:1. https://doi.org/10.1080/20008198.2021.1956746
12. Williamson AA, Zendarski N, Lange K, Quach J, Molloy C, Clifford SA, Mulraney M (2021) Sleep problems, internalizing and externalizing symptoms, and domains of health-related quality of life: bidirectional associations from early childhood to early adolescence. Sleep 44(1):zsaa139. https://doi.org/10.1093/sleep/zsaa139
13. Yang Y, Liu X, Liu ZZ, Tein JY, Jia CX (2023) Life stress, insomnia, and anxiety/depressive symptoms in adolescents: a three-wave longitudinal study. J Affect Disord 322:91–98. Epub 2022 Nov 11. https://doi.org/10.1016/j.jad.2022.11.002
14. Menghini L, Yuksel D, Prouty D, Baker FC, King C, de Zambotti M (2022) Wearable and mobile technology to characterize daily patterns of sleep, stress, presleep worry, and mood in adolescent insomnia. Sleep. Health 9:108. Epub ahead of print. https://doi.org/10.1016/j.sleh.2022.11.006
15. Büttner-Teleagă A, Kim YT, Osel T, Richter K (2021) Sleep disorders in cancer—a systematic review. Int J Environ Res Public Health 18(21):11696. https://doi.org/10.3390/ijerph182111696
16. Hansen J (2017) Night shift work and risk of breast cancer. Curr Environ Health Rep 4(3):325–339. https://doi.org/10.1007/s40572-017-0155-y
17. Richter K, Acker J, Adam S, Niklewski G (2016) Prevention of fatigue and insomnia in shift workers-a review of non-pharmacological measures. EPMA J 7(1):16. https://doi.org/10.1186/s13167-016-0064-4
18. Richter K, Acker J, Kamcev N, Bajraktarov S, Piehl A, Niklewski G (2011) Recommendations for the prevention of breast cancer in shift workers. EPMA J 2(4):351–356. Epub 2011 Dec 23. https://doi.org/10.1007/s13167-011-0126-6
19. Irwin M, Mascovich A, Gillin JC, Willoughby R, Pike J, Smith TL (1994) Partial sleep deprivation reduces natural killer cell activity in humans. Psychosom Med 56(6):493–498. https://doi.org/10.1097/00006842-199411000-00004
20. Irwin M, McClintick J, Costlow C, Fortner M, White J, Gillin JC (1996) Partial night sleep deprivation reduces natural killer and cellular immune responses in humans. FASEB J 10(5):643–653. https://doi.org/10.1096/fasebj.10.5.8621064
21. Lange T, Dimitrov S, Born J (2010) Effects of sleep and circadian rhythm on the human immune system. Ann N Y Acad Sci 1193:48–59. https://doi.org/10.1111/j.1749-6632.2009.05300.x
22. Besedovsky L, Lange T, Born J (2012) Sleep and immune function. Pflugers Arch 463(1):121–137. https://doi.org/10.1007/s00424-011-1044-0
23. Richter K, Kellner S, Hillemacher T, Golubnitschaja O (2021) Sleep quality and COVID-19 outcomes: the evidence-based lessons in the framework of predictive, preventive and personalised (3P) medicine. EPMA J 12(2):221–241. https://doi.org/10.1007/s13167-021-00245-2
24. Bloomgarden ZT (2020) Diabetes and COVID-19. J Diabetes 12(4):347–348. https://doi.org/10.1111/1753-0407.13027
25. Wilder-Smith A, Mustafa FB, Earnest A, Gen L, Macary PA (2013) Impact of partial sleep deprivation on immune markers. Sleep Med 14(10):1031–1034. https://doi.org/10.1016/j.sleep.2013.07.001
26. Huang C et al (2021) 6-month consequences of COVID-19 in patients discharged from hospital: a cohort study. Lancet 397(10270):220–232. https://doi.org/10.1016/s0140-6736(20)32656-8
27. Guo YR, Cao QD, Hong ZS, Tan YY, Chen SD, Jin HJ, Tan KS, Wang DY, Yan Y (2020) The origin, transmission and clinical therapies on coronavirus disease 2019 (COVID-19) outbreak—an update on the status. Mil Med Res 7(1):11. https://doi.org/10.1186/s40779-020-00240-0
28. Yeghiazarians Y, Jneid H, Tietjens JR, Redline S, Brown DL, El-Sherif N, Mehra R, Bozkurt B, Ndumele CE, Somers VK (2021) Obstructive sleep apnea and cardiovascular disease: a scientific statement from the American Heart Association. Circulation 144(3):e56–e67. Epub 2021 Jun 21. Erratum in: Circulation 2022 Mar 22;145(12):e775. https://doi.org/10.1161/CIR.0000000000000988

29. Makarem N, Castro-Diehl C, St-Onge MP, Redline S, Shea S, Lloyd-Jones D, Ning H, Aggarwal B (2022) Redefining cardiovascular health to include sleep: prospective associations with cardiovascular disease in the MESA sleep study. J Am Heart Assoc 11(21):e025252. Epub 2022 Oct 19. https://doi.org/10.1161/JAHA.122.025252
30. Sanche S, Lin YT, Xu C, Romero-Severson E, Hengartner N, Ke R (2020) High contagiousness and rapid spread of severe acute respiratory syndrome coronavirus 2. Emerg Infect Dis 26(7):1470–1477
31. Islam MA, Kundu S, Alam SS, Hossan T, Kamal MA et al (2021) Prevalence and characteristics of fever in adult and paediatric patients with coronavirus disease 2019 (COVID-19): a systematic review and meta-analysis of 17515 patients. PLoS One 16(4):e0249788. https://doi.org/10.1371/journal.pone.0249788
32. Islam MA, Sadia AS, Shoumik K, Tareq H, Amjad KM (2020) Cavestro Cinzia, prevalence of headache in patients with coronavirus disease 2019 (COVID-19): a systematic review and meta-analysis of 14,275 patients. Front Neurol 11:562634. https://doi.org/10.3389/fneur.2020.562634
33. Saniasiaya J, Islam MA, Abdullah B (2021) Prevalence of olfactory dysfunction in coronavirus disease 2019 (COVID-19): a meta-analysis of 27,492 patients. Laryngoscope 131(4):865–878. Epub 2020 Dec 5. https://doi.org/10.1002/lary.29286
34. Jeyasakthy Saniasiaya MD (2021) MMed, md Asiful Islam, PhD, Baharudin Abdullah, MBBS, MMed, prevalence and characteristics of taste disorders in cases of COVID-19: a meta-analysis of 29,349 patients. Otolaryngol Head Neck Surg 165(1):33–42. https://doi.org/10.1177/0194599820981018
35. Interim Clinical Guidance for Management of Patients with Confirmed Coronavirus Disease (COVID-19). U.S. Centers for Disease Control and Prevention (CDC). https://www.cdc.gov/coronavirus/2019-ncov/hcp/clinical-guidance-management-patients.html. Accessed 6 Apr 2020
36. Long COVID or Post-COVID Conditions. https://www.cdc.gov/coronavirus/2019-ncov/long-term-effects.html
37. https://www.worldometers.info/coronavirus/
38. Orbea CP et al (2021) Association of Sleep-Related Hypoxia with Risk of COVID-19 hospitalizations and mortality in a large integrated health system. JAMA Netw Open 4(11):e2134241. https://doi.org/10.1001/jamanetworkopen.2021.34241
39. https://www.alivecor.com/
40. https://www.sleepfiles.com/OSCAR/
41. The new Apple Watch says my lungs may be sick. Or perfect. It can't decide. Geoffrey A. Fowler, The Washington Post, September 23, 2020 at 7:00. https://www.washingtonpost.com/technology/2020/09/23/apple-watch-oximeter/
42. Jonasdottir SS, Minor K, Lehmann S, Zendarski N, Lange K, Quach J, Molloy C, Clifford SA, Mulraney M (2021) Gender differences in nighttime sleep patterns and variability across the adult lifespan: a global-scale wearables study. Sleep 44:zsaa139. https://doi.org/10.1093/sleep/zsaa139
43. Acker J, Golubnitschaja O, Büttner-Teleaga A et al (2021) Wrist actigraphic approach in primary, secondary and tertiary care based on the principles of predictive, preventive and personalised (3P) medicine. EPMA J 12:349–363. https://doi.org/10.1007/s13167-021-00250-5
44. Peter L, Reindl R, Zauter S, Hillemacher T, Richter K (2019) Effectiveness of an online CBT-I intervention and a face-to-face treatment for shift work sleep disorder: a comparison of sleep diary data. Int J Environ Res Public Health 16(17):3081. https://doi.org/10.3390/ijerph16173081
45. Espie CA (2022) Standard CBT-I protocol for the treatment of insomnia disorder. Book Editors: Chiara Baglioni, Colin A. Espie, Dieter Riemann, European Sleep Research Society, European Insomnia Network, European Academy for Cognitive Behavioural Therapy for Insomnia. First published: 08 July 2022. https://doi.org/10.1002/9781119891192.ch2

46. https://sleepdata.org/. Accessed 23 Oct 2022
47. Blok S, van der Linden EL, Somsen GA, Tulevski II, Winter MM, van den Born BH (2021) Success factors in high-effect, low-cost eHealth programs for patients with hypertension: a systematic review and meta-analysis. Eur J Prev Cardiol 28(14):1579–1587. Epub 2020 Sep 11. https://doi.org/10.1177/2047487320957170
48. Strausz S, Kiiskinen T, Broberg M, Ruotsalainen S, Koskela J, Bachour A et al (2021) Sleep apnoea is a risk factor for severe COVID-19. BMJ Open Respir Res 8(1):1–6
49. Ho JPTF, Donders HCM, Zhou N, Schipper K, Su N, de Lange J (2021) Association between the degree of obstructive sleep apnea and the severity of COVID-19: an explorative retrospective cross-sectional study. PLoS One 16:e0257483. https://doi.org/10.1371/journal.pone.0257483
50. Xie J, Covassin N, Fan Z et al (2020) Association between hypoxemia and mortality in patients with COVID-19. Mayo Clin Proc 95(6):1138–1147. https://doi.org/10.1016/j.mayocp.2020.04.006
51. Peker Y, Hedner J, Norum J, Kraiczi H, Carlson J (2002) Increased incidence of cardiovascular disease in middle-aged men with obstructive sleep apnea: a 7-year follow-up. Am J Respir Crit Care Med 166(2):159–165. https://doi.org/10.1164/rccm.2105124
52. Hertzog RG, Bicheru NS, Popescu DM, Călborean O, Catrina AM (2021) Hypoxic preconditioning—a nonpharmacological approach in COVID-19 prevention. Int J Infect Dis 103:415–419. https://doi.org/10.1016/j.ijid.2020.11.181
53. Punjabi NM, Caffo BS, Goodwin JL et al (2009) Sleep-disordered breathing and mortality: a prospective cohort study. PLoS Med 6(8):e1000132. https://doi.org/10.1371/journal.pmed.1000132
54. Karmouty-Quintana H, Thandavarayan RA, Keller SP, Sahay S, Pandit LM, Akkanti B (2020) Emerging mechanisms of pulmonary vasoconstriction in SARS-CoV-2-induced acute respiratory distress syndrome (ARDS) and potential therapeutic targets. Int J Mol Sci 21(21):1–21. https://doi.org/10.3390/ijms21218081
55. Potus F, Mai V, Lebret M et al (2020) Novel insights on the pulmonary vascular consequences of COVID-19. Am J Physiol Lung Cell Mol Physiol 319(2):L277–L288. https://doi.org/10.1152/ajplung.00195.20
56. Grieco DL, Menga LS, Cesarano M et al (2021) Effect of helmet noninvasive ventilation vs high-flow nasal oxygen on days free of respiratory support in patients with COVID-19 and moderate to severe hypoxemic respiratory failure: the HENIVOT randomized clinical trial. JAMA 325(17):1731–1743. https://doi.org/10.1001/jama.2021.4682
57. Smagula SF, Stone KL, Redline S et al (2016) Actigraphy- and polysomnography-measured sleep disturbances, inflammation, and mortality among older men. Psychosom Med 78(6):686–696. https://doi.org/10.1097/PSY.0000000000000312

Chronic Mental Disorders: Limitations and Perspectives of Prediction, Prevention, Diagnosis, and Personalized Treatment in Psychiatry

Joanna Rymaszewska, Karolina Fila-Pawłowska, and Dorota Szcześniak

Abbreviations

3 PM	3 Predictive, preventive and personalized medicine
aDBS	Adaptive deep brain stimulation
AI	Artificial intelligence
ALIC	Anterior Limb of Internal Capsule
aTMS	Accelerated transcranial magnetic stimulation
A-to-I RNA	Individual adenosine (A) bases in pre-mRNA are modified to yield inosine (I)
BDNF	Brain-derived neurotrophic factor
BNST	Bed nucleus of stria terminalis
CBT	Cognitive behavioral therapy
CL stimulation	Closed-loop stimulation
CSF	Cerebrospinal fluid
CSTC circuit	Cortico-striato-thalamo-cortical circuit
CYP2D6	Cytochrome P450 2D6
DALYS	Disability-adjusted life-years
DBS	Deep brain stimulation
DHT	Digital health technologies
DNA	Deoxyribonucleic acid

J. Rymaszewska (✉)
Department of Clinical Neuroscience, Wroclaw University of Science and Technology, Wroclaw, Poland
e-mail: joanna.rymaszewska@pwr.edu.pl

K. Fila-Pawłowska · D. Szcześniak
Department of Psychiatry, Wroclaw Medical University, Wroclaw, Poland
e-mail: k.fila-witkowska@umw.edu.pl; dorota.szczesniak@umw.edu.pl

H. Podbielska, M. Kapalla (eds.), *Predictive, Preventive, and Personalised Medicine: From Bench to Bedside*, Advances in Predictive, Preventive and Personalised Medicine 17, https://doi.org/10.1007/978-3-031-34884-6_15

DTI	Diffusion tensor imaging
dTMS	Deep transcranial magnetic stimulation
ECT	Electroconvulsive therapy
EEG	Electroencephalography
EMEA	European Medicines Agency
FDA	Food and Drug Administration
fMRI	Functional magnetic resonance imaging
GABAA receptors	γ-Aminobutyric acid receptors
GMF-β	Glia maturation factor beta
GTPase-activating protein	Guanosine triphosphate activating protein
HPA-axis	Hypothalamus-pituitary-adrenal axis
IL-2, IL-4, IL-6, IL-10	Interleukins 2,4,6,10
IT	Information technology
ITP	Inferior thalamic peduncle
LFP	Local field potential
MDD	Major depressive disorder
MFB	Medial forebrain bundle
ML	Machine learning
NAc	Nucleus accumbens
NGF	Nerve growth factor
NIBS	Non-invasive brain stimulation
NIH	National Institutes of Health
OCD	Obsessive-compulsive disorder
OFC	Orbitofrontal cortex
pTMS	Priming transcranial magnetic stimulation
RAB3GAP1 catalytic subunit	RAB3 GTPase Activating Protein Catalytic Subunit 1
RCT	Random clinical trials
RNA	Ribonucleic acid
rTMS	Repetitive transcranial magnetic stimulation
sgACC	Subgenual anterior cingulate cortex
SMA	Supplementary motor area
SNPs	Single nucleotide polymorphisms
sTMS	Synchronized transcranial magnetic stimulation
STN	Subthalamic nucleus
tDCS	Transcranial direct current stimulation
TMS	Transcranial magnetic stimulation
TRD	Treatment resistant depression
VC/VS	Ventral capsule/ventral striatum
WHO	World Health Organization
YLD	Years lived with disability
YLL	Years of life lost

1 Introduction

The brain is a fascinating organ of our human body. Its complexity is captivating, however, our knowledge of how it works is still significantly limited. One of the effects of this sophisticated organ is the human mind, encompassing thoughts and emotions, ongoing comprehensive mental processes. Disturbances in the functioning of the central nervous system can generate psychopathological symptoms and syndromes such as depressive, anxiety, psychotic, obsessive-compulsive episodes.

Whole generations of scientists, including psychiatrists, neurologists, psychotherapists from the clinical background, are working on the achievements of psychiatry and neuroscience. Among them are a group of distinguished and outstanding ones, as well as those whose work and contributions inspire and become the beginning for further scientific achievements. One of the great authorities is Eric Kandel, the Nobel prize winner 2000, shared with Arvid Carlsson and Paul Greengard, for his research on the physiological basis of memory storage in neurons. Despite the fact that he was working on the snail's nervous system, has contributed so much to the field of human neuroscience.

Kandel formulated five basic principles of neuroscience that directly apply to psychiatry and point the way for current research and those planned for the future. In a nutshell they sound as follows [1]:

- Principle 1. *All mental processes, even the most complex psychological processes, derive from operations of the brain.*
- Principle 2. *Genes and their protein products are important determinants of the pattern of interconnections between neurons in the brain and the details of their functioning.*
- Principle 3. *Altered genes do not, by themselves, explain all of the variance of a given major mental illness. Social or developmental factors also contribute very importantly.*
- Principle 4. *Alterations in gene expression induced by learning give rise to changes in patterns of neuronal connections.*
- Principle 5. *Insofar as psychotherapy or counseling is effective and produces long-term changes in behavior, it presumably does so through learning, by producing changes in gene expression that alter the strength of synaptic connections and structural changes that alter the anatomical pattern of interconnections between nerve cells of the brain.*

2 Severity of the Problem: Prevalence and Burden

The scale of the problem is very large. The data shows a very high prevalence of mental disorders. Long-term prospective studies indicate that with each decade the number of mental disorders is increasing. These are, of course, indicators based on recorded and recognized clinical cases.

According to the WHO data, in 2019, 1 in every 8 people, or 970 million people around the world were living with a mental disorder, with anxiety disorders (301 million people including 58 million children and adolescents) and depressive disorders the most common (280 million people living with depression, including 23 million children and adolescents). Additionally, 40 million people experienced bipolar disorder, schizophrenia affects approximately 24 million people or 1 in 300 people worldwide, 14 million people experienced eating disorders including almost three million children and adolescents [2].

Researchers from the Global Burden of Diseases 2019 group studied a range of important mental health indicators worldwide (204 countries), including the global, regional, and national prevalence, disability-adjusted life-years (DALYS), years lived with disability (YLDs), and years of life lost (YLLs) for mental disorders from 1990 to 2019 [3]. They found that between 1990 and 2019, the proportion of global DALYs attributed to mental disorders increased from 3.1% (95% UI 2.4–3.9) to 4.9% (3.9–6.1), while age-standardized DALY rates remained largely consistent. Mental disorders increased 48.1%, from 654.8 million estimated cases in 1990 and 970.1 million in 2019. It is important to mentioned that about 14.6% of global YLDs in 2019 was attributable to mental disorders, which means they remained among the top ten leading causes of burden worldwide. Moreover, mental disorders jumped from the 13th leading cause of DALYs in 1990 to the seventh position in 2019, and were the second most common cause of YLDs in both years. The largest burdens, based on the proportion of DALYs, due to mental disorders were depressive disorders (37.3%), anxiety disorders (22.9%), and schizophrenia (12.2%), across age groups. At least four groups of mental disorders that are highly challenging in psychiatry were not included in these analyses - dementias, including neurodegenerative diseases, addictions to alcohol and other substances, behavioral addictions, and personality disorders.

It is common for mental disorders to have high comorbidity. In big cohort study Lamers et al. found 67% of those with a depressive disorder also had a comorbid anxiety current problem, and 75% had one at some point in their lives. And vice versa, 63% of people with a current anxiety problem also had a current depressive condition, and 81% experienced one over their lifetime [4]. In patients with major depressive disorder (MDD) and comorbid anxiety disorders, increased rates of functional impairment and suicidality were confirmed [5]. Patients with MDD who also have concomitant anxiety disorders had greater rates of early treatment termination when receiving psychotherapy, antidepressant resistance, and poorer outcomes [6, 7]. Given the results of lower treatment effectiveness in the case of co-occurrence of two disorders, it can be concluded that the reason is not only the number of symptoms and their severity, but also perhaps the greater complexity of the causes of their origin. Thus, clinical symptoms and their composition and severity, as well as their duration, is certainly the tip of the iceberg.

Psychiatric comorbidities are frequent in patients with schizophrenia [8]. Approximately 23%–55% of patients with first episode psychosis had high rates of depressed symptoms, whereas anxiety prevalence rates in schizophrenia have been estimated to range between 35% and 65%. A study of a large cohort of patients with lifetime MDD in the US found that 40% had an alcohol use disorder and 17% had a drug use disorder. When two or more psychiatric conditions are present at the same time, the intensity of the combined condition is higher, the pharmaceutical treatment is less effective, and the risk of suicide is higher than with just one disorder. Moreover, psychiatric disorders influence on the course and prognosis of many common somatic disorders, including ischemic heart disease, obesity,and diabetes [9].

The above data clearly indicate that not only the number of people suffering from various mental disorders is increasing, but also indicates that available treatment methods are insufficiently effective.

3 Diagnostic Methods in Psychiatry

In medicine, we try to diagnose each patient's condition, its symptoms and their severity, and determine what kind of illness we are dealing with. We confirm or rule out the suspected diagnosis by performing a number of diagnostic tests (blood tests, urine tests, saliva samples, fecal samples, cerebrospinal fluid, even hair), electrocardiogram, ultrasound, and radiological studies.

In psychiatry, diagnosis is based almost exclusively on phenomenology, that is, based on psychopathological symptoms. Instead of measuring the direct link to brain function and illness, the diagnosis is dependent on descriptive data gleaned from clinical observation [10]. This is due to the fact that we understand the brain less thoroughly than we do many other aspects of medicine, where naturally, much simpler organs are the main object of study. Laboratory and neuroimaging studies are used for the most part to exclude other causes of the observed symptoms, such as endocrine disorders in the course of hypothyroidism with such patient complaints as drowsiness, lack of energy, etc. As Craddock mentioned, it is crucial to consider factors other than the diagnosis when making assessments of etiology, symptom severity and pattern, and functioning impairment (also known as the "domains of psychopathology"). The identification of biomarkers has long-term potential to improve the diagnosis and treatment of mental disorders, and diagnosis will certainly be supported by unbiased laboratory tests.

For conditions related to the central nervous system, which also include mental disorders, direct access to research material is limited. With few exceptions (such as biomarkers of Alzheimer's disease), even cerebrospinal fluid (CSF) testing does not currently offer clinically relevant markers and its collection is somewhat of a barrier in daily practice. Fortunately, it turns out that there is a close two-way interaction between the CNS and the immune system, and that link is lymphocytes. By taking blood samples from patients with mental disorders, we can study certain genes on lymphocytes, such as c-Fos protein, interleukins (IL-2, IL-4, IL-6, IL-10), nerve growth factor (NGF), brain-derived neurotrophic factor (BDNF), cannabinoid receptors, acetylcholine, GABAA receptors, B2-adrenergic receptors, glucocorticoid receptors, mineralocorticoid receptors, dopaminergic D3 receptors, and serotonin receptors. It can be said that they are peripheral biomarkers [11]. To date, inadequate knowledge of the etiopathogenesis of mental disorders, significant heterogeneity of disorders, widespread comorbidities, and low specificity of biomarkers limit research in this area and do not function as yet in everyday clinical practice [12].

Functional neuroimaging techniques have played a major role in the development of knowledge about mental disorders, making it possible to observe changes in local cerebral flow, energy metabolism, and the density and occupation of neurotransmitter receptors in the course of disorders. They are an important element in research, but nevertheless do not reach the level of nerve cell biochemistry. Functional magnetic resonance imaging (fMRI) of the brain has made it possible to understand the functional architecture, including determining in which areas of the brain functions are located. Thanks to fMRI, we know how complex the processes are in a healthy mind and to some extent in a disturbed one. Functional neuroimaging beautifully shows network connections and makes it clear that individual thought and emotional processes are not located in one specific place but are extremely complex neuronal networks. It allows a more accurate understanding of the functioning of an individual patient's brain structures in planning advanced therapies such as deep brain stimulation for treatment-resistant disorders (Fig. 1).

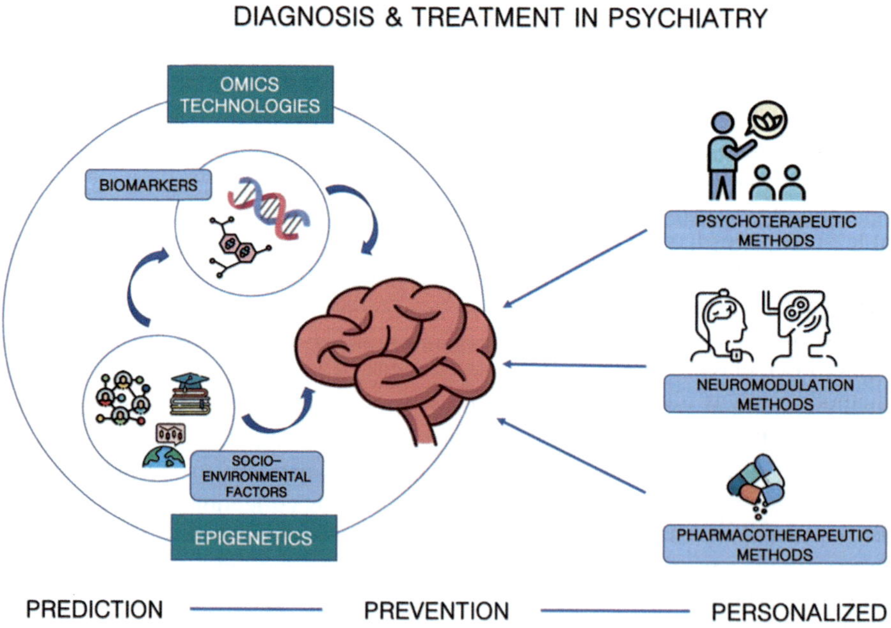

Fig. 1 Key elements of contemporary neuroscience research in the diagnosis and treatment of mental disorders

3.1 Usefulness of Biomarkers in Psychiatry

The definition of the Food and Drug Administration (FDA) in collaboration with the NIH Joint Leadership Council convened the FDA-NIH Biomarker Working Group from 2016 defined biomarker clearly: a characteristic that is measured as an indicator of normal biological processes, pathogenic processes or responses to an exposure or intervention [13]. A good biomarker should be useful in clinical practice, and therefore have such characteristics as: be detectable and measurable, has high reproducibility, and meet the criterion of dynamic and reliable modification as the clinical condition progresses. Thus, the biomarker should be available for testing, for example, as a parameter from blood plasma, genetic testing or be detectable through histological, or neuroimaging techniques. Based on their primary clinical use, this group classified various types of biomarkers into diagnostic, monitoring, pharmacodynamic/response, predictive, prognostic, safety, and susceptibility/risk biomarkers. Diagnostic biomarkers would enable the development of personalized psychiatry, increasing the effectiveness of therapeutic response. Biomarkers at the individual patient level could also play a predictive role for the outcome of a specific treatment. Studied previously, in healthy individuals they provide information about the risk of developing any disease among the population in the area of public health.

3.1.1 Diagnostic Biomarkers

Research on biomarkers in psychiatric disorders is being intensively conducted, nevertheless, it has not yet entered everyday clinical practice and are not included in international classifications of diseases. One example is the lack of use of biomarkers in the diagnosis of dementia such as the levels of A42 and total tau (T-tau) in the CSF fluid of these group of patients in a diagnostic process for Alzheimer's disease, that are still not recommended in everyday practice.

3.1.2 Monitoring Biomarkers

The increase in serum creatinine and/or potassium concentrations following a pharmacologic intervention is an illustration of a general monitoring biomarker. These values are frequently employed as indicators of the likelihood to experience side effects. A clinical intervention, such as pharmacological therapies, modifies a pharmacodynamic biomarker, which then determines the progression of treatment. It is possible to determine which patient or group of patients is more likely to have an impact as a result of a therapeutic intervention or exposure to an environmental chemical based on the presence or alteration of a predictive biomarker. This effect may manifest as a symptomatic improvement or remission, a rise in survival, or a negative occurrence. In randomized, controlled clinical trials of new medicines, predictive biomarkers are investigated. The existence of 12 single nucleotide polymorphisms (SNPs) in a Chinese community of schizophrenia patients, which were associated with increased olanzapine efficacy, is an example of a predictive biomarker. When a patient is diagnosed with an illness, a prognostic biomarker is used to determine the likelihood that a clinical event (death, disease progression, recurrence, or formation of a new disease) will occur. Prognostic biomarkers are utilized as inclusion or exclusion criteria in clinical trials. If known, can be helpful for treatment selections in therapeutic work.

For many therapies, monitoring hepatic, renal, and cardiovascular functions (safety biomarkers) have ability to detect or predict toxicity prior to initiation of therapy; onset of clinical signs and before irreversible damage. They can detect toxicity ensuring the safety of the therapy under study or identify patients in which particular therapies should not be initiated because of significant safety risks. For instance, genetic changes in CYP2D6 enzymes alter how some medications, such approximately 50% of antipsychotics, react with the body. There is a connection between the cardiac toxicity of the antipsychotic risperidone and the quantity of CYP2D6 genes that are activated. Subjects with one active CYP2D6 gene have a longer QTc interval in electrocardiography than individuals with two active genes. The research found a correlation between the number of CYP2D6 active genes and the risperidone plasma concentration when adjusted [14].

3.1.3 Risk Biomarkers

A susceptibility or risk biomarker can be used to assess the likelihood of developing a disease, such as a genetic biomarker that can be found years or even decades before the beginning of the clinical symptoms. Accordingly, Hartwig and al. found that twofold increments in circulating levels of C-reactive protein and soluble interleukin-1 receptor levels were associated with a 10% reduction and a 6% increase in the lifetime odds of developing schizophrenia respectively, possibly due to increased susceptibility to early life infection [15].

3.2 "Omics" Technologies in Psychiatry

"Omics" technologies are a relatively new field of research such as genomics, proteomics or metabolomics where information technology (IT) is at the heart of "omics" research used to analyze large amounts of data. For example, genomics as the branch of biology that studies an organism's entire genome by sequencing, combining, and analyzing the function and structure of its DNA may contribute great progress in understanding various diseases, also psychiatric. The new field of research can become the fundament for the development of more effective treatment strategies and the selection of better tools to facilitate decision-making in the personalized medicine.

"Omics" technologies are also being used in the search for biomarkers to assess risk, diagnose, monitor progression, and predict response to treatment in mental disorders. The European Medicines Agency (EMEA) defined a genomic biomarker as "a measurable deoxyribonucleic acid (DNA) and/or ribonucleic acid (RNA) characteristic that is an indicator of normal biologic processes, pathogenic processes, and/or response to therapeutic or other interventions" [16]. For example, a large study conducted in Europe, North America, and Australia identified 30 genomic loci relevant to Bipolar Disorder in European participants. Among those 30 loci eight have also been described in patients with schizophrenia. They stated that type I of bipolar disorder is strongly genetically correlated with schizophrenia, driven by psychosis, whereas type II of bipolar disorder - with major depressive disorder [17].

The studies on transcriptome defined as the complete set of all RNA molecules in one cell or a population of cells at a specific developmental stage or physiological condition, are also conducted in the field of neuroscience. As an example, we can cite Chimienti et al., who establish a direct relationship between A-to-I RNA modifications of peripheral markers and A-to-I RNA editing-related modifications in brain [18]. The researchers presented the first immune response-related brain marker for suicide. The next step will be to identify a blood-based biomarker that predicts suicidal behavior, and then the transcriptomic biomarkers can be used in prevention efforts.

As a result, blood, plasma, or serum are biological materials frequently employed for routine diagnostic analyses in clinical practice, making sample collection easier, proteomics techniques using these samples represent a highly wanted tool for biomarker profiling of mental disorders. Additionally, because of its proximity to the brain, cerebrospinal fluid (CSF) is a sample of particular interest in neuropsychiatry for the discovery of putative proteomic biomarkers.

As an illustration, a study by Rodrigues-Amorim et al. found that potential biomarkers in schizophrenia could be the glia maturation factor beta (GMF-β), the brain-derived neurotrophic factor (BDNF), and the 115-kDa isoform of the Rab3 GTPase-activating protein catalytic subunit RAB3GAP1, which showed significantly reduced levels in plasma of patients with schizophrenia [19].

The study of metabolites, or tiny molecules such as drugs, in complex matrices such as blood, urine, saliva, cerebrospinal fluid is the focus of metabolomics. The metabolome offers a direct functional measure of cellular activity and physiological condition since it is naturally more dynamic and time-sensitive than the proteome and genome. The dynamic combination of environmental, genetic, pathological, developmental, and lifestyle factors results in changes in the metabolome - a set of metabolomic biomarkers.

Recently, a study of Czysz et al. among depressive patients attempted to identify a biological predictor of recovery after escitalopram monotherapy, bupropion-escitalopram combination, or venlafaxine-mirtazapine combination. Patients' outcomes were worse when their baseline plasma concentrations of phosphatidylcholine C38:1 were higher. However, after 8 weeks of therapy, an increased ratio of hydroxylated sphingomyelins relative to non-hydroxylated sphingomyelins at baseline was associated with symptom improvement. All metabolite-based models performed superior to treatment as usual and models only using clinical and sociodemographic variables [20]. However, metabolomics biomarkers have not met the regulatory requirements for their use in clinical practice due to the lack of reliable assays for routinely quantifying putative biomarkers and because studies are heterogeneous.

3.2.1 Epigenetic in Psychiatry

Different forms of epigenetic regulation (changes of chromatin structure, without changes in sequence of DNA itself but modified the expression of genes) may provide a functional interface between genotype, environmental exposure, and phenotype.

García-Giménez et al. defined very aptly an epigenetic biomarker as "any epigenetic mark or altered epigenetic mechanism that can be measured in the body fluids or tissues defining a disease (detection); predicts the outcome of disease (prognostic), responds to therapy (predictive); monitors responses to therapy or medication (therapy monitoring) and predicts risk of future disease development (risk)" [11].

Numerous of the scientific advances so far are positive, showing important correlations between epigenetic modifications of genes controlling neurotransmission, neurodevelopment, and immunological function in mental illnesses. Returning to the extremely important phenomenon, the hypothalamus-pituitary-adrenal axis (HPA-axis), neurotrophic factors, serotoninergic, and GABAergic systems have been proposed as epigenetic biomarkers for suicide, suicide ideation, and suicide attempt.

Despite progress in neuroscience, there is still a long way to go before there is a clear biological basis underlying mental disorders and appropriate treatment choices. García-Gutiérrez et al. stressed that the clinical use of epigenetic biomarkers has been hampered by the heterogeneity of the techniques and methods employed, with a range in sensitivity for detecting effects; the absence of adjusting the genome-wide outcome to account for cell specificity; confounding variables such as patient treatment, population origin, and included phenotypes; and the absence of additional studies to demonstrate the concordance between brain–blood data.

With advances in neuroscience and other areas of research, including "omics" related to mental disorders, objectified diagnostic protocols will be established in the future. The search for biomarkers that would facilitate a more accurate diagnosis or diagnoses, allow to predict or even prevent from onset of mental disorders is ongoing. Nevertheless, there is currently a lack of indicators that would accurately pinpoint the causes of mental disorders and then more precisely treat them.

4 Treatment of Mental Disorders

Psychiatry owes its heyday to coincidence, when in the 1950s the anti-allergic drug, chlorpromazine, showed sedative effects and began to be used in patients with psychosis. However, the first modern drug in psychiatry is considered lithium carbonate (1949), which is still used today for bipolar affective disorder. Shortly thereafter, haloperidol, an antipsychotic drug, and imipramine, the first modern antidepressant, entered treatment. Parallel to the discovery of more drugs and pharmacology, psychotherapy with its various strands developed in the twentieth century. Today, we have a number of medications available that are effective in treating the symptoms of various mental disorders.

In recent years, new pharmacological solutions for treating depression have been emerging, based on long-known compounds. Among them are ketamine and compounds known as psychedelics. Since its creation in the 1960s, ketamine has been utilized as a surgical anesthetic. It has been used as a recreational drug that has the potential to have dissociative side effects, including hallucinations. Currently a novel oral or nasal formulation of ketamine seems to be promising as add-on therapy for patients with treatment-resistant depression, the same with synthetic formulation of psilocybin.

However, due to the complex causality of mental disorders and the pathomechanisms of their onset, which are not fully understood, many patients cannot currently be helped. More than 30% of patients do not respond to standard treatment, and 10% are completely resistant to conventional therapies. Resistance to treatment results in patients with a markedly reduced quality of life, a high risk of suicide, personal distress and a high likelihood of relapse. These are the most important reasons for exploring new methods of prevention and treatment of mental disorders.

Pharmacological treatment is aimed at eliminating the symptoms of disorders. The effectiveness of psychotherapeutic techniques depends largely on the basis of the disorder. Very good and good results are achieved in many anxiety disorders, some depressive disorders and sometimes personality disorders. In many cases, psychotherapy is an adjunctive therapy.

Studies demonstrate that psychotherapy can lead to structural and functional changes in the brain. Obsessive-compulsive disorder has proven to be one of the better models to provide evidence for the Kendel's 4 and 5 principles. Research findings using functional magnetic resonance imaging have consistently demonstrated lower metabolism in the right caudate nucleus as a result of cognitive behavioral therapy (CBT) for obsessive-compulsive disorder (OCD), where there is hyperactivity producing symptoms. On the same basis of suppressing overactive neurons there was less activity in the limbic and paralimbic regions after CBT for phobia. After effective treatment with antidepressants, as selective serotonin reuptake inhibitors for OCD and phobia, similar effects were seen, pointing to shared biological pathways between psychotherapy and medication [21]. Unfortunately, explanations may not be so obvious and well localized functionally and structurally in every disease entity. In the case of major depressive disorder (MDD) there are heterogeneous results across studies and also across treatment approaches. This provides further evidence of the complexity of the brain's workings and the necessity for more advanced techniques to more accurately monitor the emergence and evolution of mental disorders as they are treated.

Achievements in anatomical and functional neuroimaging studies have allowed us to take a few steps backward to move forward in psychiatry. We have seemingly moved backwards from the end level of disease expression, i.e., psychopathological symptoms, on which the diagnostic criteria for mental illnesses are still based today, to the pathomechanisms of their formation. Today, research in psychiatry is at a fascinating juncture, when from bedside to bench we are trying to figure out the causes and structural and functional errors at a very subtle and complex level of the formation of mental disorders. Thanks to modern neuroimaging research, we know that the brain functions as an extremely complex network of neuronal circuits. Thanks to a new scientific discipline, imaging genetics, it is being studied how genes affect information processing in specific brain circuits.

4.1 Development of Brain Stimulation Methods

Continuing progress in the field of neurophysiology, radiology, psychiatry, neurology, neurosurgery and biomedical engineering, which has been progressing for several decades, results in the creation of new ways of neurons stimulation. These methods significantly enrich the range of therapeutic interventions used in psychiatry, finding, apart from pharmacotherapy and psychotherapy, an increasingly wider application in the treatment of mental disorders.

The use of electricity in psychiatry stemmed from the helplessness and lack of effective treatments for patients. Electroshock was first used by Ugo Cerletti and Lucio Bini in 1938 on a patient with paranoid schizophrenia, achieving a cessation of manufacturing symptoms after several applications. The aim was not to stimulate but to induce epileptic seizures. Much earlier, in 1891, Klemens Maleszewski, a Polish physician in Vilnius, used an electric current from a galvanic cell to successfully treat a patient with catatonia [22]. Today, electroconvulsive therapy (ECT), thanks to the use of anesthesia (since 1951), is used painlessly mainly in patients with depression and schizophrenia, especially catatonic patients resistant to treatment. Its efficacy is high [23], trials among patients with treatment-resistant depression have shown pooled response rates of 60–80% and pooled remission rates of 50–60%, whereas among patients with treatment-resistant schizophrenia, ECT efficacy rates ranged from 40 to 70%. The incompletely understood mechanism of action of electroconvulsive therapy exemplifies the complexity of brain function. In depressed patients treated with ECT, structural changes were found (increased gray matter volume in frontal-limbic areas, including the hippocampus and amygdala). In turn, diffusion tensor studies showed increased integrity of white matter pathways in frontal and temporal areas [23]. Increased neurogenesis, synaptogenesis, and BDNF factor have been shown in animal models. More advanced studies are currently underway with the analysis of gene expression, use of multimodal neuroimaging, and "omics" studies [24]. The pathogenesis of mental disorders, including depression or schizophrenia, are still being investigated, and the mechanism of action of ECT, which has shown great clinical effectiveness is still not fully explored.

Nevertheless, more subtle or more precise methods of biologically affecting brain tissue have emerged in parallel. Modern psychoneuromodulation is quite a young method, when in 1995 M. George described the changes in mood after using transcranial magnetic stimulation (TMS) [25]. TMS was approved for the treatment of depression in 2008. The first deep brain stimulation (DBS) treatments of the Anterior Limb of Internal Capsule (ALIC) area were performed by Bart Nuttin in 1999 on patients with obsessive-compulsive disorder. In 2009, DBS of the ALIC area in the treatment of OCD was found to be effective [26].

4.2 Transcranial Magnetic Stimulation

The transcranial magnetic stimulation is a process in which the device creates an interaction of neurons with a strong magnetic field (with a local intensity of up to 3 tesla), generated by the magnetic coil applied to the head. The depth of such an interaction is limited (up to 4 cm), therefore, TMS can stimulate the cerebral cortex and the spinal cord only. The magnetic field induces changes in the electric field in the brain, which significantly affects the polarity and excitability of neurons. Exposure to low-frequency pulses (1–5 Hz) has an inhibitory effect on neurons, while high frequency (≥5 Hz) stimulates neurons. The studies on mechanism of magnetic stimulation showed changes at the level of individual neurons as well as on whole neural circuity. The diversity of TMS protocols are currently being tested, in which repetitive pulses of the same frequency (repetitive TMS, rTMS) or a series of high-frequency pulses and a relatively small amplitude are used (theta burst stimulation, TBS). The protocols also differ in the frequency of stimulation sessions - the accelerated TMS (aTMS) is currently investigated, in which up to four sessions per day are performed in order to obtain a rapid clinical response. Another approach is to carry out high-frequency stimulations first, before low-frequency sessions - the priming TMS (pTMS). Thanks to the progress in the reduction of artefacts in the electroencephalographic record (EEG) during TMS, the possibility of pulse synchronization with the patient's alpha rhythm synchronized TMS (sTMS) was also created [25]. Different designs of coil shape allow an influence on larger group of neurons or the inclusion of deeper brain structures into the magnetic field. The H-coil in the shape of a helmet, which allows a stimulation of up to approximately 5 cm deep into the brain tissue, the deep TMS (dTMS). Recurrent depression and schizophrenia are the primary psychiatric indications for TMS use, although the range of uses is expanding as new TMS protocols are developed and research into the pathophysiology of mental diseases advances.

TMS, on the other hand, is a non-invasive method of brain stimulation that is very well tolerated, with few transient side effects like headache and very rare complications. Thanks to advances in the development of new therapeutic protocols, TMS is finding clinical application in an ever-widening spectrum of psychiatric disorders such as recurrent depression, bipolar affective disorder, schizophrenia, cognitive dysfunction, and post-traumatic stress disorder.

Last meta-analyses proved that patients with different mental disorders may benefit from non-invasive brain stimulation (NIBS), which includes transcranial magnetic stimulation (TMS) and transcranial direct current stimulation (tDCS). Based on 208 RCTs, Hyde et al. conducted a number of random effects meta-analyses to evaluate the effectiveness of NIBS in comparison to sham. In generalized anxiety disorder, obsessive-compulsive disorder, and unipolar depressive symptoms, they confirmed significant favorable effects of TMS; in substance use disorder, they confirmed significant positive effects of tDCS. There was only conclusive evidence for tDCS to enhance attention and working memory in schizophrenia patients in terms of neurocognitive outcomes [26].

4.3 Deep Brain Stimulation

Deep brain stimulation (DBS), unlike various methods of transcranial stimulation, requires a high degree of individualization. DBS involves using a pacemaker-like device to deliver constant electrical stimulation by electrodes to problematic areas within the brain.

Nowadays treatment-resistant obsessive-compulsive disorder (OCD) remains a main psychiatric indication for DBS. Many studies focus on the assessment of efficacy and safety of this method in different mental disorders, including depressive disorders, Alzheimer's disease, anorexia nervosa, Tourette syndrome, substance addiction or aggressive behaviors. Single cases of successful treatment in bipolar disorder, schizophrenia, and post-traumatic stress disorder also emerged in recent years. During recent years, many different brain regions have been suggested as possible targets for stimulation. In OCD striatal targets consist of ALIC, nucleus accumbens (NAc) [28], ventral capsule/ventral striatum (VC/VS), and ventral area of caudate nucleus. Another possible target is subthalamic nucleus (STN). Recent years brought proposition of new targets: bed nucleus of stria terminalis (BNST), inferior thalamic peduncle (ITP), and supero-lateral branch of the medial forebrain bundle (MFB) [27].

Personalized management at the preoperative stage of DBS involves, for example, the use of preoperative diffusion tensor imaging (DTI) within the structures planning to be stimulating, due to the considerable individual variability of particular brain areas (Fig. 2). Personalization of every combined therapy with DBS is necessary with exploration of individual factors as past traumas and personality traits and comorbidity [29].

Recently, it was suggested that the implementation of an adaptive DBS (aDBS) system should be taken into consideration. A prototype of such a system is currently being developed and tested; it is able to monitor local field potentials during DBS treatment and adjust stimulation parameters to further reduce obsessive ideations

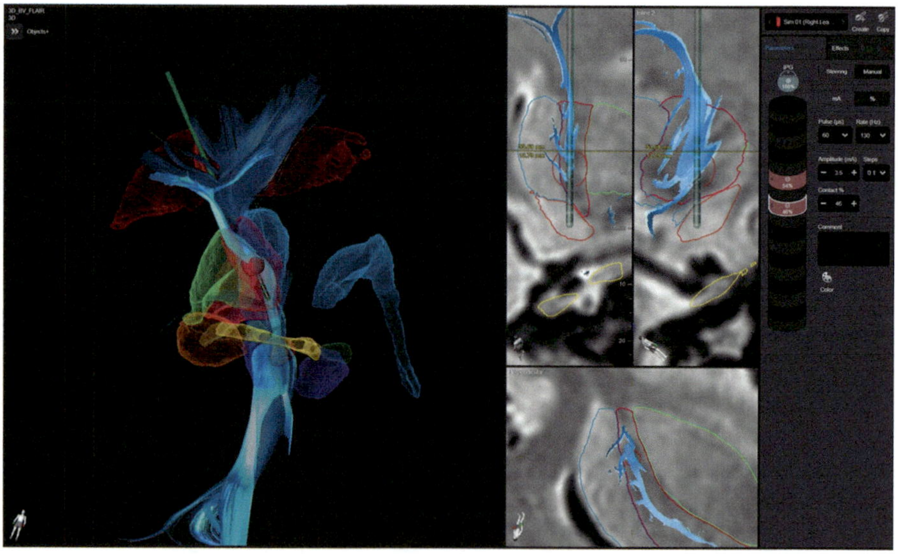

Fig. 2 Planning of deep brain stimulation in obsessive-compulsive disorder (OCD) using neuroimaging technics, structures of the basal nuclei, the Neurosurgery Clinic of the Wroclaw University Clinical Hospital (Fiber bundles of MFB in blue, optic chiasm in yellow, red sphere – activation field from the electrode)

and compulsive behaviors, as well as to lower the risk of adverse effects in the form of acute mood changes, including hypomania. Utilizing an automated facial recognition tool will help quickly identify mood swings. Whereas the dynamic nature of mental disorders is not adequately addressed by tonic continuous stimulation; symptoms may change over the course of minutes to days.

There has also been some focus on improving DBS treatment through the addition of postoperative cognitive behavioral therapy (CBT). Many patients claim that during stimulation they are able to engage in CBT exercises, which have an even greater impact in terms of OCD symptom reduction, even though the majority of patients are either unable to get CBT before DBS therapy or it is unsuccessful.

We know that most of the neuroanatomical centers regulating mood, affect, and motivation are interconnected. Neuromodulatory methods, even as seemingly locally acting as DBS, can affect, regardless of the immediate target, distant centers thanks to the interconnections of neuronal networks. On the one hand, this is an advantage, and on the other hand, a great difficulty in the unambiguous assessment of the mechanisms of action. This represents one of the most important research challenges in neuromodulation. The exact mechanism of stimulation's effect on neurons is still under investigation. Changes occur at the level of individual neurons, as well as within the entire neuronal network, and involve neurotransmitters as well as neuroplasticity. In addition, effects occurring immediately after stimulation, as well as deferred in time, are observed. Both of these facts testify to the high complexity of the effects of these methods as well as the pathomechanisms of mental disorders. Despite much research and initial enthusiasm, to date DBS in depression is not a method recognized as fully effective, and the most appropriate stimulation areas and their parameters are still being sought. Tractography and functional neuroimaging techniques can provide valuable information for treatment planning and monitoring during the stimulation period. Identification of individual clinical characteristics and biomarkers of treatment response requires research.

Considering that mental disorders are neural network disorders of brain function with very complex causes, research is being conducted on stimulation involving more and more new hypotheses and solutions, including machine learning (ML). These may in time not only lead to greater effectiveness of the stimulations used, but also uncover pathomechanisms of disorders. Evidence from studies of DBS for treatment-resistant depression shows that antidepressant effects happen in two stages: a rapid shift in depressive mood and psychomotor retardation with initial bilateral stimulation at the optimized target within the white matter, and a slower, more gradual improvement in symptom ratings over weeks to months that, if achieved, is usually maintained long-term.

Changes in the severity of depressive symptoms and their significant periodic dynamics are typical of the natural course of this disorder. High variability in recovery trajectories is also frequently observed in DBS patients [29]. Neuman et al. evaluated usefulness of patterns of local field potential (LFP) activity in the limbic system of MDD and OCD patients with DBS. They found that α-activity in the limbic system may serve as a potential state biomarker for closed-loop DBS in MDD but not in OCD [30].

Through the combination of recording behavioral changes (self-report scales), imaging and electrophysiological techniques (e.g., intracranial electrophysiology data) that record daily or weekly online psychopathological symptoms of the patient, it will be possible in the future to adjust stimulation parameters in a more precise way.

The physiological or behavioral markers to monitor this variation in recovery trajectories by understanding the changes in brain activity that underlie sustained recovery will be very useful [31]. Additionally, the markers will be very important in relation to adaptive neurotechnologies for closed-loop (CL) stimulation.

Large volumes of multimodal data have been gathered due to the growing interest in adaptive neuromodulation, and machine learning approaches have been used to provide insight [32]. During annual DBS Think Tank in 2022 researchers discussed about the "explainable artificial intelligence (xAI)" approaches, which can be introduced to analyze the complex data to identify potential biomarkers in complex neuromodulation therapies [31].

In addition to engaging machine learning and artificial intelligence to analyze big data, researchers are looking for single markers to implement adaptive BS using close-loop stimulation. Clark et al. [33] pointed out to a unique role for beta rhythms in the subgenual anterior cingulate cortex (sgACC), which is central to emotion processing circuits and exhibits hyperactivity in treatment-resistant depression (TRD). However, it is currently unknown how the spectrum pattern found relates to the high-frequency stimulation used to treat TRD and whether abnormal beta oscillations would return to normal following a successful DBS of the sgACC. Large-scale longitudinal studies are necessary to confirm if beta rhythms may eventually become a biomarker for regional hyperactivity and for responsive closed-loop neuromodulation systems.

The research group of Mayberg et al. presented the first longitudinal observations of local field potentials (LFP) from the subcallosal cingulate region outside the postoperative period. Their findings specifically showed that right hemisphere recordings appear sensitive to mood state. The frequency-domain 1/f activity is measurable in a combined DBS-LFP recording system, it can be potential biomarker considered in ongoing efforts to develop adaptive DBS delivery systems in mental disorders [34].

Attempts to implement DBS as a treatment for psychiatric disorders show the extraordinary complexity of the brain's functioning and the long road ahead leading to knowledge of this complexity. A sample of illustrating this complexity can be a clinical case study at the same meeting of researchers. A specific cortico-striato-thalamo-cortical (CSTC) circuit, which includes the orbitofrontal cortex (OFC), head of the caudate, and dorsomedial nucleus of the thalamus, is linked to obsessive-compulsive disorder and hyperconnectivity. This hyperconnectivity is thought to be disrupted by traditional DBS at the FDA-approved ventral capsule/ventral striatum (VC/VS) target for treatment-resistant OCD. Using bilateral cortical leads at the supplementary motor area (SMA) and the standard VC/VS target, researchers attempted to desynchronize this CSTC circuit. The results showed an immediate improvement in subjects' perceptions of their ability to focus away from obsessions. DBS for treatment-resistant OCD may be successful with multi-site stimulation with rather hypo-functioning CSTC loops augmented, than a disruption of a hyper-connected loop [31].

One of the authorities and leading DBS researchers, Prof. Helen Meyberg and colleagues recently published an article with the much-talked-about title: *From bed to bench side: Reverse translation to optimize neuromodulation for mood disorders* [35]. They stated that although DBS and other new neuromodulation techniques have showed a lot of promise, they have been slow to develop and there are still many unanswered concerns regarding how they work. They even content that reverse translation to nonhuman primates, which have a high degree of similarity to humans, is necessary for their continuous evolution. Using an animal model, specifically intracerebral microinfusions with cardiovascular and behavioral monitoring in marmoset monkeys Aleksander et al. demonstrated a causal role for primate sgACC/ area 25 over-activity in selective aspects of impaired reward processing translationally relevant to anhedonia, a core symptom of depression [36]. It is still unknown how chronically induced hyper- or hypo-activity of subcallosal ACC alters activity in related brain regions, but doing so may disclose biomarkers that could be utilized to regulate DBS stimulation adaptively. Neurostimulation methods represent a promising therapeutic approach related to intervention at the neuronal level of generating mental disorders. Perhaps they will become an alternative form of treatment, a therapy for treatment-resistant patients, and possibly a form of prevention. Given the 3 PM (predictive, preventive, and personalized medicine) concept, bench-to-bedside research in psychiatry should also focus on predicting individual predisposition to disorders, response to treatment, and relapse. The wide variation in the level of effectiveness of neuromodulation methods in psychiatric disorders indicates the need for a personalized approach to method selection and personalized treatment algorithms tailored to the individual. The effectiveness of neuromodulation methods will certainly depend on the identification of an individualized patient profile. Neuromodulation can also become one of the methods to protect the patient from another episode in the future. However, in order to fully realize the potential of neuromodulatory methods in the prevention and personalized treatment of mental disorders, close cooperation between researchers in the clinical and basic sciences is essential.

5 Current and Future Perspectives in Neuropsychiatry

In psychiatry, we have a rather unique situation where, based on clinical symptoms and medical history, we diagnose mental disorders without a clear and full understanding of the pathomechanism and the cause. Then we implement treatment—mainly psychotherapy or/and pharmacotherapy, and those therapeutic methods are often effective, but to varying degrees. We do not fully know the mechanisms of action of these methods, or know only partially. It is not always possible to link the mechanism of action of the applied therapy with the pathomechanism of the disease, or they overlap only partially. Pharmacotherapy in mental disorders is also a kind of neuromodulation method. After several decades of development of psycho-pharmacotherapy, we have a number of doubts that need to be resolved in further scientific research.

In recent years, there has been considerable debate about antidepressant drugs summarized by Prof. Fava. According to him, antidepressant therapy can activate processes that are in opposition to the drug's initial, health impacts. In some cases, important clinical reactions can be observed during or after antidepressant treatment such as 1) early phase of treatment up to 6 weeks - paradoxical effects, switching to bipolar course, 2) during long-term treatment phase - same as in short term and additionally loss of antidepressant efficacy, delayed side effects, refractoriness) and in post-treatment phase - new withdrawal reactions, switching and persistent post-withdrawal disorder, resistance [37]. The oppositional model of tolerance proposed by Fava still awaits adequate pre-clinical and clinical research testing. This model provides a conceptual framework for unifying adverse clinical phenomena that may occur in some, not all, patients. Investigating the variables that are associated with the occurrence of adverse consequences of pharmacotherapy in certain patients will allow the implementation of predictive factors in the selection of the appropriate treatment method. According to Fava, it can be one of the most important tasks of current therapeutic research.

The reasons for the incomplete effectiveness of the therapies used are increasingly being sought. While constructing studies of the effectiveness of therapeutic methods, at the same time, individualized characteristics or factors are sought to predict a better or worse response to a particular treatment method.

One of the challenges in psychiatry is the different background of the same symptoms. Again, depression is a good example. The heterogeneity of the cause and course of depressive disorders clearly suggests different etiology and pathogenesis of these disorders. At the same time, this variation complicates therapeutic decision-making. Attempts have been made to use symptom profiles and look for biomarkers to develop clinically useful prognostic factors. So far, not enough have been clearly defined to enter the standards of practice [38]. Kessler et al. used ML models developed from self-reports of disease episode characteristics and comorbidities among respondents with major depressive disorder (MDD) over a lifetime. The authors claim that they predicted the persistence, chronicity, and severity of MDD with good accuracy and are superior to conventional methods.

According to Menke and many other previously mentioned researchers, machine learning or artificial intelligence could be a helpful solution for psychiatry [39]. The development of mental disorders is probably determined by combined effects of genetic predisposition and environmental adversity, which can alter gene regulation. These effects can lead to changes in functioning of cells and organs, including brain.

The idea of using artificial intelligence methods is to incorporate genetic variants contributing to the mental disorder, drug response, gene–environment interactions, biomarkers from blood, results of neuropsychological tests, and data from electronic health records. Important factors include also early life adversity and stressful life events as well as factors based on lifestyle, nutrition, and sport activity.

There are also proposals to use data from social media and smartphones (such as language, face reactions, monitoring behavior) to predict people at high risk of depression, suicide or psychosis, monitor well-being, etc. [39].

Social networking, virtual reality, digitally-delivered psychological therapies, chatbots, and other new technological advancements are already reshaping mental health services in unexpected ways [40]. Efforts should be directed toward the necessity for stronger evidence base of digital health technologies (DHTs) for privacy and security rules and for DHT efficacy and effectiveness in RCT studies toward proper validation, implementation, and clinical integration.

6 Conclusion and Recommendations

At this stage of knowledge we have, we can speak of psychiatry entering a new era of research. Neuroscience studies in psychiatry have brought it into the field of translational medicine [40]. Dealing with mankind mental problems, social relationship dysfunctions, and disturbances in the control emotions and behavior, psychiatry, and psychology has come a long way. This path has led from psychoanalysis and dissociation from medicine, through becoming enthralled with the first possibilities of pharmacotherapy, experiencing disappointment with the lack of sufficiently satisfying efficacy of drugs, psychotherapy, and new neuromodulatory methods to opening up to numerous fields of knowledge seemingly distant from psychiatry.

Research in the area of etiopathogenesis and pathomechanisms of mental disorders should and must open up to collaboration with basic science researchers. Large-scale research is needed that, relying on new technologies of machine counting and AI, will be able to make appropriate use of large databases. Otherwise, it will not be possible to accurately predict the onset and monitor the course of mental disorders and also to introduce effective prevention plans.

For a better understanding of the functioning of the mind, it is necessary to develop neuroimaging techniques and make them more widely available for clinical research.

The rapid development of new technological solutions based on digital health technologies and their rapid, widespread availability, in turn, may lead to haphazard and unsupported clinical research use in therapy and self-therapy. It can result in a delay in receiving the correct diagnosis and treatment for a person with a mental disorder.

Reaching again to a psychiatry that is personalized and oriented to the unique complexity of the human mind, recognizing its individuality, psychiatry with psychology draw from various fields related to neuroscience. We look forward to further scientific evidence allowing psychiatry to insert itself more boldly and fully into the modern therapy of accurately diagnosed mental problems, psychiatry having greater certainty of predictive, preventive, and personalized management of mental disorders.

References

1. Kandel ER (1998) A new intellectual framework for psychiatry. Am J Psychiatry 155(4):457–469. https://doi.org/10.1176/ajp.155.4.457
2. Institute of Health Metrics and Evaluation. Global Health Data Exchange (GHDx). https://vizhub.healthdata.org/gbd-results/. Accessed 14 May 2022
3. GBD (2019) Mental Disorders Collaborators. Global, regional, and national burden of 12 mental disorders in 204 countries and territories, 1990–2019: a systematic analysis for the Global Burden of Disease Study 2019. Lancet Psychiatry 10:2022. https://doi.org/10.1016/S2215-0366(21)00395-3
4. Lamers F, van Oppen P, Comijs HC et al (2011) Comorbidity patterns of anxiety and depressive disorders in a large cohort study: The Netherlands study of depression and anxiety (NESDA). J Clin Psychiatry 72:341. https://doi.org/10.4088/JCP.10m06176blu
5. Seo HJ, Jung YE, Kim TS, Kim JB, Lee MS, Kim JM, Lim HW, Jun TY (2011) Distinctive clinical characteristics and suicidal tendencies of patients with anxious depression. J Nerv Ment Dis 199(1):42–48. https://doi.org/10.1097/NMD.0b013e3182043b60
6. Chen LC, Chen YH, Bai YM, Chen TJ, Chen MH, Su TP (2020) Antidepressant resistance in adolescents with major depressive disorder: a nationwide longitudinal study. J Affect Disord 262:293–297. https://doi.org/10.1016/j.jad.2019.11.038
7. Furukawa TA, Efthimiou O, Weitz ES, Cipriani A, Keller MB, Kocsis JH, Klein DN et al (2018) Cognitive-behavioral analysis system of psychotherapy, drug, or their combination for persistent depressive disorder: personalizing the treatment choice using individual participant data network Metaregression. Psychother Psychosom 87(3):140–153. https://doi.org/10.1159/000489227
8. Wilson RS, Yung AR, Morrison AP (2020) Comorbidity rates of depression and anxiety in first episode psychosis: a systematic review and meta-analysis. Schizophr Res 216:216322–216329. https://doi.org/10.1016/j.schres.2019.11.035
9. Rahe C, Khil L, Wellmann J, Baune B, Arolt V, Berger K (2016) Impact of major depressive disorder, distinct subtypes, and symptom severity on lifestyle in the BiDirect study. Psychiatry Res 245:164–171. https://doi.org/10.1016/j.psychres.2016.08.035
10. Craddock N, Mynors-Wallis L (2014) Psychiatric diagnosis: impersonal, imperfect and important. Br J Psychiatry 204(2):93–95. https://doi.org/10.1192/bjp.bp.113.133090
11. Biomarker Working Group F-N (2016) In: Spring S (ed) BEST (biomarkers, endpoints, and other tools) resource. FDA-NIH, Silver Spring, MD
12. Llerena A, Berecz R, Dorado P, de la Rubia A (2004) QTc interval, CYP2D6 and CYP2C9 genotypes and risperidone plasma concentrations. J Psychopharmacol 18(2):189–193. https://doi.org/10.1177/0269881104042618
13. Hartwig FP, Borges MC, Horta BL, Bowden J, Smith GD (2017) Inflammatory biomarkers and risk of schizophrenia: a 2-sample Mendelian randomization study. JAMA Psychiatry 74(12):1226–1233. https://doi.org/10.1001/jamapsychiatry.2017.3191
14. European Medicines Agency (EMA) (2007) ICH Topic E15 Definitions for genomic biomarkers, pharmacogenomics, pharmacogenetics, genomic data and sample coding categories
15. Stahl EA, Breen G, Forstner AJ, McQuillin A, Ripke S, Trubetskoy V et al (2019) Genome-wide association study identifies 30 loci associated with bipolar disorder. Nat Genet 51:793–803. https://doi.org/10.1038/s41588-019-0397-8
16. Chimienti F, Cavarec L, Vincent L, Salvetat N, Arango V, Underwood MD et al (2019) Brain region-specific alterations of RNA editing in PDE8A mRNA in suicide decedents. Transl Psychiatry 9(1):91. https://doi.org/10.1038/s41398-018-0331-3
17. Rodrigues-Amorim D, Rivera-Baltanás T, Vallejo-Curto MDC, Rodriguez-Jamardo C, De las Heras E, Barreiro-Villar C et al (2019) Proteomics in schizophrenia: a gateway to discover potential biomarkers of psychoneuroimmune pathways. Front Psych 10:885. https://doi.org/10.3389/fpsyt.2019.00885
18. Czysz AH, South C, Gadad BS, Arning E, Soyombo A, Bottiglieri T, Trivedi MH (2019) Can targeted metabolomics predict depression recovery? Results from the CO-MED trial.

Transl Psychiatry 9:11. PMID: 30664617; PMCID: PMC6341111. https://doi.org/10.1038/s41398-018-0349-6
19. García-Giménez JL, Seco-Cervera M, Tollefsbol TO, Romá-Mateo C, Peiró-Chova L, Lapunzina P, Pallardó FV (2017) Epigenetic biomarkers: current strategies and future challenges for their use in the clinical laboratory. Crit Rev Clin Lab Sci 54(7–8):529–550. https://doi.org/10.1080/10408363.2017.1410520
20. Malhotra S, Sahoo S (2017) Rebuilding the brain with psychotherapy. Indian J Psychiatry 59(4):411–419. https://doi.org/10.4103/0019-5545.217299
21. Nasierowski T (2002) Klemens Maleszewski – pionier terapii elektrowstrząsowej w psychiatrii polskiej. Psychiatr Pol 36:259–269
22. Espinoza RT, Kellner CH (2022) Electroconvulsive therapy. N Engl J Med 386(7):667–672. https://doi.org/10.1056/NEJMra2034954
23. Li M, Yao X, Sun L, Zhao L, Xu W, Zhao H et al (2020) Effects of electroconvulsive therapy on depression and its potential mechanism. Front Psychol 11:80. https://doi.org/10.3389/fpsyg.2020.00080
24. Wieczorek T, Kobyłko A, Stramecki F, Fila-Witecka K, Beszłej J, Jakubczyk M, Piotrowski P, Senczyszyn A, Siwicki D, Szcześniak D, Rymaszewska J (2021) Transcranial magnetic stimulation (TMS) in treatment of psychiatric disorders - review of current studies. Psychiatr Pol 55(3):565–583. https://doi.org/10.12740/PP/OnlineFirst/115556
25. Beszłej JA, Wieczorek T, Kobyłko A, Piotrowski P, Siwicki D, Weiser A, Fila-Witecka K, Rymaszewska J, Tabakow P (2019) Deep brain stimulation: new possibilities for the treatment of mental disorders. Psychiatr Pol 53(4):789–806. https://doi.org/10.12740/PP/OnlineFirst/103090
26. Hyde J, Carr H, Kelley N, Seneviratne R, Reed C, Parlatini V et al (2022) Efficacy of neurostimulation across mental disorders: systematic review and meta-analysis of 208 randomized controlled trials. Mol Psychiatry 27(6):2709–2719. https://doi.org/10.1038/s41380-022-01524-8
27. Beszłej JA, Siwicki D, Fila-Witecka K, Wieczorek T, Piotrowski P, Weiser A, Tabakow P, Rymaszewska J (2019) Deep brain stimulation in obsessive-compulsive disorder—case report of two patients. Psychiatr Pol 53(4):807–824. https://doi.org/10.12740/PP/104643
28. Rymaszewska J, Wieczorek T, Fila-Witecka K, Smarzewska K, Weiser A, Piotrowski P, Tabakow P (2023) Various neuromodulation methods including deep brain stimulation of the medial forebrain bundle combined with psychopharmacotherapy of treatment-resistant depression-case report. Front Psych 13:1068054. https://doi.org/10.3389/fpsyt.2022.1068054
29. Neumann WJ, Huebl J, Brücke C, Gabriëls L, Bajbouj M, Merkl A, Schneider GH, Nuttin B, Brown P, Kühn AA (2014) Different patterns of local field potentials from limbic DBS targets in patients with major depressive and obsessive compulsive disorder. Mol Psychiatry 19(11):1186–1192. https://doi.org/10.1038/mp.2014.2
30. Wong JK, Deuschl G, Wolke R, Bergman H, Muthuraman M, Groppa S et al (2022) Proceedings of the ninth annual deep brain stimulation think tank: advances in cutting edge technologies, artificial intelligence, neuromodulation, Neuroethics, pain, interventional psychiatry, epilepsy, and traumatic brain injury. Front Hum Neurosci 16:813387. https://doi.org/10.3389/fnhum.2022.813387
31. O'Shaughnessy M, Canal G, Connor M, Rozell C, Davenport M (2020) Generative causal explanations of black-box classifiers. Adv Neural Inf Proces Syst 33:5453–5467
32. Clark DL, Brown EC, Ramasubbu R, Kiss ZHT (2016) Intrinsic local Beta oscillations in the Subgenual cingulate relate to depressive symptoms in treatment-resistant depression. Biol Psychiatry 80(11):e93–e94. https://doi.org/10.1016/j.biopsych.2016.02.032
33. Veerakumar A, Tiruvadi V, Howell B, Waters AC, Crowell AL, Voytek B, Riva-Posse P, Denison L, Rajendra JK, Edwards JA, Bijanki KR, Choi KS, Mayberg HS (2019) Field potential 1/*f*activity in the subcallosal cingulate region as a candidate signal for monitoring deep brain stimulation for treatment-resistant depression. J Neurophysiol 122(3):1023–1035. https://doi.org/10.1152/jn.00875.2018
34. Rudebeck PH, Rich EL, Mayberg HS (2019) From bed to bench side: reverse translation to optimize neuromodulation for mood disorders. Proc Natl Acad Sci U S A 116(52):26288–26296. https://doi.org/10.1073/pnas.1902287116

35. Alexander L, Gaskin PLR, Sawiak SJ, Fryer TD, Hong YT, Cockcroft GJ, Clarke HF, Roberts AC (2019) Fractionating blunted reward processing characteristic of anhedonia by over-activating primate Subgenual anterior cingulate cortex. Neuron 101(2):307–320.e6. https://doi.org/10.1016/j.neuron.2018.11.021
36. Fava GA (2020) May antidepressant drugs worsen the conditions they are supposed to treat? The clinical foundations of the oppositional model of tolerance. Ther Adv Psychopharmacol 10:1–11. https://doi.org/10.1177/2045125320970325
37. Menke A (2018) Precision pharmacotherapy: psychiatry's future direction in preventing, diagnosing, and treating mental disorders. Pharmgenomics Pers Med 11:211–222. https://doi.org/10.2147/PGPM.S146110
38. Nobis A, Zalewski D, Waszkiewicz N (2020) Peripheral markers of depression. J Clin Med 9(12):3793. https://doi.org/10.3390/jcm9123793
39. Torous J, Bucci S, Bell IH, Kessing LV, Faurholt-Jepsen M, Whelan P, Carvalho AF, Keshavan M, Linardon J, Firth J (2021) The growing field of digital psychiatry: current evidence and the future of apps, social media, chatbots, and virtual reality. World Psychiatry 20(3):318–335. https://doi.org/10.1002/wps.20883
40. Češková E, Šilhán P (2021) From personalized medicine to precision psychiatry? Neuropsychiatr Dis Treat 17:3663–3668. https://doi.org/10.2147/NDT.S337814

Development of Artificial Intelligence Algorithms to Analyse Weather Conditions for the Prediction of Cerebrovascular Accidents

Artur Kwiatkowski, Oliwer Sobolewski,
Agnieszka Wyłomańska, Marek Sawicki, Piotr Zieleń,
Adam Druszcz, and Mariusz Ptak

Abbreviations

ADAM	Adaptive Moment Estimation
AI	Artificial intelligence
AIM	Artificial Intelligence in Medicine
ALS	Amyotrophic lateral sclerosis
CNN	Convolutional neural networks
DL	Deep learning
EBM	Evidence-based medicine
NLP	Natural Language Processing
PPPM/3PM	Predictive, preventive, and personalised medicine
SGM	Stochastic gradient descent

A. Kwiatkowski · A. Druszcz
Department of Neurosurgery, Provincial Specialist Hospital in Legnica, Legnica, Poland
e-mail: artur.kwiatkowski@szpital.legnica.pl; adam.druszcz@szpital.legnica.pl

O. Sobolewski · M. Sawicki · M. Ptak (✉)
Faculty of Mechanical Engineering, Wroclaw University of Science and Technology, Wroclaw, Poland
e-mail: 247291@student.pwr.edu.pl; sawicki.marek@pwr.edu.pl; mariusz.ptak@pwr.edu.pl

A. Wyłomańska · P. Zieleń
Faculty of Pure and Applied Mathematics, Wroclaw University of Science and Technology, Wroclaw, Poland
e-mail: agnieszka.wylomanska@pwr.edu.pl; 255752@student.pwr.edu.pl

H. Podbielska, M. Kapalla (eds.), *Predictive, Preventive, and Personalised Medicine: From Bench to Bedside*, Advances in Predictive, Preventive and Personalised Medicine 17, https://doi.org/10.1007/978-3-031-34884-6_16

1 Introduction

Human life and health are undoubtedly the two most important values in the modern world. In order to provide better and better means of protecting them, medicine must constantly develop. It is, therefore, not surprising that modern research methods are increasingly being used to understand the functioning of the human body better. Neural networks have turned out to be one of the most effective tools to support decision-making regarding human health, as their operation is similar to the reasoning of doctors making a diagnosis. As a result of the rapid development of artificial intelligence algorithms over the last decade, the application of artificial intelligence-based medical systems in practice is constantly growing and bringing more and more benefits to humanity.

In the practice of medical doctors dealing with the treatment of vascular diseases analysed in this work, i.e., cardiologists, neurologists, neurosurgeons, angiologists, vascular surgeons, there is a belief that some cases co-occur with weather conditions. Higher than usual incidence rates are sometimes observed during the passage of a weather front, yet the association of an increased incidence of vascular events with the passage of a weather front has never been scientifically fully established. This study is one of the first in the literature to demonstrate weather parameter correlations with cerebrovascular accidents. To date, there is a limited number of publications where machine learning is used to analyse weather conditions in predicting cerebrovascular accidents—the recent works of Wlodaczyk and Molek et al. shall be acknowledged [1, 2].

1.1 Artificial Intelligence in Medicine

Despite the fact that artificial intelligence algorithms have been known since the 1950s, machine learning methods became popular in medicine only a dozen years ago. The limits imposed by early models made them useless in medicine, because the degree of complexity of phenomena occurring in living organisms was too high for them. Only the development of algorithms allowing for self-learning networks and the concept of deep neural networks in the early twenty-first century caused the abolition of these limits, allowing artificial intelligence algorithms to be widely used in medicine, also in the context of predictive, preventive, and personalised medicine (PPPM/3PM) [3, 4]. Methods from the field of artificial intelligence AI pose a great opportunity to drive the transition toward the PPPM paradigm [5]. Another factor driving research in this area of knowledge was the increase in computing power and memory in computers used for calculations, in accordance with Moore's law, as well as the exponential growth of statistical data collected by various authorities, serving as input data sets for model training.

Artificial intelligence in medicine (AIM) has evolved significantly over the last 50 years. Thanks to the advent of deep learning (DL) algorithms, the current field of AIM applications has greatly expanded, allowing the creation of personalised and dynamically responsive therapies instead of universal and static, based on rigid treatment algorithms used so far. Another application of AIM is the creation of predictive models used to diagnose diseases, predict treatment effects, and estimate the chances of occurrence of a given disease entity. Artificial intelligence can also contribute to improving the accuracy of diagnoses, increase the efficiency of clinical trials of drugs, as well as provide better monitoring of the course of diseases and the general health of patients. This paper addresses an important and timely topic of using artificial intelligence to create a predictive model that will be able to assess the risk of vascular incidents based on the collected environmental data.

1.2 The History of the Development of Artificial Intelligence in Medicine

The very idea of using computers to simulate intelligent life appeared in the 1950s, thanks to Alan Turing. In the book "Computing machinery and intelligence," he tried to answer the question "can machines think?" thus developing the assumptions for the famous "Turing test" [6]. This test, called by the author himself "the game of imitation," consists in asking questions by the interrogator to two individuals—another human and a machine. The machine passes the test, and therefore "has human intelligence," if the interrogator is unable to determine with certainty which of the interrogated persons is human. Unquestionably, at that time, there were no machines or algorithms that could even take part in such a test, but the interesting fact is that even today no artificial intelligence algorithm has fully passed the Turing test. This may suggest that the creation of "real" intelligence is still a distant task for humanity.

Among researchers, it is generally accepted that artificial intelligence was born together with the first robots [7]. In fact, to this day, artificial intelligence is inseparably associated with robotics for most people, mainly due to popular science-fiction movies and books. Of course, this assumption is not unfounded, because early discoveries in the field of AI were focused precisely on the development of machines with the ability to make decisions that previously only humans could make.

The first industrial robot, "Unimate," began working on the General Motors production line in 1961, where it was used to automate the die-casting process. Just 3 years later, in 1964, Joseph Weizenbaum created the first social robot named Eliza. Eliza was able to communicate using pattern matching and substitution algorithms to mimic human conversations. This way of superficial communication is at the heart of today's chatterbots [8].

In 1966, "Shakey" was created, often referred to as "the first electronic person." Unlike Unimate, this mobile robot was able to interpret complex commands and create an algorithm from simple instructions that must be performed to fulfill the given command. It was a milestone in both robotics and artificial intelligence [9].

Unfortunately, it was also the beginning of the almost two-decade "AI Winter." At that time, AI lost interest in most of the scientific community due to the lack of development of solutions to the limitations and problems of neural networks discovered in the late 1960s—mainly the lack of self-learning capabilities—and later due to the high cost of maintaining huge databases needed to effectively train models.

However, the development of AI did not stop completely, and it was then that the idea of using its methods in medicine was born. In 1976, a consultation program for patients with glaucoma was created using the CASNET (Casual-Associative Network) model. This program was able to analyse the data from the patient's observations and link them with the information stored in the database regarding the patient's disease, and then advise the doctor on the next steps to be taken with the patient [10].

In a similar period, the expert artificial intelligence system with backward chaining MYCIN was developed. Backward reasoning is similar in concept to the technique people use to solve problems by testing hypotheses [11]. An example is a doctor who, suspecting certain problems in a patient, makes hypotheses about his disease and tries to prove them by looking for specific symptoms. The MYCIN system worked in the same way—using information about the patient from the preliminary research and a knowledge base of around 600 rules, the algorithm could generate a list of potential bacterial pathogens and recommend an appropriate course of antibiotics based on the patient's age and weight. This system operated on a similar level of competence as human blood infection specialists and was usually even better than general practitioners. The MYCIN systems and their successor EMYCIN had a significant impact on the development of artificial intelligence, because they were the pioneer structures of the rule-based expert system, which is still widely used in various industries today [12].

In 1986, the DXplain decision support system was developed at the University of Massachusetts. This program is an excellent learning tool for internists, because it is able to generate a differential diagnosis based on the symptoms observed in the patient, and at the same time it acts as an electronic encyclopaedia of diseases. At the time of its launch, the system contained information on about 500 diseases, and today the database has been extended to over 2400 different diseases [8].

The next 20 years did not bring any significant applications for artificial intelligence in medicine. However, in 2007 IBM created a question-answering system called Watson, and interest in using AI in the medical community increased again [13]. The breakthrough of the Watson system was moving away from the idea of backward reasoning and abandoning the rule-based system, and adopting the new, rapidly developing DeepQA technology. This technology uses Natural Language Processing (NLP) methods and various search algorithms to analyse unstructured data to generate likely answers. It was quickly noticed that DeepQA technology could be used to process information contained in electronic health records of patients and obtain evidence-based conclusions (Evidence-Based Medicine–EBM). This paved the way for evidence-based clinical decision support systems. Such systems quickly became popular, and one of their greatest successes was the identification of new RNA-binding proteins found in amyotrophic lateral sclerosis (ALS).

Taking advantage of the success of new artificial intelligence technologies, as well as modern and very fast computer equipment, digital medicine has become much more accessible, and artificial intelligence systems in medicine have started to develop rapidly. As a result, recent years have brought many medical applications for artificial intelligence methods. The trend of using CNNs (convolutional neural networks) to analyse images in order to report the health of patients and detect signs of disease is particularly noticeable. Practically implemented algorithms have improved the accuracy, consistency, and efficiency of X-ray and MRI image analysis. An example of this type of system is CardioAI, the first product of the American company Arterys and at the same time the first DL system supporting clinical decision-making approved by the US Food and Drug Administration. CardioAI analyses magnetic resonance spectroscopy images of the heart in seconds, almost instantly providing the cardiologist with all the information necessary to make a diagnosis.

Artificial intelligence has come a very long way since its inception, and its incredibly dynamic development in recent years offers an exciting vision of automating many areas of life that previously seemed impossible to automate. Such as area is medicine—replacing a doctor with a robotic assistant is an idea straight from a science-fiction book, and the current trend of AIM development shows more and more that it can come true. Figure 1 depicts the timeline of the development of artificial intelligence in medicine. A slightly more mundane and realistic vision is to use AI to facilitate the work of doctors, especially in tasks involving data analysis and drawing conclusions based on them. The prediction model created as part of this diploma thesis is part of both of these ideas to some extent—linking environmental data with the occurrence of a given disease entity can help doctors assess the number of patients, allowing them to prepare for their admission, and at the same time helps patients from the risk group to take appropriate health decisions.

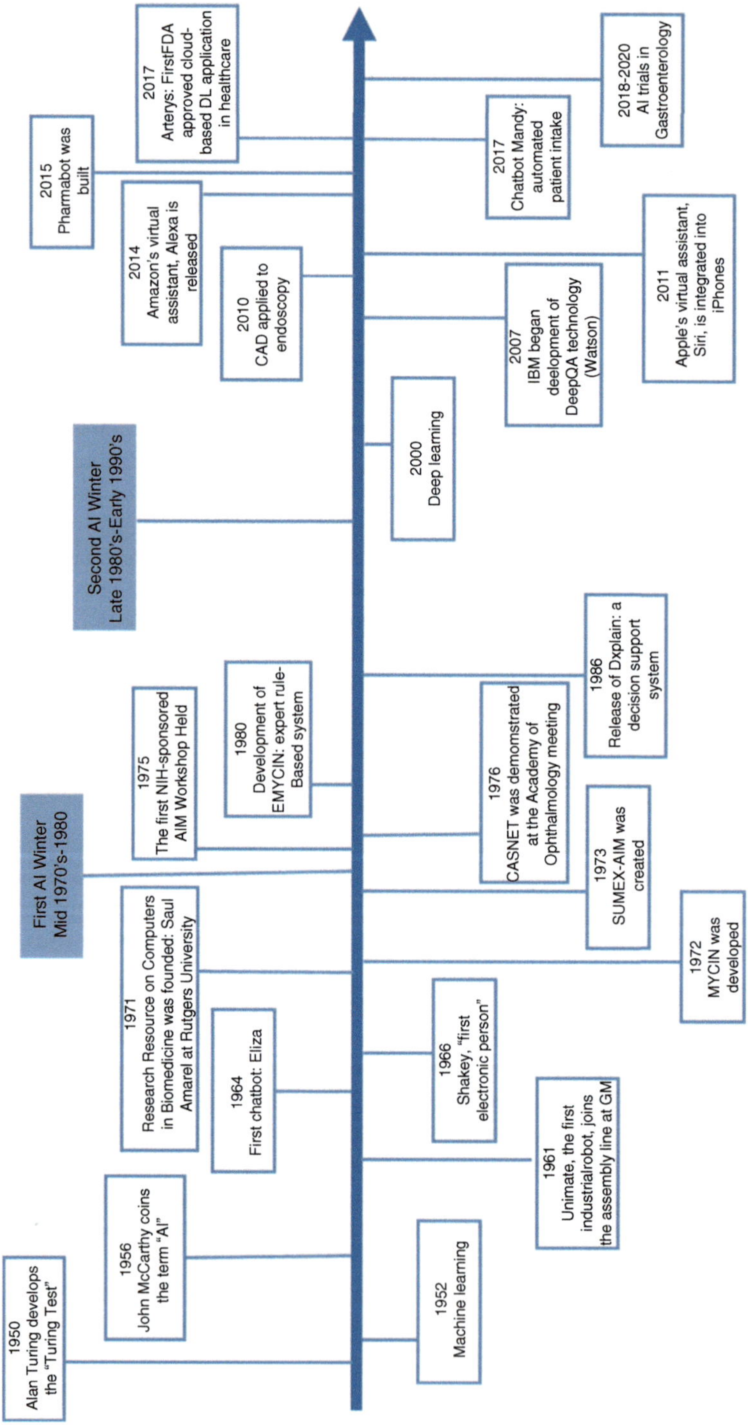

Fig. 1 Timeline of the development of artificial intelligence in medicine, based on [14]

2 Pathophysiology of Vascular Diseases

The main aim of the work is to determine the strength of the influence of environmental conditions on the occurrence of vascular diseases. In order to properly understand this impact and the implications of the predictive model, it is first necessary to understand the mechanisms behind these diseases and their consequences. In the human body, blood circulation in two independent circuits is forced by the work of the heart. The heart cycle consists of a synchronised contraction of the atria, which pumps blood into the ventricles, followed by a contraction of the ventricles 120–220 ms later, which pumps blood to the pulmonary arteries and aorta. Backflow of blood is prevented by valves between the atria and the ventricles and between the main ventricles by the arteries coming from the heart. The small blood circulation begins in the right ventricle, from which blood is pumped through the pulmonary arteries to the capillaries of the lungs. There, it is oxygenated, releases carbon dioxide previously collected from the tissues, and then returns through the pulmonary veins to the heart, to the left atrium. The large circulation of blood begins in the left ventricle, from which the aorta pumps blood to the peripheral arteries of all the organs of the body. After flowing through the capillary network and other specialised arteriovenous connections, it returns through the veins to the right atrium of the heart.

The rate of blood circulation is reflexively regulated by modifying the frequency of heart contractions and the tension of the elastic walls of arterial and venous vessels. The heart rate, depending on the body's energy needs, ranges from 50 to over 200 beats/min. The arterial blood pressure in adults at rest is between 90 and 140 mmHg during systole and between 60 and 90 mmHg during diastole. The difference between the systolic and diastolic pressures creates a pulse wave traveling from the heart along the arteries and creates positive pressure in the veins. Due to the fact that the heart as a pump does not have a suction phase, but only fills under the influence of the pressure prevailing in the venous system, the veins below the level of the right atrium are equipped with valves that prevent the backflow of blood under the influence of gravity [15].

2.1 The Structure of Arterial and Venous Walls and Normal Blood Pressure in Arteries and Veins

Due to the large differences between the pressure values prevailing in various segments of the circulatory system, the structure of the vessel walls and their mechanical properties correspond to the performed functions. A section through the arterial wall reveals its layered structure. From the outside, this wall consists of:

1. Adventitia—collagen tissue surrounding the arteries, which performs supporting functions, and in larger arteries, also nourishing functions.
2. The middle layer—smooth muscle fibres arranged circularly, which, under the influence of nerve and hormonal impulses, allow you to change the diameter of

the vessel, as well as the susceptibility of the wall to pulse waves—blood pressure regulation.
3. The inner layer, which is made of endothelial cells that ensure proper conditions for laminar blood flow in the vessel. Under normal conditions, this layer prevents blood coagulation by constantly secreting substances that inhibit thrombocyte aggregation and fibrinogen. When the endothelium is damaged, an enzymatic cascade reaction and blood coagulation occurs.

Apart from the essential cells of each layer, the vessel wall is reinforced with layers of elastic membrane. Compared to arteries, venous vessels have a much smaller layer of smooth muscles, their lumen is more susceptible to deformation caused by pressure from the outside, they can collapse under conditions of low pressure inside and expand under the influence of greater blood inflow. This construction enables a large range of regulation of the volume of blood returning to the heart during the work cycle (the so-called venous return), it is one of the mechanisms regulating the efficiency (amount of blood flow) in the circulatory system per unit of time.

Small arterial and venous vessels, as well as the smallest capillaries, consisting only of the endothelial layer, form an extensive network supplying blood to the tissues, where they form extensive surfaces for the exchange of gases and other substances [16, 17].

2.2 Pathophysiology of Atherosclerotic Plaque

The atherosclerotic process is a slow, multi-stage disease affecting the entire vascular system, but atherosclerosis of the aorta, coronary vessels, cerebral arteries, and arteries of the extremities has the greatest clinical significance. Damage to these vessels most often cannot be compensated by collateral circulation and leads to hypoxia and tissue necrosis of the corresponding organs.

The initiation of the atherosclerotic process is most often caused by local damage to the vessels caused by prolonged increased blood pressure, the presence of free radicals, and other toxic substances. Leukocytes, inflammatory mediators, and lipid compounds accumulate at the site of injury. The pathological inflammatory reaction causes muscle hypertrophy, aggregation of proteoglycans, and lipids. The inflammatory process leads to the death of the cells of the vascular wall, and their remnants form a necrotic core, which in a stable atherosclerotic plaque is covered with a layer of endothelium. As a result of the formation of atherosclerotic plaque, the lumen of the vessel is narrowed (internal remodelling) or the external perimeter is enlarged with relative preservation of the lumen (external remodelling) [18]. Often both processes run in parallel.

The narrowing of the lumen of the vessel causes an increase in blood flow velocity, turbulence, and also an increase in pressure in the part in front of the atherosclerotic plaque. The formation of vessel thickening, even without narrowing its lumen, has a negative impact on mechanical parameters. In the advanced stage, often under the influence of an internal impulse (e.g., a spike in blood pressure) or an external stimulus (e.g., mechanical trauma), plaque ruptures damaging the inner layer of the vessel. This leads to the formation of a blood clot, and then either a local narrowing of the lumen or detachment of the embolic material and further blockage of the vessel. If the plaque is stiff, its cracking may cause tearing of the entire vessel wall and cause massive haemorrhage. Such an event lead to an organ stroke, ischemic (aka infarction) or haemorrhagic, respectively [19].

3 Analysed Vascular Diseases

3.1 Myocardial Infarction, Heart Attack

In developed societies, vascular diseases, including coronary atherosclerosis and myocardial infarction, are the most common cause of death. Medical classifications distinguish different clinical forms: transmural infarction and subendocardial infarction. The most dangerous and at the same time the most associated with atherosclerotic plaque rupture is transmural infarction, which occurs as a result of occlusion of a large coronary vessel. Due to the heart's high demand for oxygen, the closure of the blood supply quickly leads to damage to the heart's muscle cells (cardiomyocytes). The optimal method of treatment is to unblock the vessel as soon as possible, most often by balloon angioplasty in the haemodynamic laboratory of the hospital. The time of performing this procedure is a critical parameter of treatment success and in medical analyses it is measured in minutes that elapsed between the arrival of the patient in the hospital and the expansion of the balloon in the vessel and the restoration of blood flow (door-to-balloon time). Proper preparation of the hospital and emergency teams, and earlier allocation of additional resources in situations of an increased number of myocardial infarctions, are of key importance for survival and avoiding disability in patients.

3.2 Cerebral Infarction, Ischemic Stroke

Ischemic stroke occurs both as a result of rupture of the atherosclerotic plaque, in a mechanism similar to myocardial infarction, and as a result of the ingress of embolic material from other parts of the vascular system. Closing a large vessel within a few minutes leads to irreversible hypoxia of the neurons. The areas of cerebral vascularisation partially overlap in such a way that in the event of a stroke, around the irreversibly damaged focus, there is an oxygen-depleted area, which, due to the proper blood flow in the adjacent vessels, is possible to save (so-called penumbra). Proper diagnosis and prompt treatment can save patients from death and severe neurological complications.

3.3 Haemorrhagic Stroke

The rupture of the vessel together with the plaque and haemorrhage into the brain tissues leads to the formation of an intracerebral hematoma. Extravasated blood damages the brain tissue both directly at the site of bleeding and in more distant areas as a result of compression and pressure increase in the closed space of the cranial cavity. Extensive bleeding is most often associated with irreversible disability and can lead to brain swelling and death of the patient. If treated promptly, the secondary effects of bleeding are somewhat alleviated.

3.4 Aortic and Peripheral Vascular Aneurysms

Disturbances in the structure of collagen, aging of collagen fibres in the vascular wall and high blood pressure that persists for years can lead to pathological vasodilatation, usually most visible in the area of the aorta and its largest branches. Uneven distribution of stress and different susceptibility of individual vessel layers, combined with locally very stiff, calcified atherosclerotic plaques, create conditions for vessel rupture—aneurysm rupture or internal damage to individual layers, their dissection and formation of an abnormal channel within the wall.

3.5 Pathophysiology of Intracranial Aneurysms

At rest, about 20% of the blood leaving the left ventricle is directed to the cerebral vessel. Due to the high flow through the cerebral vessels, their structure and functioning is slightly different than that of other peripheral arteries peripheral [20]. Two main pairs of vessels nourishing the brain: the internal carotid arteries and the vertebral arteries, have a sigmoid section at the entrance to the cranial cavity, and their internal structure differs from that of the other vessels, mainly in terms of the elastic and muscular layers. Aneurysms arising on cerebral vessels are mainly caused by genetic abnormalities in the synthesis of elastic fibres [21]. Then the weakened vessel wall bulges locally and an aneurysm sac is formed. In addition to genetic factors, the formation and enlargement of aneurysms is also influenced by environmental conditions, such as smoking, high blood pressure or amphetamine use [22]. As the aneurysm expands, its wall becomes thinner and more prone to rupture. This is usually triggered by an abrupt rise in the pressure gradient over the weakest point. Bleeding from a ruptured cerebral aneurysm is often a catastrophic event and leads to death or permanent disability.

All the described events have a well-known correlation with the arterial blood pressure. Any significant rise of this pressure may lead to the failure of the arteries previously damaged by chronic diseases. Arterial pressure is mostly related to the internal factors of the human body but there is also a possibility that external pressure changes may be the trigger, especially near the threshold levels.

4 Artificial Neural Networks

Artificial neural networks are the quintessence of deep learning models. To illustrate the difference between machine learning models and deep learning models, it is best to use the diagram shown in Fig. 2. It shows that the basic difference is the presence of additional layers of the model, whose task is to automatically detect

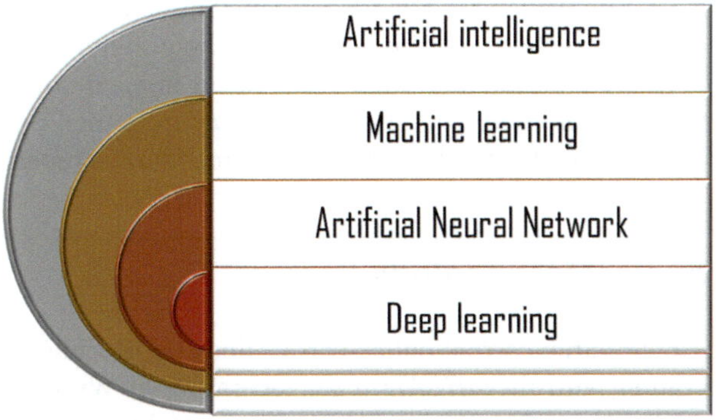

Fig. 2 Diagram showing the interrelationships between different concepts related to Artificial Intelligence. Deep learning is a subset of feature learning, which in turn is a subset of machine learning, which is used for many, but not all, approaches to implementing artificial intelligence

simple features and build on their basis more complex abstract features in subsequent layers. The number of parameters that need to be trained in a deep learning model is therefore much greater than in the case of a classic machine learning model.

The most basic model of neural networks are feedforward *neural networks*, specifically multilayer *perceptrons* (MLP). They are one-way because the flow of information is one-way—the function $f$is defined on the basis of data $x$whose output is y. In such a model, there is no feedback loop by which the output is fed back into the algorithm. Models that have feedback are called recurrent neural *networks*.

One-way neural networks are networks because they are represented as a network of interconnected functions. Their model is related to a directed acyclic graph describing the mutual relations of given functions. For example, the three functions $f^{(1)}$, $f^{(2)}$, and $f^{(3)}$are chained together to form the function $f(x) = f^{(3)}(f^{(2)}(f^{(1)}(x)))$. The chain structure is the most commonly used neural network structure - in this case, the function $f^{(1)}$is the first layer of the network, the function$f^{(2)}$ the second layer of the neural network, and the function$f^{(3)}$ third layer. The total number of features (string length) is called the depth of the model. The last layer of the neural network is the output layer of the model. The main task of the neural network is to approximate a certain function f^*, which is a real function describing the object. For this purpose, when training the model, it has the task of matching its function $f$to the function as much as possiblef^*. Each training example $x$has a label $y$for which $y \approx f^*(x)$. Thanks to this relationship, the network knows what the expected value $y$of the output layer is for each training example. The behavior of all other layers is not directly related to the training data—the model must independently use individual layers to create the best possible representation of the function f^*. Since the training data has an expected value only for the output layer, all other layers whose desired output values are unknown are called hidden layers.

Neural networks are called *neural networks* because they are loosely related to the neurological workings of the brain. Each hidden layer is typically a function vector. The dimensions of the hidden layers indicate the width of the model. Each element of the hidden layer vector can be interpreted as a single neuron, analogous to a biological neuron. These elements of the layer vector are simple functions and are called units. The units work in a similar way to neurons in the sense that they receive inputs from many other units of the previous layer and calculate their activation value based on them. Each unit in the layer runs in parallel and represents a function whose input is a vector of the previous layer's output and whose output is a single scalar. The values calculated in each unit are then placed in the output vector (feature vector) of the layer, which is then passed to each unit of the next layer in the chain, where the whole procedure is repeated.

5 Methodology

The research carried out as part of this engineering thesis was carried out in cooperation with the *aHEAD* team, operating at Wrocław University of Science and Technology [23]. Their main goal was to link environmental data, and more precisely, meteorological data, with the occurrence of vascular diseases. For this purpose, the appropriate data for the analysis was obtained, a machine learning model was designed and a neural network was trained. The obtained results were then analysed with statistical tools in order to calculate model quality indicators. The individual steps will be described in detail later in this chapter, yet the vision of data management utilised for the study is depicted in Fig. 3.

5.1 Data Acquisition

Designing any machine learning model starts with data acquisition. It was no different in this case. The data acquisition process began in June 2021 and took a few months. Gaining access to medical data has proven to be the most challenging task, as medical data is confidential. In order to obtain them, a method of providing them in an anonymous form had to be developed - this method will be described below.

5.2 Meteorological Data

The weather data were obtained from the Institute of Meteorology and Water Management and contain detailed weather data on environmental conditions over the years 2018–2019 for all weather stations in Poland (Fig. 4). The data was made available

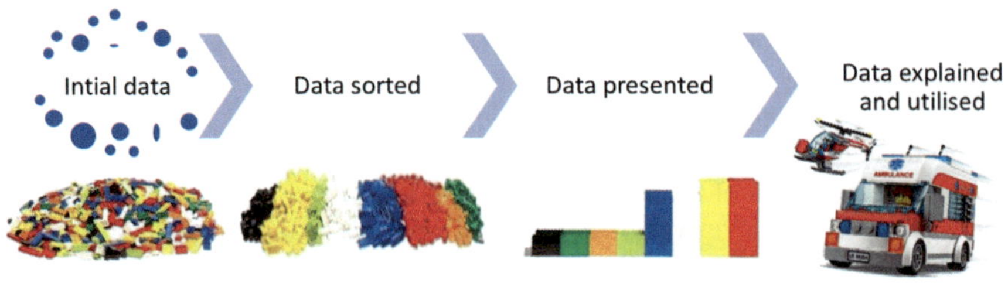

Fig. 3 The vision of data management utilised for the study

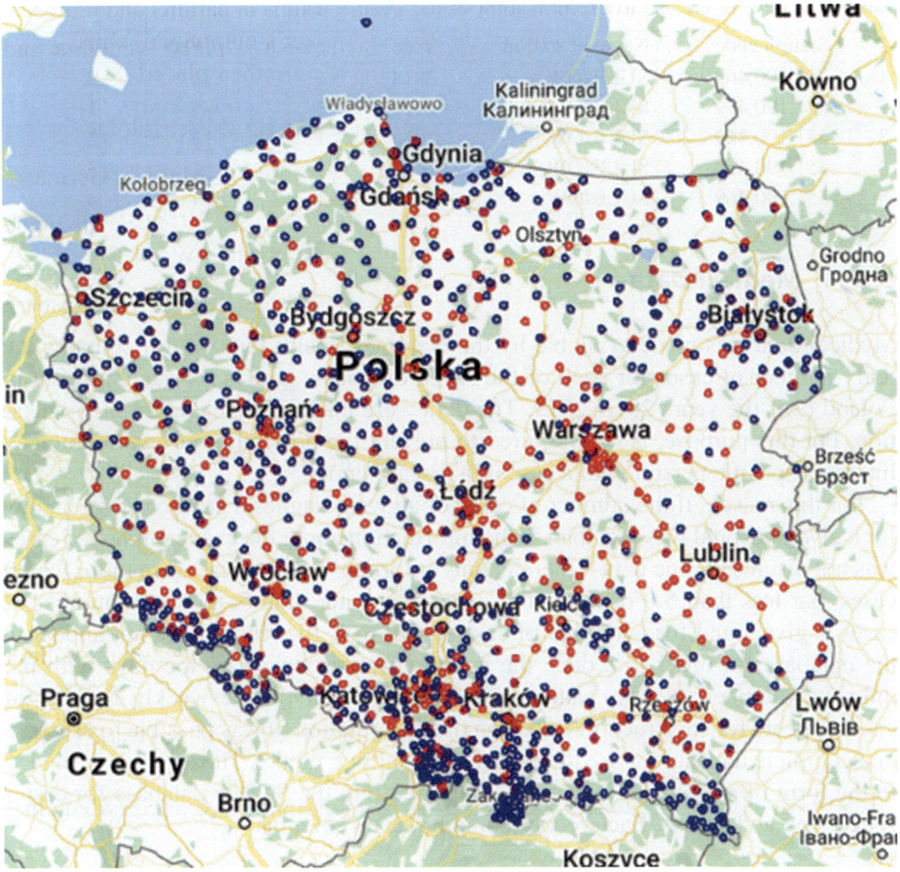

Fig. 4 Visualisation of the location of weather stations (blue) and hospitals (red) from which the data was obtained in Poland

in the form of CSV files that were imported into the SQLite database for easier processing and access. Each record in the created database contains 109 columns, namely:

1. Measurement index
2. Station code
3. Station name
4. Year of measurement
5. Month of measurement
6. Measurement day
7. Time of measurement
8. Detailed weather data

The weather database contains 84,814 records from the regions which are depicted in Fig. 4. Below is an array of the first five records (Table 1):

Table 1 A table of the first five records from shared weather data

#	Station code	Name of station	Year	Month	Day	Time
1	351,190,469	SULEJÓW	2018	1	1	0
2	351,190,469	SULEJÓW	2018	1	1	1
3	351,190,469	SULEJÓW	2018	1	1	2
4	351,190,469	SULEJÓW	2018	1	1	3
5	351,190,469	SULEJÓW	2018	1	1	4

5.3 Medical Data

Medical data was made available by the National Health Fund and it contains the daily number of cases for each of the seven diagnosis groups for each hospital in Poland over the years 2018–2019. The data were made available after anonymisation. For this purpose, it was required to prevent the possibility of unambiguously linking a specific person with a case of a disease entity.

For this reason, if the number of cases of a given diagnosis group on a given day for a given hospital was less than 5, the information about the exact number of cases was not disclose in the data—there is only information that there were more than 0 cases, but less than 5. For a number of cases greater than 5, the exact number of cases is given, and for a number of cases equal to 0, the record does not appear in the database. In order to reduce the uncertainty introduced by the days with the unknown number of cases, additional information about the weekly number of cases appears for each record. Based on this information, it was possible to estimate and complete the data for use in the machine learning model. The data was provided in the form of a CSV file, which was imported into the SQLite database for easier processing and access. Each record contains seven columns:

1. Adoption date in the format *dd/mm/yyyy*.
2. Group of diagnoses from 1 to 7—compare Fig. 5.
3. Hospital location: TERYT code (National Official Register of the Territorial Division of Poland)
4. Daily number of cases
5. Weekly number of cases
6. Week
7. Year

In total, the database contains 405,853 records. Table 2 shows the view of the first five records:

5.4 Initial Analysis of the Input Data

In order to use the acquired data as input to a machine learning model, it needs to be properly processed. The initial analysis of the data to be used in the neural network

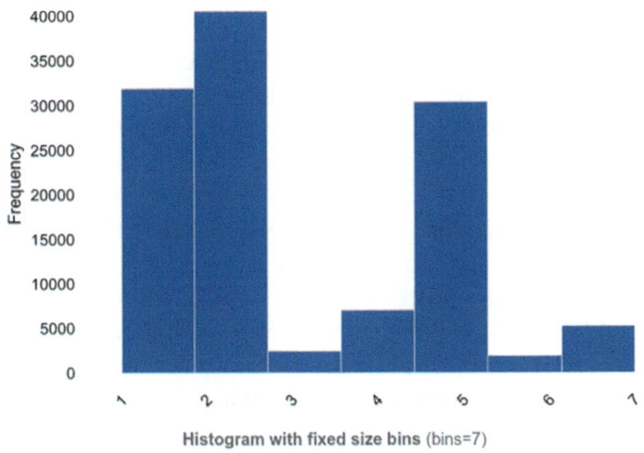

Fig. 5 Histogram with the number of record occurrences for each recognition group. Group 1: Full-thickness myocardial infarction and other heart attacks; Group 2: Pulmonary oedema; Group 3: Cerebral aneurysm haemorrhage; Group 4: Spontaneous brain haemorrhage (rupture of a vessel); Group 5: Ischemic stroke (rupture of the atherosclerotic plaque, blockage of the vessel); Group 6: Vascular events involving the aorta; Group 7: Vascular events involving peripheral arteries

Table 2 A table of the first five records from shared medical data

Group	Location	D note	week note	week	Year
2	0604011_1	<5	16	01	2018
2	0663011_4	<5	16	01	2018
2	2861011_1	<5	6	01	2018
2	0606011_1	<5	12	01	2018
2	0607011_1	<5	14	01	2018

allows making decisions related to its architecture, which is why it is an essential element of the machine learning algorithm creation process.

5.5 Combining Medical Data with Weather Data

The model data is divided into two separate databases, so it was important to find the right key and combine them together to get a pair of input $\boldsymbol{x}$ vector and output vector $\boldsymbol{y}$. Each element $\boldsymbol{x}$ was to be an example containing data on the weather conditions at the hospital location on a given day, and each element a $\boldsymbol{y}$ label containing data on the number of cases for a given group of diagnoses for a given example. Based on the columns described in the previous section, it was known that in the medical database there is a location column containing the TERYT code of a given hospital, and in the weather database there is a station code that uniquely defines the city in which it is located. These locations could not be directly connected because the station code and the TERYT code are not dependent on each other.

In order to obtain the geographical location of each hospital, appropriate queries had to be made to the database of the General Statistical Office, which, based on the TERYT code sent, returned the geographical location and name of the commune in which the given hospital was located. If there was more than one hospital in the commune, each of them contained an additional index after the TERYT code, e.g., 351190469 _ 1. The longitude and latitude were obtained from the query to the Google Maps API. The location of each hospital along with its name and TERYT code, was added as a new table to the SQLite database for easy access in later calculations. The geographical location of each weather station was provided by the Meteorology and Water Management office. Station data with the completed location has also been added to the SQLite database as a new table. Afterwards, to connect each hospital to the nearest station, a distance measurement script using the *haversine* algorithm was utilised.

5.6 Data Analysis Using the *pandas_profiling* Library

Initial data analysis was performed using Python 3 and the *pandas_profiling library*. The combined input and output data were retrieved from the SQLite database by executing the appropriate query combining the previously created tables. This data was then placed in a *DataFrame* provided by the *pandas* library. This structure represents a two-dimensional array and provides the ability to perform operations on cells, rows, and columns. The *DataFrame* created in this way was passed to the ProfileReport function from the *pandas_profiling* library for preliminary statistical analysis of the data. Figure 5 presents the histogram with the number of record occurrences for each recognition group, which are explained below the figure. There is a noticeable difference between the number of cases in each group which is expected due to differences in morbidities.

Analysing the received report, the following conclusions were drawn:

- The daily number of cases correlation with any other column is always very close to 0. This means that there is no direct relationship between any component of weather data (e.g., pressure, temperature) and the number of cases.
- Most records have a case count of “<5” (depicted in Fig. 5). In order to obtain valuable results, the daily data should be supplemented as much as possible based on the weekly number of cases.
- Individual groups of recognition may have a different relationship to environmental data. In order to obtain unambiguous results, the model must be trained separately for each of the seven recognition groups.
- The number of cases varies from hospital to hospital, for example, due to population density. Therefore, the number of cases should be averaged for each hospital to make the data independent of external factors such as hospital size and population density.

5.7 Data Preprocessing

Preprocessing was carried out in the Python 3 programming language with the use of tools included in the *pandas*, *numpy*, and *sklearn* libraries. Again, the combined inputs and outputs were taken from an SQLite database and placed in a *DataFrame*.

5.8 Binarisation of Output Data

Finally, it was decided that the model would solve the problem of **anomaly** detection. This means that the task of the neural network will be able to identify examples for which the daily number of examples is unusually high. To do this, you need to create two categories of labels. Category "0" means no anomaly and category "1" means detected anomaly. Since the vast majority of examples are characterised by a number of cases equal to 0, it was assumed that an anomaly means a record in which the number of cases is higher than the average value.

5.9 Standardisation of Input Data

The weather data, which is the input to the model, is presented in ambiguous scales. Pressure, represented by numerical values in the thousands, and temperature, represented by numerical values in the tens, must be brought to a common scale. Otherwise, features expressed in larger numbers will be much more important for the machine learning model than features represented by fractional values. It is also important that the mean of each feature in the input data set is 0, and the standard deviation is 1. To do this, standardise the input data. Standardisation was carried out using the *StandardScaler* tool from the *sklearn* library, which greatly facilitated this procedure.

5.10 Creating a Sequence for a Recursive Network

The final network architecture is a recursive network - this means that instead of a single data vector, each example must contain a sequence of weather data vectors from several days. In other words, each example, $x^{(i)}$in addition to the weather data vector for the day it originally described, also contains vectors of the $t - 1$ days before it, where t is the length of the sequence.

5.11 Data Division into Training and Test Sets and Selection of the Model Architecture

The last stage of data processing is their division into training and test sets. In this case, a 7:3 division was adopted. It should be remembered that a set of validation data was separated from the training data.

Initially, it was assumed that the task of the neural network model would be to determine the predicted number of cases based on weather data - so it was supposed to be a regression problem. For this purpose, a sequential model of a multilayer perceptron was constructed, but the results were not satisfactory. It was quickly noticed that it would be most valuable for the network to indicate the days for which the risk of a case would be the highest. The risk in this case can be approximated by the daily number of cases - if there were a relatively large number of cases, the risk is high. Due to the fact that for the vast majority of examples the daily number of cases is 0, detecting high-risk days is an anomaly detection problem. Based on the existing network models used in the industry, it is known that the best network architecture for this task are recursive networks. For this reason, the classic *MLP* architecture was abandoned and a recursive network architecture was used instead.

5.12 Model Training

The cross-entropy loss function was used to train the model. The adaptive algorithm of stochastic gradient descent *ADAM* (*adaptive moment estimation) was* used as the teaching method, which is the best *SGD* optimisation for a large amount of data. Accuracy, precision, and recall were used as indicators of model quality, which will be presented in the next section. The series size is 128 and the number of epochs is 10. These hyperparameters were determined on the basis of repeated training of the network.

The learning process for recognition group 1 and sequence length will be shown below $t = 11$. Then the phenomenon of overfitting begins to occur in the model. In order to assess the quality of the model, appropriate metrics must be defined. Before doing so, however, it is necessary to introduce the concepts of errors that are used in the definition of metrics for the binary categorisation problem:

- **False positive** (*FP*), i.e., an example classified by the network as an anomaly (cat. 1) when its true label is no anomaly (cat. 0).
- **False negative** (*FN*), i.e., an example classified by the network as no anomaly (cat. 0) when its true label is an anomaly (cat. 1).
- **True positive** (*TP*), i.e., an example classified by the network as an anomaly (cat. 1) when its true label is an anomaly (cat. 1).
- **True negative** (*TN*), i.e., an example classified by the network as no anomaly (cat. 0) when its true label is no anomaly (cat. 0).

In the previous section, it was noted that the metrics used to evaluate the designed neural network model are as follows:

Accuracy, i.e., the ratio of well-classified examples to all examples. Thus, it answers the question of what percentage of examples have been correctly classified. Accuracy can be determined by the formula:

$$\text{Accuracy} = \frac{\text{TP} + \text{TN}}{\text{TP} + \text{FP} + \text{TN} + \text{FN}}$$

Precision, i.e., the ratio of well-classified anomalies to all examples classified as anomalies. Thus, it answers the question of what percentage of anomalies identified by the network were well classified. Precision is expressed by the formula:

$$\text{Precision} = \frac{\text{TP}}{\text{TP} + \text{FP}}$$

Recall, which is the ratio of well-classified anomalies to all real examples of anomalies. Thus, it answers the question of what percentage of all anomalies were well classified. Precision is expressed by the formula:

$$\text{Recall} = \frac{\text{TP}}{\text{TP} + \text{FN}}$$

Accuracy and *recall* are important metrics for this machine learning model, as cases classified as anomaly tend to be far fewer. In the case where 10% of the real cases are anomalies, it would be enough to classify each test example as category 0 to get 90% accuracy. Watching at least two of these metrics at the same time ensures that the network is functioning properly. In the same case as above, if the network achieves an accuracy of 90% and a *recall* of 80%, it means that it is doing very well—out of 100 test examples, 82/90 examples of category 0 and 8/10 cases of category 1 were indicated correctly. In the problem of anomaly detection, the most important metric is *recall*—the most important thing is to detect all anomalies.

6 Results and Implementation in 3P-Medicine

Table 3 presents a summary of model quality metrics for all seven recognition groups and three different sequence length values *t*, determined on the basis of examples from the test set. The column "Actual % of anomalies" indicates the

Table 3 Obtained results of the designed machine learning model

Group	Group description	Accuracy	Recall	Precision	Actual % of anomalies
1	Group 1: Full-thickness myocardial infarction and other heart attacks	88.6%	76.7%	73.5%	22.7%
2	Group 2: Pulmonary oedema	86.2%	76.7%	73.3%	27.1%
3	Group 3: Cerebral aneurysm haemorrhage	98.4%	68.1%	84.0%	3.4%
4	Group 4: Spontaneous haemorrhage (rupture of a vessel)	98.0%	80.5%	92.3%	7.3%
5	Group 5: Ischemic stroke (rupture of the atherosclerotic plaque, blockage of the vessel)	89.3%	75.0%	68.6%	17.9%
6	Group 6: Vascular events involving the aorta	98.9%	65.0%	82.3%	2.3%
7	Group 7: Vascular events involving peripheral arteries	98.1%	75.1%	92.2%	6.1%

number of examples with the actual label category "1," out of all examples. For all recognition groups, the model performed best with sequence length $t = 11$. The diagnosis group for which the model works best is group 4, i.e., spontaneous haemorrhages. This means that the diseases associated with this group of diagnoses are most dependent on weather conditions, and the designed model reflects this relationship very well.

Prevention is the most efficient way of dealing with vascular incidents [24]. Obesity, smoking, uncontrolled hypertension, untreated diabetes and mental stress are the most common risk factors of atherosclerosis [25]. Despite the fact that risk factors are identified, and methods of elimination are straightforward, the application of preventive measures is still not easy. Levels of inadequate blood pressure control in the hypertensive population are high despite the availability of good and affordable medications [26, 27].

One of the possible applications of our work aims to aid with fighting harmful habits of the people at risk of atherosclerosis. Personalised web and mobile applications warning patients at risk about perilous environmental conditions in real time may help with better control of taken medications, closely following the doctor's advice and avoiding risky behaviour in harsh weather conditions. Such software may be of help, especially in groups averting ordinary medical check-ups and overestimating their health fitness.

7 Conclusion and Recommendations

The main objective of the study was to determine the impact of environmental conditions on the occurrence of vascular incidents and to develop a mathematical model capable of detecting atmospheric conditions that increase the risk of vascular incidents. To this end, the authors reviewed the literature sources, on the basis of which we developed an approach to machine learning algorithms and diseases of the vascular system. Furthermore, we obtained the required weather and medical data from the relevant institutions. These data were statistically analysed and supplemented to best prepare them for use in the machine learning model. Based on the accumulated theoretical knowledge, the architecture of a recursive neural network was developed, and its hyperparameters were determined experimentally. The designed network was finally trained separately for each of the seven reconnaissance groups.

The results obtained by the authors give reason to believe that there is indeed a relationship between environmental conditions and the occurrence of vascular events. The *recall values* obtained for most diagnosis groups reach 75%, which is enough to confirm this hypothesis. It is probably impossible to obtain better quality metrics because more external factors than the weather alone can influence the occurrence of vascular events. Such factors may be, for example, the day of the week or the holiday season. The model itself also needs some improvements, for example, a better definition of anomaly categories. The model achieved the best results for group 4, i.e., spontaneous haemorrhages. This means that the diseases associated with this group of diagnoses are most dependent on weather conditions, and the designed model reflects this relationship very well. The presented technological solutions play a great role in prediction, prevention, and a personalised approach to a patient.

The biggest problem encountered in the implementation of the work was incomplete medical data provided by the National Health Fund. However, this data had to be incomplete in order to ensure their anonymity. In the future, steps will be taken to obtain more complete data, at the cost of extending the area of aggregation of the daily number of cases to the entire commune or even the powiat/county.

It is interesting that the results obtained by the model become much better with the length of the sequence. It would be a natural guess that the occurrence of vascular events is most influenced by a sharp change in weather from day to day. Based on the fact that the model obtained the best results for 11 days in sequence, it can be concluded that in fact the general weather has the greatest impact on the occurrence of the above-mentioned incidents. It is also surprising that the *recall* and *precision* values obtained are very similar for all recognition groups. This would mean that all vascular incidents are similarly dependent on meteorological conditions. The confirmation of the existence of a connection between specific weather conditions and vascular incidents can help not only medical facilities but also patients. Thanks to such forecasting methods, hospitals could prepare for periods of an expected increased number of patients requiring urgent help.

References

1. Wlodarczyk A, Molek P, Bochenek B, Wypych A, Nessler J, Zalewski J (2022) Machine learning analyzed weather conditions as an effective means in the predicting of acute coronary syndrome prevalence. Front Cardiovasc Med 9:830823
2. Molek P, Wlodarczyk A, Bochenek B, Wypych A, Nessler J, Zalewski J (2020) The artificial intelligence system in prediction of the prevalence of acute coronary syndromes based on weather conditions. Eur Heart J 41:3456
3. Zheng Y, Guo Z, Zhang Y, Shang J, Yu L, Fu P et al (2022) Rapid triage for ischemic stroke: a machine learning-driven approach in the context of predictive, preventive and personalised medicine. EPMA J 13:285–298
4. Bauer J, Hoq MN, Mulcahy J, Tofail SAM, Gulshan F, Silien C et al (2020) Implementation of artificial intelligence and non-contact infrared thermography for prediction and personalized automatic identification of different stages of cellulite. EPMA J 11:17–29
5. Birkenbihl C, Emon MA, Vrooman H, Westwood S, Lovestone S, Hofmann-Apitius M et al (2020) Differences in cohort study data affect external validation of artificial intelligence models for predictive diagnostics of dementia—lessons for translation into clinical practice. EPMA J 11:367–376
6. Turing AM (2012) Computing machinery and intelligence. Mach Intell Perspect Comput Model 49:1–28
7. Hamet P, Tremblay J (2017) Artificial intelligence in medicine. Metabolism 69:S36–S40
8. Kaul V, Enslin S, Gross SA (2020) History of artificial intelligence in medicine. Gastrointest Endosc 92:807–812
9. Muthukrishnan N, Maleki F, Ovens K, Reinhold C, Forghani B, Forghani R (2020) Brief history of artificial intelligence. Neuroimaging Clin N Am 30:393–399
10. Weiss SM, Kulikowski CA, Amarel S, Safir A (1978) A model-based method for computer-aided medical decision making, vol 11, p 145

11. Al-Ajlan A (2015) The comparison between forward and backward chaining. Int J Mach Learn Comput 5:106
12. Daniel M, Hajek P, Nguyenb PH (1997) Artificial intelligence in medicine CADIAG-2 and MYCIN-like systems. Artif Intell Med 9:241
13. Marshall TE, Lambert SL (2018) Cloud-based intelligent accounting applications: accounting task automation using IBM Watson cognitive computing. J Emerging Technol Account 15:199–215
14. Kurzweil R (1985) What is artificial intelligence anyway. Am Sci 73:258
15. Bott R (2014) Guyton and hall textbook of medical physiology, 13th edn. W. B. Saunders, Philadelphia
16. Mescher AL (2019) Junqueira's basic histology: text atlas, 15th edn. McGraw Hill, New York
17. Putz R, Sobotta J, Pabst R (2008) Sobotta atlas of human anatomy: head, neck, upper limb, thorax, abdomen, pelvis, lower limb. Elsevier, Amsterdam
18. Bodle JD, Feldmann E, Swartz RH, Rumboldt Z, Brown T, Turan TN (2013) High-resolution magnetic resonance imaging: an emerging tool for evaluating intracranial arterial disease. Stroke 44:287–292
19. Seidman MA, Mitchell RN, Stone JR (2014) Pathophysiology of atherosclerosis. In: Cellular and molecular pathobiology of cardiovascular disease, pp 221–237
20. Faraci FM, Heistad DD (1990) Regulation of large cerebral arteries and cerebral microsvascular pressure. Circ Res 66:8–17
21. Brega KE, Seltzer WK, Munro LG, Breeze RE (1996) Genotypic variations of type III collagen in patients with cerebral aneurysms. Surg Neurol 46:253
22. Connolly ES, Poisik A, Winfree CJ, Kim LJ, Huang J, McMahon DJ et al (1999) Cigarette smoking and the development and rupture of cerebral aneurysms in a mixed race population: implications for population screening and smoking cessation. J Stroke Cerebrovasc Dis 8:248
23. Ptak M et al (2022) aHEAD Project. www.aheadproject.org. Accessed 15 Oct 2022
24. Arnett DK, Blumenthal RS, Albert MA, Buroker AB, Goldberger ZD, Hahn EJ et al (2019) 2019 ACC/AHA guideline on the primary prevention of cardiovascular disease: executive summary. J Am Coll Cardiol 74:1376–1414
25. Knoflach M, Kiechl S, Kind M, Said M, Sief R, Gisinger M et al (2003) Cardiovascular risk factors and atherosclerosis in young males. Circulation 108:1064–1069
26. Banegas JR, Segura J, Sobrino J, Rodríguez-Artalejo F, de la Sierra A, de la Cruz JJ et al (2007) Effectiveness of blood pressure control outside the medical setting. Hypertension 49:62–68
27. Mancia G, Sega R, Milesi C, Cessna G, Zanchetti A (1997) Blood-pressure control in the hypertensive population. Lancet 349:454–457

Periodontal Health Status Is Pivotal for an Effective Disease Prediction, Targeted Prevention and Personalised Treatments of Associated Pathologies

Vadim V. Tachalov, Tatyana V. Kudryavtseva, Irina V. Berezkina, Maka G. Pachkoriia, Ekaterina S. Loboda, Liudmila Yu. Orekhova, and Olga Golubnitschaja

1 Why Predictive, Preventive and Personalised Medicine Is Considered an Optimal Approach in Oral Cavity Healthcare?

Oral cavity health plays a key role in predicting and preventing periodontal and dental diseases which frequently cascade systemic effects such as chronic inflammation and associated pathologies [1–6]. Individualised patient profiling is instrumental for implementing 3PM strategies in periodontology and dentistry [7–9]. To this end, suboptimal health conditions demonstrating a reversible damage to health are in focus of primary healthcare promoting targeted prevention against health-to-disease transition that is pivotal for the cost-effective healthcare meeting needs of the society at large [5, 7, 10, 11].

V. V. Tachalov · T. V. Kudryavtseva · I. V. Berezkina · M. G. Pachkoriia
Therapeutic Dentistry and Periodontology Department, Pavlov First Saint Petersburg State Medical University, St. Petersburg, Russia

E. S. Loboda · L. Y. Orekhova
Therapeutic Dentistry and Periodontology Department, Pavlov First Saint Petersburg State Medical University, St. Petersburg, Russia

City Periodontology Centre, "PAKS", St. Petersburg, Russia

O. Golubnitschaja (✉)
Predictive, Preventive, Personalised (3P) Medicine, Department of Radiation Oncology, University Hospital Bonn, Rheinische Friedrich-Wilhelms-Universität Bonn, Bonn, Germany
e-mail: olga.golubnitschaja@ukbonn.de

H. Podbielska, M. Kapalla (eds.), *Predictive, Preventive, and Personalised Medicine: From Bench to Bedside*, Advances in Predictive, Preventive and Personalised Medicine 17, https://doi.org/10.1007/978-3-031-34884-6_17

2 Periodontal Diseases Affect Majority of Adult Populations

Periodontal diseases (PDs) affects up to over 50% of populations in developed and developing countries worldwide. The entire age spectrum from adolescence to elderly is affected that makes PDs to a global challenge [12]. An extensive destruction of connective tissues of the periodontium and alveolar bone is characteristic for PDs and has been associated in a reciprocal manner with cascading systemic diseases including cardiovascular diseases, diabetes mellitus type 2 with complications, liver and chronic obstructive pulmonary diseases as well as several types of malignancies [13–15].

3 Risk Factors, Pathomechanisms and Systemic Effects of the Chronic Periodontitis

Chronic periodontitis (CP) is a bacterial inflammatory disease damaging oral cavity health and teeth structures [16, 17]. CP creates tremendous socio-economic burden to populations and requires in-depth understanding of risk factors and treatments tailored to the person [18]. Most prominent risk factors comprise both non-modifiable such as ageing and medication, and modifiable, i.e., preventable ones such diabetes mellitus type 2, inadequate oral hygiene and dental care, smoking, and stress overload [8]. Individually and synergistically the risks promote CP development [12]. Proposed pathmechanisms are based on bacteraemia and systemic inflammation indicated by elevated C-reactive protein patterns and highly increased oxidative stress [3, 15]. Despite local symptoms of the CP, inflammatory mediators produced as well as subgingival species and shifted microbiome become spread systemically leading to cascading extra-oral pathological changes at molecular, cellular, and organ levels [19]. To this end, CP associated carcinogenesis is relevant for both – the oral cavity and extra-oral sites typical for the orodigestive cancers extended to the oral, oesophageal, gastric, colorectal, and pancreatic malignancies [19]. There is an evident reciprocal relationship between CP development and severe systemic diseases which an altered microbiome and chronic inflammation are relevant for [3, 8, 15, 20]. For example, CP significantly increases risks of cardiovascular complications and concomitant mortality in the diabetic patient cohort, while diabetic history is in turn a well-acknowledged risk factor of CP [19]. Clinically established CP has been, further, associated with maternal infections, foetal growth restriction, preterm birth, and strong predisposition to preeclampsia—all demonstrated as life-long health risks of mother and offspring [11].

4 Patient Stratification Is a Multi-Factorial Approach in Periodontology

Our recent study performed at the Periodontology Department, Pavlov First Saint Petersburg State Medical University, has analysed prevalence of chronic disorders in the age-stratified patient groups such as diabetes mellitus type 2, cardiovascular and gastrointestinal diseases, chronic kidney and liver diseases, amongst others. High prevalence of collateral pathologies has been demonstrated for patients diagnosed with periodontitis: 87.5% in the age group between 61 and 75 years old followed by 75.8% in the age group between 45 and 60 years old.

Age is a multi-faceted determinant for the patient stratification and tailored 3 PM strategies.

An important aspect is the age-specific behavioural patterns towards healthcare measures, offered services, their duration, quality, and costs. From this point of view, elderly is associated with challenging care and strong socio-economical limitations. Contextually, highly specific medical, mental, social, and financial aspects should be carefully considered for this sub-population optimally meeting its needs [21–26]. Essential expertise carries a multi-professional character including geriatrics and gerontology preventing oral dryness / dry mouth syndrome, tongue-lip motor, masticatory and swallowing dysfunction – all together leading to the oral hypofunction which is characteristic for elderly and other vulnerable groups in the population [27–29].

5 Challenges of Participatory Medicine

Inadequate periodontal health services provided to the population may be caused by several deficits such as insufficient awareness of corresponding impacts in affected subpopulations and subpopulations in suboptimal health conditions, low educational level with consequent ignorance towards the periodontal health, low socio-economic status of affected individuals, lack of the relevant insurance, insufficient density of specialised medical units, amongst others [8, 30, 31]. Contextually, to raise awareness towards periodontal health and corresponding services is pivotal to advance health quality in the population [8, 32, 33]. This is the task for participatory medicine focused on the active participation of populations in maintaining satisfactory health status. Promoting participatory medicine in the population, generally it should be kept in mind that healthcare remains unsatisfactory as long as the patient does not feel responsible for their health condition [34]. This conclusion can be well exemplified by chronically diseased patients observed in periodontology [8].

6 Virome–Microbiome Axis: A Vicious Circle in Disease Promotion

An association between periodontal diseases, viral and bacterial overload with poor outcomes is clearly demonstrated in several studies [27, 35]. The human body hosts vast microbial and viral communities collectively termed "**microbiome**" and "**virome,**" respectively. The human virome is complex consisting of about 10^{13} particles per individual [36]. Both human virome and microbiome are highly heterogeneous. Depending on individual profiles of microbial and viral communities, they can be associated with adverse outcomes for the human host, whereas other states are characteristic of health. Furthermore, there are evident synergies in the host–virome–microbiome interactions in health and disease. To this end, during the past influenza outbreaks, such as influenza in 1918, H1N1 influenza in 2009 these interactions have been demonstrated for the respiratory viruses, in turn associated with bacterial superinfections as the main risk of a severe disease course and death [37]. Periodontopathic microfora is implicated in systemic microbiome composition alterations promoting chronic inflammation, systemic health-to-disease transition leading to sepsis, pneumonia development, and death. The dual antiviral and antibiotic medication is considered optimal to protect human body against pathologic shift in the virome–microbiome axis leading to the vicious circle in disease promotion.

7 Periodontal Disease as the Clue to the COVID-19-Associated Poor Outcomes

Clear association has been demonstrated between clinically manifested periodontitis in COVID-19 infected patients and high risk of their admission to intensive care units and related death [28]. The absolute majority of the affected patients exhibited bacterial superinfections and severe disease course as demonstrated in the UK study of COVID-19-infected individuals [27]. Patients with poor COVID-19 outcomes demonstrated high levels of periodontopathic bacteria communities comprising Prevotella, Staphylococcus, and Fusobacterium. For 80% of patients treated at intensive care units, a particularly high periodontal bacterial was characteristic. Noteworthy, advanced age, diabetes mellitus, and cardiovascular diseases are frequently associated with both poor periodontal health and poor outcomes of the COVID-19 infection. In common are significantly shifted virome–microbiome profiles and systemic inflammation [29]. Suggested pathomechanisms include virome–microbiome–host interactions in the respiratory and gastrointestinal tracts [37]. On the molecular level, the overexpression of angiotensin-converting enzyme 2—the receptor for SARS-CoV-2—and production of inflammatory cytokines in the lower respiratory tract are characteristic for poor outcomes in COVID-19 infected individuals. To this end, an aspiration of periodontopathic bacteria induces the angiotensin-converting enzyme 2 actively contributing therefore to the cytokine storm typical for the COVID-19 aggravation and associated severe disease course [38]. Contextually, periodontal health is crucial for the cost-effective primary prevention, improved individual outcomes, and reduced morbidity under pandemic conditions [27, 39]. Application of oral probiotics is strongly recommended to stabilise the gut–lung axis and health microflora [40].

8 Individualised Patient Profiling: Risk Factors and Big Data Analyses Exemplified by "Dry Mouth" Syndrome Phenotype

Implementation of individualised patient profiles (IPP) is strongly recommended for protective periodontal care. Phenotyping and genotyping are instrumental for IPP and demand big data analysis comprising non-modifiable (e.g., genetic predisposition) and modifiable risk factors such as behavioural and dietary habits. Relevant surveys have been developed, for example, to identify individuals with the dry mouth syndrome phenotype. To this end, dry mouth syndrome is highly relevant for xerostomia-associated disorders such as periodontitis and systemic inflammation predisposition to which can be detected early in life [4]. Predisposition to xerostomia in otherwise healthy young individuals can be further associated with the stress overload that is well detectable using non-sophisticated health risk assessment tools [5] followed by the targeted primary prevention [5, 41–44]. Health risk assessment under stress condition is further discussed by Golubnitschaja O. in the book chapter dedicated to the mitochondrial health.

References

1. Beck JD, Ofenbacher S (2005) Systemic effects of periodontitis: epidemiology of periodontal disease and cardiovascular disease. J Periodontol 76(11 Suppl):2089–2100. https://doi.org/10.1902/jop.2005.76.11-S.2089
2. Larsen T, Fiehn NE (2017) Dental bioflm infections—an update. APMIS 125(4):376–384. https://doi.org/10.1111/apm.12688
3. Sanz M, Marco Del Castillo A, Jepsen S, Gonzalez-Juanatey JR, D'Aiuto F, Bouchard P, Chapple I, Dietrich T, Gotsman I, Graziani F, Herrera D, Loos B, Madianos P, Michel JB, Perel P, Pieske B, Shapira L, Shechter M, Tonetti M, Vlachopoulos C, Wimmer G (2020) Periodontitis and cardiovascular diseases: consensus report. J Clin Periodontol 47(3):268–288. https://doi.org/10.1111/jcpe.13189
4. Kunin A, Polivka J Jr, Moiseeva N, Golubnitschaja O (2018) "Dry mouth" and "Flammer" syndromes—neglected risks in adolescents and new concepts by predictive, preventive and personalised approach. EPMA J 9(3):307–317. https://doi.org/10.1007/s13167-018-0145-7
5. Kunin A, Sargheini N, Birkenbihl C, Moiseeva N, Fröhlich H, Golubnitschaja O (2020) Voice perturbations under the stress overload in young individuals: phenotyping and suboptimal health as predictors for cascading pathologies. EPMA J 11(4):1–11. https://doi.org/10.1007/s13167-020-00229-8
6. Ma X, Wang Y, Wu H, Li F, Feng X, Xie Y, Xie D, Wang W, Lo ECM, Lu H (2021) Periodontal health related-inflammatory and metabolic profiles of patients with end-stage renal disease: potential strategy for predictive, preventive, and personalized medicine. EPMA J 12(2):117–128. https://doi.org/10.1007/s13167-021-00239-0
7. Pei J, Li F, Xie Y, Liu J, Yu T, Feng X (2020) Microbial and metabolomic analysis of gingival crevicular fuid in general chronic periodontitis patients: lessons for a predictive, preventive, and personalized medical approach. EPMA J 11(2):197–215. https://doi.org/10.1007/s13167-020-00202-5
8. Tachalov VV, Orekhova LY, Kudryavtseva TV et al (2021) Making a complex dental care tailored to the person: population health in focus of predictive, preventive and personalised (3P) medical approach. EPMA J 12:129–140. https://doi.org/10.1007/s13167-021-00240-7
9. Golubnitschaja O, Liskova A, Koklesova L, Samec M, Biringer K, Büsselberg D, Podbielska H, Kunin AA, Evsevyeva ME, Shapira N, Paul F, Erb C, Dietrich DE, Felbel D, Karabatsiakis A, Bubnov R, Polivka J, Polivka J Jr, Birkenbihl C, Fröhlich H, Hofmann-Apitius M, Kubatka P (2021) Caution, "normal" BMI: health risks associated with potentially masked individual underweight-EPMA position paper 2021. EPMA J 12(3):243–264. https://doi.org/10.1007/s13167-021-00251-4
10. Wang W, Yan Y, Guo Z, Hou H, Garcia M, Tan X, Anto EO, Mahara G, Zheng Y, Li B, Kang T, Zhong Z, Wang Y, Guo X, Golubnitschaja O (2021) Suboptimal health study consortium and European Association for Predictive, preventive and personalised medicine. All around subop-

timal health - a joint position paper of the suboptimal health study consortium and European Association for Predictive, preventive and personalised medicine. EPMA J 12(4):403–433. https://doi.org/10.1007/s13167-021-00253-2
11. Evsevieva M, Sergeeva O, Mazurakova A, Koklesova L, Prokhorenko-Kolomoytseva I, Shchetinin E, Birkenbihl C, Costigliola V, Kubatka P, Golubnitschaja O (2022) Pre-pregnancy check-up of maternal vascular status and associated phenotype is crucial for the health of mother and offspring. EPMA J 13(3):351–366. https://doi.org/10.1007/s13167-022-00294-1
12. Nazir MA (2017) Prevalence of periodontal disease, its association with systemic diseases and prevention. Int J Health Sci (Qassim) 11(2):72–80
13. Lalla E, Papapanou PN (2011) Diabetes mellitus and periodontitis: a tale of two common interrelated diseases. Nat Rev Endocrinol 7(12):738–748. https://doi.org/10.1038/nrendo.2011.106
14. Ide M, Linden GJ (2014) Periodontitis, cardiovascular disease and pregnancy outcome–focal infection revisited? Br Dent J 217(8):467–474. https://doi.org/10.1038/sj.bdj.2014.903
15. Kitamura M, Mochizuki Y, Miyata Y, Obata Y, Mitsunari K, Matsuo T, Ohba K, Mukae H, Yoshimura A, Nishino T, Sakai H (2019) Pathological characteristics of periodontal disease in patients with chronic kidney disease and kidney transplantation. Int J Mol Sci 20(14):3413. https://doi.org/10.3390/ijms20143413
16. Kinane DF (2000) Causation and pathogenesis of periodontal disease. Periodontol 2000 2001(25):8–20. https://doi.org/10.1034/j.1600-0757.2001.22250102.x
17. Yu JC, Khodadadi H, Baban B (2019) Innate immunity and oral microbiome: a personalized, predictive, and preventive approach to the management of oral diseases. EPMA J 10(1):43–50. https://doi.org/10.1007/s13167-019-00163-4
18. Cafero C, Matarasso S (2013) Predictive, preventive, personalised and participatory periodontology: 'the 5Ps' age has already started. EPMA J 4(1):16. https://doi.org/10.1186/1878-5085-4-16
19. Hoare A, Soto C, Rojas-Celis V, Bravo D (2019) Chronic infammation as a link between periodontitis and carcinogenesis. Med Inform 2019:1029857. https://doi.org/10.1155/2019/1029857
20. Konkel JE, O'Boyle C, Krishnan S (2019) Distal consequences of oral infammation. Front Immunol 10:1403. https://doi.org/10.3389/fmmu.2019.01403
21. Johnson RJ, Wolinsky FD (1994) Gender, race, and health: the structure of health status among older adults. Gerontologist 34(1):24–35. https://doi.org/10.1093/geront/34.1.24
22. Locker D, Gibson B (2006) The concept of positive health: a review and commentary on its application in oral health research. Community Dent Oral Epidemiol 34(3):161–173. https://doi.org/10.1111/j.1600-0528.2006.00263.x
23. MacEntee MI (2006) An existential model of oral health from evolving views on health, function and disability. Community Dent Health 23(1):5–14
24. Brondani MA, MacEntee MI, Bryant SR, O'Neill B (2008) Using written vignettes in focus groups among older adults to discuss oral health as a sensitive topic. Qual Health Res 18(8):1145–1153. https://doi.org/10.1177/1049732308320114
25. Kop WJ, Gottdiener JS, Tangen CM, Fried LP, McBurnie MA, Walston J, Newman A, Hirsch C, Tracy RP (2002) Inflammation and coagulation factors in persons > 65 years of age with symptoms of depression but without evidence of myocardial ischemia. Am J Cardiol 89(4):419–424. https://doi.org/10.1016/s0002-9149(01)02264-0
26. Xue QL, Bandeen-Roche K, Varadhan R, Zhou J, Fried LP (2008) Initial manifestations of frailty criteria and the development of frailty phenotype in the Women's health and aging study II. J Gerontol A Biol Sci Med Sci 63(9):984–990. https://doi.org/10.1093/gerona/63.9.984
27. Sampson V, Kamona N, Sampson A (2020) Could there be a link between oral hygiene and the severity of SARS-CoV-2 infections? Br Dent J 228(12):971–975. https://doi.org/10.1038/s41415-020-1747-8
28. Marouf N, Cai W, Said KN, Daas H, Diab H, Chinta VR, Hssain AA, Nicolau B, Sanz M, Tamimi F (2021) Association between periodontitis and severity of COVID-19 infection: a case-control study. J Clin Periodontol 48:483. https://doi.org/10.1111/jcpe.13435

29. Pitones-Rubio V, Chávez-Cortez EG, Hurtado-Camarena A, González-Rascón A, Serafín-Higuera N (2020) Is periodontal disease a risk factor for severe COVID-19 illness? Med Hypotheses 144:109969. https://doi.org/10.1016/j.mehy.2020.109969
30. Vujicic M (2015) Solving dentistry's 'busyness' problem. J Am Dent Assoc 146(8):641–643. https://doi.org/10.1016/j.adaj.2015.06.001
31. Waldman HB, Perlman SP (2016) Ethics, economics and dentistry for individuals with disabilities in New York state. N Y State Dent J 82(2):38–42
32. Tavakol M, Torabi S, Lyne OD, Zeinaloo AA (2005) A quantitative survey of intern's knowledge of communication skills: an Iranian exploration. BMC Med Educ 5(1):6. https://doi.org/10.1186/1472-6920-5-6
33. Abraham JA, Golubnitschaja O, Akhmetov I et al (2016) EPMA-world congress 2015. EPMA J 7(Suppl). https://doi.org/10.1186/s13167-016-0054-6
34. Golubnitschaja O, Baban B, Boniolo G, Wang W, Bubnov R, Kapalla M, Krapfenbauer K, Mozaffari MS, Costigliola V (2016) Medicine in the early twenty-first century: paradigm and anticipation—EPMA position paper 2016. EPMA J 7(1):23. https://doi.org/10.1186/s13167-016-0072-4
35. Cox MJ, Loman N, Bogaert D, O'Grady J (2020) Co-infections: potentially lethal and unexplored in COVID-19. Lancet Microbe 1(1):e11. https://doi.org/10.1016/S2666-5247(20)30009-36
36. Liang G, Frederic D, Bushman FD (2021) The human virome: assembly, composition and host interactions. Nat Rev Microbiol 8:514–527. https://doi.org/10.1038/s41579-021-00536-5
37. Xiang Z, Koo H, Chen Q, Zhou X, Liu Y, Simon-Soro A (2020) Potential implications of SARS-CoV-2 oral infection in the host microbiota. J Oral Microbiol 13(1):1853451. https://doi.org/10.1080/20002297.2020.1853451
38. Takahashi Y, Watanabe N, Kamio N, Kobayashi R, Iinuma T, Imai K (2020) Aspiration of periodontopathic bacteria due to poor oral hygiene potentially contributes to the aggravation of COVID-19. J Oral Sci 63(1):1–3. https://doi.org/10.2334/josnusd.20-0388
39. Botros N, Iyer P, Ojcius DM (2020) Is there an association between oral health and severity of COVID-19 complications? Biomed J 43(4):325–327. https://doi.org/10.1016/j.bj.2020.05.016
40. Baindara P, Chakraborty R, Holliday ZM, Mandal SM, Schrum AG (2021) Oral probiotics in coronavirus disease 2019: connecting the gut-lung axis to viral pathogenesis, infammation, secondary infection and clinical trials. N Microb N Infect 40:100837. https://doi.org/10.1016/j.nmni.2021.100837
41. Golubnitschaja O (2019) Flammer syndrome—from phenotype to associated pathologies, prediction, prevention and personalisation. Flammer Syndr 11. ISBN 978-3-030-13549-2; ISBN 978-3-030-13550-8 (eBook). https://doi.org/10.1007/978-3-030-13550-8
42. Koklesova L, Liskova A, Samec M, Qaradakhi T, Zulli A, Smejkal K, Kajo K, Jakubikova J, Behzadi P, Pec M, Zubor P, Biringer K, Kwon TK, Büsselberg D, Sarria GR, Giordano FA, Golubnitschaja O, Kubatka P (2020) Genoprotective activities of plant natural substances in cancer and chemopreventive strategies in the context of 3P medicine. EPMA J 11(2):261–287. https://doi.org/10.1007/s13167-020-00210-5
43. Qian S, Golubnitschaja O, Zhan X (2019) Chronic infammation: key player and biomarker-set to predict and prevent cancer development and progression based on individualized patient profles. EPMA J 10(4):365–381. https://doi.org/10.1007/s13167-019-00194-x
44. Maturo MG, Soligo M, Gibson G, Manni L, Nardini C (2019) The greater infammatory pathway-high clinical potential by innovative predictive, preventive, and personalized medical approach. EPMA J 11(1):1–16. https://doi.org/10.1007/s13167-019-00195-w

Does the Evaluation of Ocular Blood Supply Play a Role in Glaucoma Diagnostics and Prognosis of Progression?

Natalia I. Kurysheva, Vitaliy Yu. Kim, and Valeria E. Kim

Abbreviations

ANS	Autonomic nervous system
ARI	Autonomic regulation index
BP	Blood pressure
CDI	Color Doppler imaging
CPT	Cold provocation test
CRA	Central retinal artery
CV	Coefficients of variation
EPS	Enhanced polarization-sensitive
FLV	Focal loss volume
FR	Functional reserves
FS	Functional status
GCC	Ganglion cell complex
GLV	Global loss volume
GON	Glaucomatous optic neuropathy
HF	High-frequency range
HRV	Heart rate variability
HTG	High tension glaucoma
ILM	Internal limiting membrane
IOP	Intraocular pressure
IPL	Inner plexiform layer

N. I. Kurysheva (✉) · V. Y. Kim · V. E. Kim
Medical Biological University of Innovations and Continuing Education, Burnazyan Federal Biophysical Center, Federal Medical and Biological Agency, Moscow, Russian Federation

Ophthalmological Center, Burnazyan Federal Biophysical Center, Federal Medical and Biological Agency, Moscow, Russian Federation

H. Podbielska, M. Kapalla (eds.), *Predictive, Preventive, and Personalised Medicine: From Bench to Bedside*, Advances in Predictive, Preventive and Personalised Medicine 17, https://doi.org/10.1007/978-3-031-34884-6_18

LF	Low-frequency range
MD	Mean deviation
MOPP	Mean ocular perfusion pressure
MvD	Microvasculature dropout
NFI	Nerve fiber indicator
NTG	Normal tension glaucoma
OCTA	Optic coherence tomography angiography
ONH	Optic nerve head
OPP	Ocular perfusion pressure
PACG	Primary angle closure glaucoma
PERG	Pattern electroretinogram
pfVD	Perifoveal vessel density
POAG	Primary open-angle glaucoma
PPPM	Predictive preventive personalized medicine
PVD	Primary vascular dysregulation
PVEP	Pattern visual evoked potential
RGC	Retinal ganglion cells
RI	Resistivity index
RMSSD	Parameter of parasympathetic autonomic regulation activity
RNFL	Retinal nerve fiber layer
ROP	Rate of progression
SAP	Standard automated perimetry
SDNN	Standard deviation of NN-interval
SD-OCT	Spectral-domain optic coherence tomography
SNA	Sympathetic neural activity
SPCA	Short posterior ciliary artery
SSADA	Split-spectrum amplitude-decorrelation angiography
TP	Total spectral power
VD	Vessel density
VF	Visual fields
VFI	Visual field index
wiVD	Whole image vessel density

1 Introduction

Primary open-angle glaucoma (POAG) is a neurodegenerative disease characterized by a progressive course and an irreversible blindness worldwide.

Accurate prediction of optimal treatment beneficial and adverse effects could improve the results of therapy. The early detection of the specific features of the patient is a key point of the personalized approach in glaucoma treatment. Individualized patient profiling is an instrumental for implementing 3PM strategies in glaucoma management [1, 2].

It is believed that there are two groups of factors responsible for the development of glaucomatous optic neuropathy (GON): (1) vascular dysregulation associated with the decrease of ocular blood flow of the optic nerve disc [3] and (2) mechanical dysregulation associated with the scleral membrane damage and infringement of the optic nerve axons. According to well-known Flammer syndrome, patients with an instable ocular blood flow respond stronger to psychological stress as it has been described in patients with primary vascular dysregulation (PVD) [4, 5]. It has also been emphasized that any psychological stress leads to vascular dysfunction [6]. PVD is believed to be a main cause of local vasospasm and impaired autoregulation as well as a possible contributing factor in glaucoma pathogenesis [7, 8]. It has been shown that PVD patients have stronger reaction to psychological stress than non-PVD subjects. It is known that any psychological stress leads to vascular dysfunction and may become a risk factor of glaucoma development and progression.

The small branches of the central retinal artery provide the blood supply of the superficial ONH layer. The prelaminar region (a small area anterior to the lamina cribrosa), however, is mainly supplied by branches from the choroidal arteries and directly from the short posterior ciliary arteries [9]. As the choroidal microcirculation is regulated by the autonomic nervous system (ANS), the ANS dysfunction is involved in glaucoma pathogenesis.

Indeed, there is a growing body of evidence suggesting that glaucoma pathogenesis is related to vascular dysfunction [10–16]. The consensus on this issue, however, still has not been found due to the lack of adequate techniques for the study of ocular blood flow despite of different measurement tools [17–20]. Therefore, it highly recommended to search for new visualization methods of the vascular bed for early diagnosis and monitoring of glaucoma. Optical coherence tomography (OCT) is a common tool for diagnosis and treatment of glaucoma disease. Doppler OCT has been used to obtain precise measurements of total retinal blood flow [21]. Although Doppler OCT may be effectively used to detect blood flow in the large vessels around the optic disc, it is not sensitive enough for the accurate measurement of low velocities in the small vessels forming the disc microcirculation. The same refers to the most widely used method—color Doppler imaging (CDI). A new method—OCT angiography (OCT-A)—has been recently introduced. This method allows measuring vessel density in the retina and choroid in the peripapillary and macular areas using high-speed OCT to perform quantitative angiography.

This book chapter will primarily discuss a role of heart rate variability (HRV) assessment and OCTA in glaucoma diagnostics and monitoring.

2 Heart Rate Variability in Glaucoma Patients

According to the literature sources, patients with cardiovascular diseases have 2.33 times more rapid glaucoma progression despite significantly lower intraocular pressure (IOP) values [22]. Moreover, the concept that vascular changes in the eye may be an early indicator of heart diseases is also discussed in literature [23].

Recent studies have shown the role of vascular disturbances and vascular dysregulation in glaucoma [24–29]. This makes glaucoma common with such forms of pathology as arterial hypertension/hypotension, migraine, and vascular spasm [29].

According to the existing literature, POAG patients have significantly smaller diameter of the arterial and venous retinal vessels compared to the control subjects. Nevertheless, both venous and arterial dilatation was normal during the activation of neurons, despite their smaller diameter. The dilatation varied among patients and did not depend on the visual field deterioration. This fact was explained by chronic vasoconstriction leading to the limited energy flow to the retinal and brain neurons, followed by hypometabolism (so-called, silent neurons) and, finally, by the death of neurons [30].

Excessive activity of the sympathetic ANS is among the possible causes of ONH blood supply violation and decreased ocular perfusion pressure (OPP) in the optic nerve and choroidal vessels. Moreover, it has been demonstrated that excessive activity of the sympathetic link of the ANS is associated with glaucoma progression due to instability of the ocular blood flow [26].

Cold stimulation, or cold provocation test (CPT) is a well-established provocation test used for detecting abnormal vascular reactivity in patients with autonomic failures [31]. The testing procedure is rather simple: a patient's hand is dipped into cold water (+4 ° C) with small pieces of ice for 30 seconds and the cardiovascular response is registered (Fig. 1). It has been revealed that the cold provocation test (CPT) may increase the ET-1 level in plasma in glaucoma patients reflected their vascular dysregulation [22]. This phenomenon may also indicate the imbalance of ANS that is manifested mostly during provocation tests, including CPT [33].

Altered ocular blood flow or reduced visual field sensitivity during sympathetic provocation tests has been demonstrated in POAG patients [34–36].

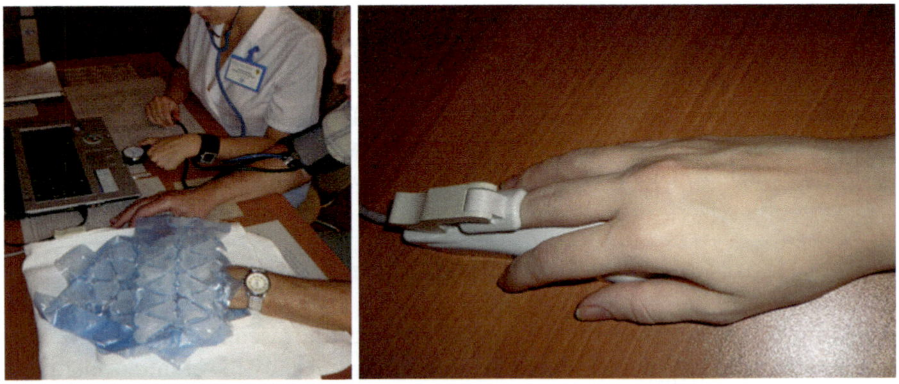

Fig. 1 Cold provocation test (CPT). Photoplethysmography with infrared sensor records from a phalanx with an infrared sensor, located in the microprocessor module of data on HRV and peripheral blood flow [32]

2.1 HRV Assessment

HRV assessment is a standard method to evaluate ANS function. The lower the HRV, the more severe the ANS dysfunction with sympathetic predominance [37].

Compared with other methods of assessing autonomic dysfunction, which include cardiovascular reflex tests, sudomotor tests, Valsalva maneuver, the tilting test, HRV assessment is simpler and non-invasive. Numerous studies have validated HRV as a reliable measure of ANS function in cardiac and non-cardiac diseases. The studies showed that POAG patients had autonomic dysfunction characterized by a HRV drop [32, 38].

We have introduced a special hardware–software complex Rhythm-MET that is based on a comprehensive analysis of HRV, systemic hemodynamics, and vegetative regulation [32].

Photoplethysmograms showing the blood flow measurements in a phalanx were recorded using an infrared detector, located in the microprocessor module of data input and processing, and served as the source of HRV and supplemental blood inflow data. Cardiointervals obtained from photoplethysmograms is processed in accordance with the recommendations for the assessment of HRV parameters and their subsequent generalization, including hemodynamics parameters, and for assessment of the functional status (FS) and functional reserves (FR) of the cardiovascular system according to the results of the examination at rest and after CPT in order to form groups homogeneous in both FS and FR.

The ensuing characteristics should be considered in agreement with the transnational standard:

- Standard divagation of NN-interval (SDNN) is the HRV parameter characterizing the total effect of autonomic blood circulation regulation. A reduction in SDNN reflects low HRV indicating a high tone of heart sympathetic exertion. The drop in SDNN reflects a drop in HRV, which indicates an increase in the heart sympathetic exertion tone.
- The parameter of parasympathetic autonomic regulation exertion (RMSSD).
- Total spectral power (TP) is the parameter of absolute exertion level of non-supervisory systems.
- Power in the high-frequency range (HF) is the parameter of the spectral power of heart rate respiratory undulations reflecting the exertion position of respiratory center. The high-frequency band reflects rapid changes in beat-to-beat variability due to parasympathetic exertion.
- Power in the low-frequency range (LF). The low-frequency band is considered to be a fair approximation of sympathetic exertion. The low-frequency band reflects substantially sympathetic stimulation.
- The low/high-frequency rate is a rate of low-frequency to high- frequency power (LF/HF). An advanced rate indicates increased sympathetic exertion or reduced parasympathetic exertion.
- The number of pairs of successive NN-intervals is the parameter of ascendance degree of parasympathetic regulation over sympathetic one (pNN50).

- Autonomic regulation indicator (ARI) is the parameter for assessment and exertion of ANS. The increased ARI shows the activation of sympathetic regulation, but the decreased ARI shows the activation of parasympathetic regulation.
- Variation range characterizing the degree of HRV (TINN).

SDNN is a representative parameter of HRV. The lower HRV is associated with enhanced SNS exertion, which may be characterized by ANS dysfunction [37].

2.2 The Results of HRV Assessment in High Tension Glaucoma (HTG) and Normal Tension (NTG) Glaucoma

The strict definition of POAG includes HTG and NTG. As far as HTG and NTG are concerned, they appear to be a continuum of glaucomatous process, in which the underlying mechanisms shifts from predominantly elevated IOP in HTG to hemodynamic change in NTG. In other words, both HTG and NTG are related to hemodynamics, but it was hypothesized that the evidence of vascular dysfunction would be more pronounced in NTG patients. One of the possible reasons for this is autonomic dysfunction that may contribute to unstable or fluctuating blood pressure and thereby may induce the dysfunction of autoregulation leading to glaucoma development and progression [3].

Some authors report on autonomic dysfunction in HTG with short term and daily analysis of heart rate variability [26, 34, 38–40]. However, the existing data on autonomic dysfunction in HTG and HTG are contradictory. According to Riccadonna M. et al., HRV and nocturnal diastolic BP variability were reduced in NTG compared to HTG [39]. Furthermore, these differences were more prominent in more severe clinical forms of NTG. The authors suggested a correlation between the extent of autonomic dis-order and severity of glaucoma.

Brown et al. assessed the baroreflective control of the blood and heart vessels using sinusoidal cervical aspiration and showed that the ANS response in healthy subjects was significantly higher than in glaucoma patients. However, they did not detect any difference between NTG and HTG. According to their data, the decreased sympathetic and parasympathetic modulation during baroreceptor stimulation in the patients with HTG and NTG suggested that autonomic dysfunction that may contribute to the pathogenesis of both diseases [40].

Mroczkowska et al. compared NTG and HTG patients with early glaucoma using 24-h outpatient blood pressure monitoring and measurement of peripheral pulse-wave analysis and thickness of the intima-media complex of the carotid arteries. The authors also evaluated reactivity of retinal vessels to flickering of light. Similar changes in systemic and ocular circulation were observed in glaucoma patients of both groups compared to healthy subjects, but no significant differences were revealed in nocturnal blood pressure, arterial or venous retinal atrial fibrillation, systemic arterial stiffness, and intima-media thickness between patients with NTG and HTG [41].

Bossuyt et al. reported on significantly reduced OPP in patients with HTG and NTG compared to the control healthy subjects. They suggested that perfusion-associated vascular changes play an important role in the pathogenesis of both conditions [42].

On the other hand, there are some important differences between HTG and NTG. The nature of VF progression in HTG differs from other types of glaucoma [43]. It is worth noting that NTG of the eye usually progressed in the central region of the VF, and this response was associated with unstable or strong fluctuations in the average 24-h ocular perfusion pressure and excessive nocturnal drops in systemic arterial blood pressure [26, 44]. Consequently, the division into NTG and HTG in clinical practice is still accepted [45].

A significant decrease in retrobulbar blood flow in HTG is described in the literature [46, 47]. Furthermore, Kaiser et al. revealed that ocular blood flow was decreased both in patients with NTG and HTG who progressed despite normal IOP values [46].

Vascular risk factors varied in HTG and NTG [7, 23, 25]. It was hypothesized in the literature that the vascular dysfunction would be more pronounced in NTG patients compared to HTG [7, 31, 48]. However, some authors reported on similar changes in systemic and ocular circulation in the early stages of the disease in patients with HTG and NTG [41].

The decrease in arterial ocular blood flow was more significant in HTG than in NTG, while lower venous blood flow was detected in patients with NTG [47]. It was emphasized in the literature that decreased blood flow rates in the central retinal artery and central retinal vein were significantly associated with the glaucoma progression both in patients with NTG and HTG with well-controlled IOP (21 mmHg or less) [46]. Circulatory disorders can occur in both NTG and HTG, regardless of the IOP level. One of the reasons is increased sympathetic nervous activity (SNA). This leads to increased vascular resistance and, especially in conditions of endothelial dysfunction, may have consequences for blood circulation related to the pathogenesis of glaucoma. The SNA activation causes an increase in stroke volume, heart rate, and vasoconstriction, as well as regulates circadian blood pressure fluctuations, and it is closely related to night dives.

Recently, we compared the shift in HRV indicators in patients with NTG and HTG after a cold provocation test (CPT). MOPP, 24-h blood pressure and HRV were studied in 30 NTG, 30 patients with HTG and 28 healthy individuals. The cardiovascular system condition was assessed before and after CPT. We applied a method of comparing regression lines to identify the differences between groups. Minimum daily diastolic blood pressure and MOPP were reduced in patients with HTG and NTG in comparison with healthy subjects. There were no differences in MOPP between HTG and NTG before CPT. However, all HRV parameters reflected the predominance of sympathetic innervation in glaucoma patients compared to healthy subjects ($p < 0.05$). Up to CPT standard deviation of NN intervals (SDNN) HRV was lower at HTG compared to NTG, 27.2 ± 4.1 ms and 35.33 ± 2.43 ms ($P = 0.02$), respectively. After CBT, SDNN decreased in NTG by 1.7 ms and increased in HTG and healthy individuals by 5.0 ms and 7.09 ms, respectively ($P < 0.05$). Analysis of the relative shift of other HRV parameters after CPT also revealed a significant difference between NTG and HTG in relation to the predominance of sympathetic innervation in NTG compared to HTG. The conclusion was made that NTG patients had a more pronounced violation of ANS than HTG patients, which was manifested by sympathetic nervous system activation in response to CPT. This discovery relates to the pathogenesis of NTG and suggests the use of HRV assessment in the diagnosis and monitoring of glaucoma [32].

Besides, we observed a significant dipping of diastolic BP both in NTG and HTG patients compared to healthy subjects. Probably, this was a consequence of the sympathetic innervation activation. There is evidence of the presence of a choroidal nerve plexus, represented by numerous internal autonomic ganglia forming an autonomous perivascular network around choroidal vessels [49]. It is considered that it plays a vasodilating function aimed at increasing ocular blood flow. Apparently, vascular mechanisms of optic nerve and retinal trophic disorders and their autonomic regulation play an important role in the ocular pathophysiology and physiology in general and in glaucoma. Vasoconstriction occurs against the background of the predominance of sympathoadrenal effects on arterioles and capillaries, as well as due to a decrease in the activity of parasympathetic effects on retinal vessels.

The abovementioned study contained the evidence of altered MOPP both in HTG and NTG patients compared to healthy subjects. However, there were no difference in the MOPP between HTG and NTG that is consistent with the results of previous studies [35, 39, 41]. The obtained results demonstrate that there may be a significant overlap in the development of NTG and HTG, especially at early glaucoma stage [41, 50]. From this point of view, it has been assumed that provocation tests may be used to reveal alterations in cardiovascular function in NTG patients [42]. Prior to CPT, there was a significant difference in all HRV parameters at rest both between glaucoma patient's groups and between HTG patients and control subjects. CPT confirmed a significant difference between the control group and glaucoma patients. In the present study we described a significant increase in the activity of the sympathetic ANS in NTG patients in response to CPT. Changes in the main HRV parameters (SDNN, HF, LF, S, and ARI) after CPT emphasize a significant difference between HTG and NTG patients. It is a well-known fact that PVD people have an increase in sympathetic ANS as a response to provocation tests. The NTG development is associated with the presence of PVD [7, 23]. But currently, this fact is not absolutely reliable, and therefore NTG is considered to be a form of open-angle glaucoma. Although the role of PVD in the pathogenesis of GON has been discussed for many years, only recent studies due to the use of modern technologies could prove that patients with NTG, but not healthy individuals, suffer from the retinal blood flow autoregulation failure in the conditions of provocation tests [51]. From this point of view, the dysfunction of the autonomic blood flow regulation seems to be of high importance and its study attracts attention of the researches. Wierzbowska et al. revealed that the sympathovagal balance of ANS in NTG patients shifted towards sympathetic exertion with no change of 24-h pattern of BP variability as compared to the control healthy group [34]. Na et al. demonstrated significantly reduced SDNN values in NTG [38].

There are new highly relevant data indicating the influence of vascular factors on the NTG development. It can be concluded that the disorders of autonomic innervation underlying PVD lead to the development of NTG, but not its specific feature. The presence of ANS imbalance in POAG patients, including HTG, can also be considered as a risk factor for an unfavorable course of GON. In any case, the obtained results demonstrate the significant role of PVD in the pathogenesis of NTG. The results of our study demonstrating the ascendance of SNA in NTG can be useful for distinguishing HTG and NTG.

This conclusion has an important practical implication for detecting NTG (or if it is suspected), determining the prognosis and choosing more appropriate therapy, as well as making recommendations to patients concerning the proper lifestyle. Further studies are needed to verify our findings as well as studies on any therapies that favorably influence ANS activity in patients with glaucoma.

2.3 The Effect of Autonomic Nervous System Dysfunction on the Progression of Primary Open-Angle Glaucoma

Patients with systemic autonomic dysfunction might be at higher risk for glaucoma progression due to higher susceptibility of the optic nerve to fluctuations of IOP or MOPP.

Park et al. in their study described NTG patients with different types of HRV and reported on the fact that the VF progression in patients with sympathetic predominance occurs faster than in patients with higher HRV. The authors concluded that autonomic dysfunction, especially a decrease in SDNN, is a predictor of the progression of central VF in NTG [26]. This study concluded that IOP-independent risk factors, such as orthostatic hypotension, migraine, and autonomic dysfunction, are associated with the progression of central VF.

In another retrospective study of 40 cases of POAG patients who underwent regular reexamination with heart rate variability (HRV) assessment for more than 3 years Liu and co-authors revealed that patients with POAG in the lowest HRV group showed a faster thinning rate of RNFL than those in the highest HRV group. The progression was accompanied by greater fluctuation of intraocular pressure and a decrease of blood pressure and ocular perfusion pressure. Moreover, thinning rate of RNLF was negatively correlated with SDNN values: the more severe the ANS dysfunction is, characterized, the faster the glaucoma progression in POAG patients. The authors explained this by the enhanced activity of the sympathetic tone and concluded that the treatment of ANS may be useful in glaucoma [37].

3 Vascular, Structural, and Functional Deterioration in Glaucoma

3.1 The Association of Vascular, Structural, and Functional Parameters in Glaucoma

For many years, there has been a debate concerning the issue which parameters—structural or functional—have the greatest diagnostic value in glaucoma [52]. Perimetry was considered a golden standard for the diagnosis of primary open-angle glaucoma (POAG) for a long time. The peripapillary retinal nerve fiber layer (RNFL) and the layer of macular ganglion cells are described in the existing literature as the most significant structural markers for the glaucoma diagnosis [53]. Some authors also reported that the molecular parameters have a high discriminating ability and high reproducibility for the early detection of glaucoma compared to the parameters of the peripapillary RNFL [54].

According to our recent studies, the circulatory parameters serve as diagnostic glaucoma markers [55]. Reduction of retinal hemoperfusion in glaucoma has been repeatedly mentioned in the literature [10, 11]. Nowadays, there is much data on hemodynamic disorders in retina, ONH, and retrobulbar circulation in glaucoma [49, 56–58]. Moreover, several authors have concluded that color Doppler imaging is associated with a prognostic value for damage to visual function in glaucoma patients [59, 60].

However, it is not clear yet if reduced blood flow is the cause or the consequence of glaucoma damage secondary to retinal ganglion cell (RGC) death. This issue can be solved only due to long-term observation of patients by using available methods of clinical examination of retinal vessels, optic nerve, and choriocapillaris. One of the candidates for this method is optical coherence tomography angiography.

3.2 Optical Coherence Tomography Angiography in Glaucoma Diagnostics and Monitoring

Optical coherence tomographic angiography (OCTA) is a new non-invasive diagnostic technique to study the microcirculation in optic nerve, retina, and choroid. OCTA opens up new prospects for examining the blood supply to main structures usually affected by glaucoma (peripapillary retina, optic disc, and internal macular layers) [61]. The studies have consistently demonstrated reduced ONH [61, 62], peripapillary [63], and macular [63–67] perfusion in glaucoma patients using OCTA.

The cross coefficients of variation (CV) range from 3.2% to 9.0% for the global OCT-A parameters of the macular and peripapillary regions [62] and from 5.0% to 6.9% for the peripapillary region [68]. According to the results of some studies, OCTA measurements of vascular density may complement the existing structural parameters for glaucoma detection and its progression by detecting changes in the microcirculatory bed supplying ganglion cells and axons before changes in structural thickness measurements [12, 65–67, 69–71]. OCTA has opened the prospects for novel imaging of retinal and ONH microcirculation [72]. OCTA is based on a new three-dimensional angiography algorithm called amplitude-decorrelation angiography with a split spectrum (SSADA), comparing successive B-scans at the same location to detect blood flow using motion contrast. The reproducibility of OCTA has been reported in several studies [61, 73, 74].

Reduced ONH and peripapillary perfusion parameters have been reported by different authors in subjects with glaucoma measured by OCTA [61, 64, 72–75]. The decreased vessel density (VD) was significantly associated with the severity of visual field damage independent of the structural loss [76, 77].

Different authors have found a significant decrease in IOP in patients with glaucoma compared with healthy people. Wang et al. reported reduced blood flow index in the entire optic disc and inferotemporal segment of the optic disc [73]. The study by Chichara et al. demonstrated the priority of detecting superficial peripapillary retinal VD to differentiate between glaucoma and ophthalmic hypertension and healthy eyes [78]. Liu et al. in their study revealed that there was a significant decrease in peripapillary VD in glaucoma patients compared to healthy subjects of the same age [74]. According to the authors, this indicator had a high diagnostic value for the early detection of glaucoma. Some other studies reported that quantitative OCT-A analysis made it possible to distinguish eyes with glaucoma from healthy eyes by evaluating the entire peripapillary vascular network, from the ILM to the Bruch membrane [76]. According to Yarmohammadi et al., the decreased VD was significantly associated with the severity of visual field damage independent of the structural loss, and whole image vessel density (wiVD) of the disc scan showed the best AUC in their study (AUC: 0.94) [77].

Previously, we have reported better diagnostic accuracy by using capillary density in the macular area over the peripapillary area and the optic disc in the early glaucoma detection [64]. These data are consistent with the literature data on early macular lesions with a high concentration of RGC in glaucoma and explain the localization of the vulnerable area of the retina affected at the very beginning of glaucoma [79, 80].

The functional activity of retinal ganglion cells can be measured using a pattern electroretinogram (PERG). The other objective method of checking visual function is the pattern of visual evoked potentials (PVEP). Glaucomatous changes in PVEP and PERG were reported before the appearance of anomalies in the peripapillary retina and ONH [80–86]. Moreover, PVEPs were used to assess reversible ganglion cell damage in the studies of neuroprotective agents for glaucoma treatment [87, 88].

Having compared the diagnostic ability of the vascular, structural, and functional parameters in differentiation between the normal eyes, early glaucoma, and moderate to severe glaucoma, we have revealed that the results of the electrophysiological testing along with the retinal microcirculation measured by OCTA demonstrated superiority over the structural variables in early glaucoma detection (Fig. 2) [89].

According to our study, a strong correlation between the amplitude of the P100 PVVP and the density of vessels in the ZEN and peripapillary retina, on the one hand, and a correlation between the density of vessels in the superficial macular plexus and the GCC thickness in inferior hemisphere, on the other hand, were

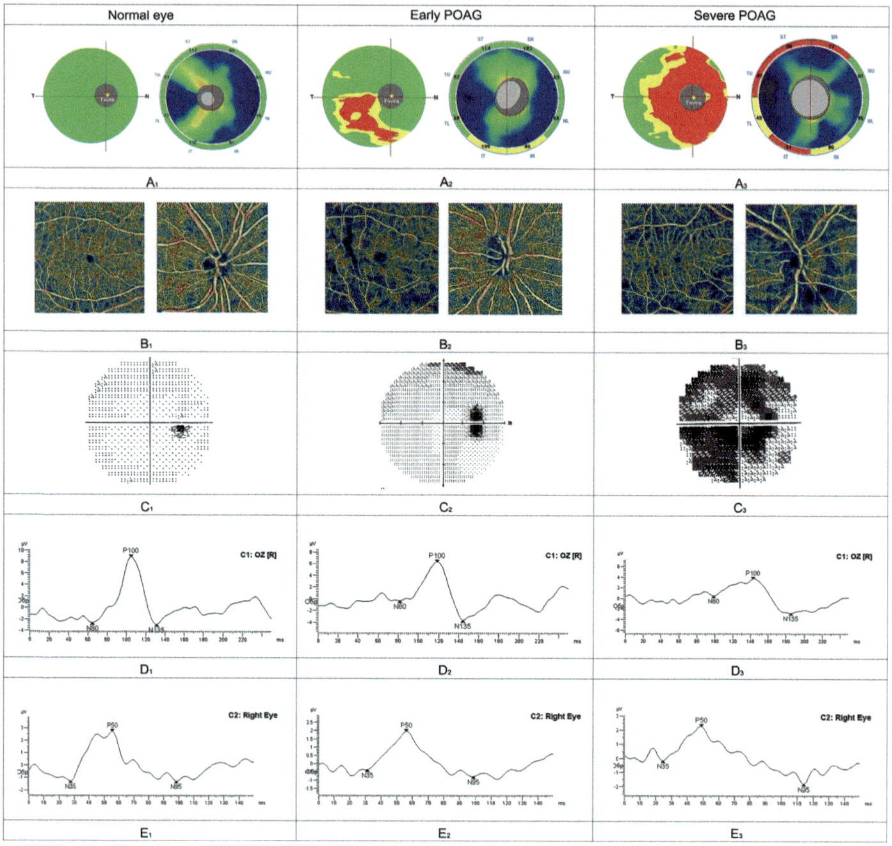

Fig. 2 Clinical examples of the normal controls, early glaucoma, and severe glaucoma. GCC map and RNFL thickness map (**a**), SAP visual field results showing corresponding visual field defects (**c**), PVEP-protocols (**d**), PERG-protocols (**e**). Figure **b** show a stepwise decrease of vessel density both in the circumpapillary VD map and Fovea and circum parafovea VD map (wiVD Disc is reduced from 54.25% (normal eye) to 52.26% (early glaucoma) to 42.17% (severe glaucoma); wiVD Macula Superficial is reduced from 52.56% (normal eye) to 41.95% (early glaucoma) to 41.29% (severe glaucoma). Figure **d** show a stepwise decrease of the amplitude and prolonged latency of P100 component of PVEP and **e** show a decrease of the amplitude and prolonged latency of N95 component of PERG in glaucoma eyes compared to normal eye. (*Modified from the National Journal of Glaucoma (RUS), 2019 with permission*)

revealed. It can be concluded that the damage of ganglion cells may be associated with decreased blood supply to the retina. It was shown that the macular capillary vessel area density strongly correlated with inferior hemimacula or structural damage [65]. Inferior hemimacular retinal structure is subject to a decrease in the area of the capillary vessels of the retina in eyes with glaucoma. Moreover, the blood flow parameters in ophthalmic artery, central retinal artery, and short posterior ciliary arteries in early glaucoma significantly correlate with the retinal thickness in the inferior hemisphere [90].

The existing results of studies demonstrate the importance of microcirculation parameters of the peripapillary retinal and macular region, PERGs and PVEPs, for early detection and monitoring of glaucoma.

3.3 The Detection of Glaucoma Progression Using OCTA

Successful monitoring of POAG depends on early detection of the disease progression. An individual treatment plan should be based on the risk factors and specific clinical markers that allow predicting the rate of disease progression and avoiding unreasonable prescriptions.

Increased intraocular pressure (IOP) [91–95] and its fluctuations [96] are commonly considered to be the main recognized factors for POAG progression. However, there is an increasing interest in the influence of other factors as it is known that the disease can progress at normal IOP [27, 97, 98]. These factors include a thin cornea [93, 99], low corneal hysteresis [100], optic disc hemorrhages [95, 101], peripapillary atrophy of the choroid [91, 100], age of patients [91, 95, 102], female sex [95, 103], presence of pseudoexfoliation [92], late detection of glaucoma [93], and arterial hypotension [104, 105] or/and hypertension [103, 106]. Nevertheless, researchers disagree on many issues regarding progression risk factors and recommend to take into account only highly reliable results concerning significant parameters [95, 107].

A number of studies demonstrate the importance of using OCT angiography for the detection of glaucoma progression. Moghimi S et al. showed that a higher rate of RNFL thinning was associated with an initially reduced density of macular and peripapillary vessels in glaucoma patients [70]. An increase in the area of depletion of vascular macular blood flow, according to the literature, significantly correlates with the presence of structural and functional markers of glaucoma progression, such as the appearance of visual field defects and thinning of the RNFL [69]. According to literature, there is a direct relationship between the vascular, structural, and functional changes in patients with advanced glaucoma [108]. Figure 3 demonstrates a clinical example of the structural and vascular loss that is accompanied by the functional deterioration.

Retinal microvascular loss may be detected more often than structural ones due to the presence of the so-called floor effect in the late stages of the disease, which certainly puts the use of OCT angiography in the forefront in assessing progression of glaucomatous optic neuropathy [109]. Thus, in advanced glaucoma, the measurement of parameters of the microvascular superficial parafoveal vessel density is more prognostic due to the lack of "floor effect" [110].

According to Kwon and co-authors, the visual field progression rate was significantly faster in eyes with parapapillary deep layer microvasculature dropout detected by OCT-A than in those without dropout, and the location of dropout and VF progression was spatially correlated. These findings implicate dropout as a structural parameter suggestive of past glaucomatous VF progression [111].

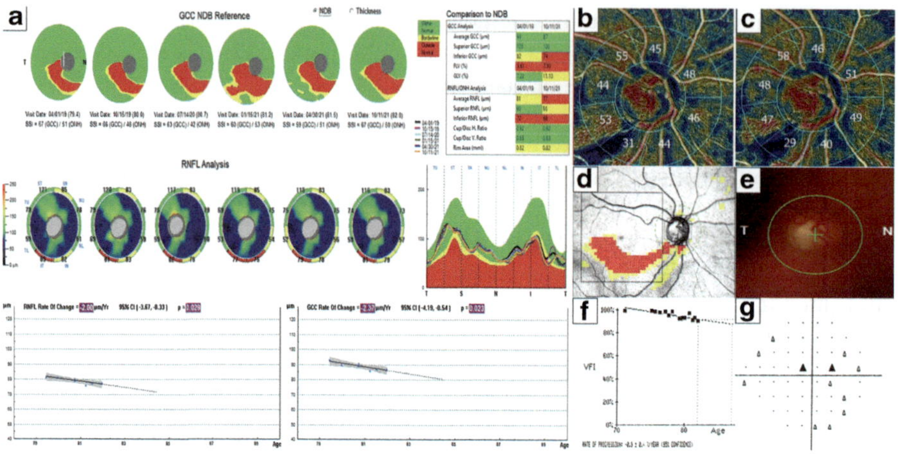

Fig. 3 Association of structural, functional progression with the decrease of microvascularity in the patient with early glaucoma. (**a**) Progressive RNFL and GCC loss; (**b**, **c**) A decrease of vessel density in the circumpapillary VD map; (**d**) A decrease of thickness of GCC and ONH corresponding to the loss of vessel density; (**e**) Fundus visualization of ONH; (**f**, **g**) SAP visual field results

An analysis of FAZ in glaucoma monitoring revealed that, as it manifested, there was a significant thinning of the RNFL and GC-IPL, while no changes in perimetric data were observed [112].

3.4 Role of the Peripapillary Choriocapillaris Loss in Glaucoma Development and Progression

Choroid is another important structure for OCTA assessment. It has the highest blood flow compared to any other tissue in the body [113]. The choriocapillary layer is formed from small arteries and veins, which then break up into many capillaries, passing several red blood cells in one row, which allows more oxygen to enter the retina. The choriocapillary layer of the choroid plays a crucial role in supplying oxygen and nutrition to the outer cells of the retina, especially the retinal pigment epithelium [114]. It should be emphasized that a lesion of blood flow in the choriocapillary layer in the area of the peripapillary retina leads to damage to the lamina cribrosa of sclerae, resulting in a weakening of the structures of the latter.

Optical coherence tomography and angiography mode have opened up new prospects in the study of choriocapillaris blood flow, or rather, the loss of choriocapillaris of the peripapillary retina in glaucoma (Fig. 4).

According to literature, more than the half of patients with primary open-angle glaucoma have a choriocapillary dropout in the beta zone of the ONH [115].

Also, during the examination of 118 patients, scientists revealed that with primary open-angle glaucoma and the presence of defects in the lamina cribrosa

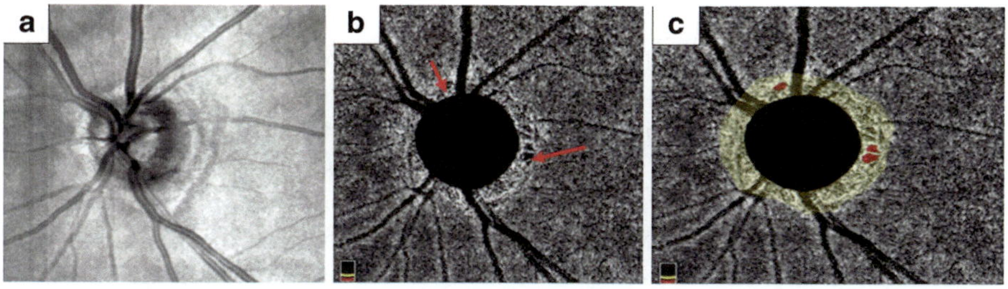

Fig. 4 (**a**, **b**, **c**). Determination of the area and localization of choriocapillary dropout within the beta zone on the density map using RTVue XR Avanti («Optovue», USA). On scans of 4.5 × 4.5 mm of ONH (**a**) at the level of the choroid inside the beta zone, the total dropout of choriocapillaris is determined (**b**: red arrows), with the help of ImageJ program, the area of choriocapillaris dropout in mm^2 inside the beta zone is calculated by pixels (**c**: red areas)

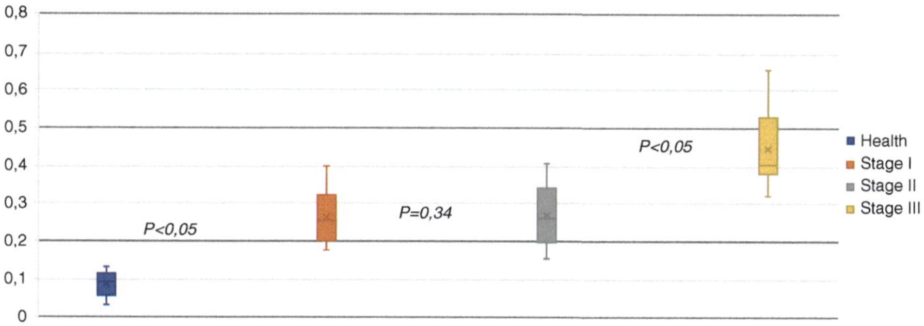

Fig. 5 Peripapillary microvasculature dropout area as a reflection of glaucoma severity

sclerae (59 patients), the frequency of detection of choriocapillary dropout was more frequent than in patients with glaucoma without defects in the lamina cribrosa sclerae (59 patients) [116].

The study by Eun Ji Lee et al. found out that larger lamina cribrosa curvature index (LCCI), disc hemorrhage, and the presence of cMvD were associated with faster global RNFL thinning in multivariate regression analysis. The regression tree analysis revealed three stratified groups based on the RNFL thinning rate divided into LCCI and the presence of cMvD. Eyes with LCCI ≥11.87 had the fastest RNFL thinning (−2.4 ± 0.8 microns/year). Among the eyes with LCCI <11.87, the presence of cMvD was the strongest factor influencing the faster thinning of RNFL (−1.5 ± 0.8 microns/year). Eyes with LCCI <11.87 and without cMvD showed the lowest RNFL thinning (−0.8 ± 0.9 μm/year) [117].

In a recent study, we also showed that the higher the stage of glaucoma, the larger the area of loss of choriocapillaris measured in mm^2 (Fig. 5).

Youn Hye Jo in their study showed that the initial parameters of choroidal microvasculature dropout (CMvD) can be predictors of the rapid development of visual field defects [118].

We have been obtaining glaucoma patients with the fast thinning of choroid that was associated with the rapid visual field deterioration despite the normal IOP (Fig. 6).

A thin peripapillary choroid is also considered a predictor of glaucoma progression [119]. The study by Kim et al. reported that the eyes with the loss of capillaries in the lower temporal quadrant of the peripapillary vasculature have more pronounced visual field damage compared to the eyes with preserved peripapillary choroidal microcirculation. Kim et al. noted an inverse relation between the VD in the peripapillary vasculature and the SNVS thickness [120]. The data of the present study on the prognostic role of the thickness of the peripapillary vasculature are consistent with these results.

Two-year observational study by Park H. et al. revealed the prolapse of peripapillary choroidal microvessels (MvD) in glaucomatous eyes with or without disc hemorrhage (DH). The authors demonstrated that MvD was significantly higher in patients with progressive glaucoma than in stable patients in both the DH and no-DH groups. Park H. et al. concluded that MvD is associated with progressive RNFL thinning. They suggested that OCTA was a new biological marker for glaucoma progression, and this biomarker is a peripapillary choroidal microvascular system [69]. The authors explained this phenomenon is caused by choroidal vascular insufficiency, which may play a significant role in the lack of prelaminar nutrition of the optic nerve during the progression of glaucoma.

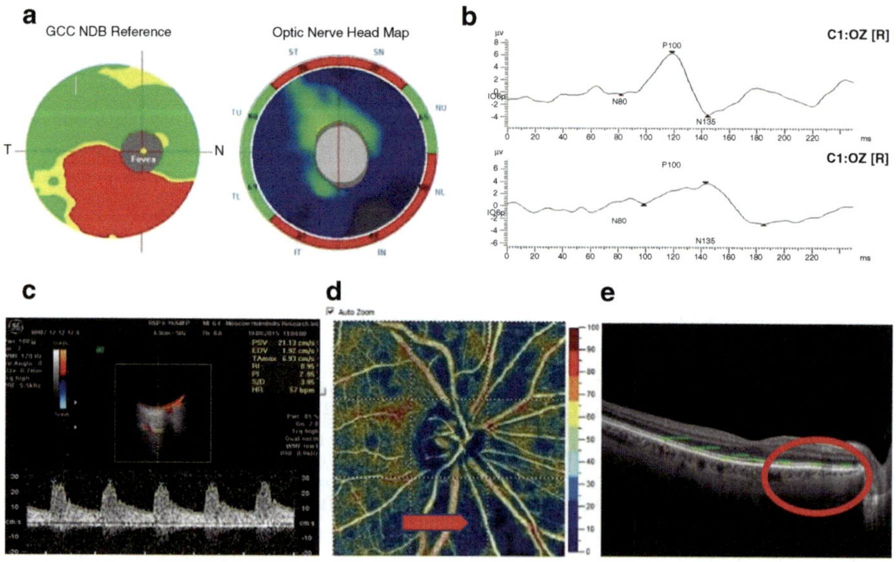

Fig. 6 Clinical example of the choroidal thinning in correspondence with structural, functional and vascular deterioration. (**a**) A decrease of thickness of RNFL and GCC; (**b**) A decrease of amplitude of PVEP; (**c**) A decrease of end-diastolic velocity in the short posterior artery; (**d**) A deep layer microvasculature dropout; (**e**) Decrease of the peripapillary choroidal thickness

3.5 The Prognosis of Glaucoma Progression on the Basis of Functional, Structural, and Circulatory Data

It is rather complicated to define glaucoma progression, since many various factors influence the course of glaucoma [92, 103]. The study by De Moraes reported on the fact that combining data can be useful when discussing risks and treatment options with individual patients, as well as when standardizing the quantitative assessment of the risk of progression in treated patients with glaucoma [100]. From this point of view, the application of new biomarkers as the vessel density, measured by OCTA, may improve the prediction of glaucoma progression.

We conducted a comparative study of microcirculation parameters, predictors of glaucoma progression, and other clinical data [121]. The following results were obtained: decreased blood circulation, including regional microcirculation and retrobulbar blood flow, is associated with the progression of glaucoma. According to the multilevel analysis of models of mixed effects, four predictors were revealed: parafoveal superficial plexus vessel density, the end-diastolic velocity of the central retinal artery, the volume of focal loss of the ganglion cell complex and the peak follow-up IOP. The rate of disease progression expressed as a change of perimetric index MD of visual field and RNFL thinning correlated with the peak follow-up IOP and the end-diastolic velocity in posterior ciliary arteries. A positive correlation was also observed between the thickness of the retinal inner layers in parafovea and the parafovea vessel density in superficial layer. Mean ocular perfusion pressure (MOPP) correlated with the average ganglion cells complex thickness and its focal loss volume [121].

The present study concluded that only a decrease in parafoveal VD in the superficial layer was associated with the glaucoma progression, which was confirmed by both functional and structural disorders in all statistical models. Several existing studies have shown that OCTA makes it possible to detect the disease at the preperimetric stage, and OCTA parameters correlate better with functional parameters, including electrophysiological parameters, than with structural ones [61, 77, 89].

Some authors have reviled that the disease progression is mainly associated with low end-diastolic velocity in short posterior ciliary arteries [59] and the high resistive index in central retinal artery [122].

A decrease in OCTA VD may actually precede both structural and functional losses and, therefore, may be useful in the diagnosis and monitoring of glaucoma at the earliest stages [123, 124]. This decrease detected at early glaucoma stages may be used as a glaucoma progression predictor.

Generally speaking, the role of OCTA in identifying glaucoma progression predictors and the dynamic range of vascular density is insignificant. Moreover, the study conducted by Moghimi and co-authors also has underlined that the correlation between the rate of RNFL loss and VD measurements was not strong. However, Moghimi et al. concluded that the OCTA parameters can predict RNFL loss during the long-term follow-up. The authors reported that OCTA may provide the data concerning early RGCs dysfunction with lower metabolic needs.

According to our study, a decrease in parafoveal vessel density can serve as a predictor of death of cells and subsequent tissue thinning with functional loss. The inferior sector of the macula as a vulnerable region for glaucoma damage makes sense, since most of the nerve fibers of the lower macula are projected into the lower quadrant of the optic disc, an area that is particularly susceptible to glaucomatous damage. Hood et al. described that thinning of RGC and the nerve fiber layer is already present in preperimetric glaucoma patients and progresses with increasing loss of mean deviation (MD) [79]. Lommatzsch et al. confirmed first that the VD of the inferior perimacular sector is lower than in all other sectors, and that this value decreases in early forms of glaucoma with progressive losses with worsening of progressive losses with deteriorating MD [125]. The recent study showed that a decrease in VF MD for every 1 dB was associated with a decrease in macular wiVD by 0.43% and pfVD by 0.46%. According to their study, the correlation between macular vessel density and MD of the visual field in the whole image was stronger than ONH whole image capillary density and GCC and RNFL thicknesses [108]. However, the authors did not sufficiently study the reasons for early macula damage in glaucoma. This fact is probably due to retinal ischemia with increased metabolic needs of the area with the highest concentration of RGC. According to the results of our study, the thickness of the RGC and its characteristics (GLV and FLV) correlated with the average ocular perfusion pressure.

The assessment of macular VD in glaucoma monitoring also makes it possible to determine the disease progression in such cases when structural parameters are unacceptable due to the presence of floor effect. According to Moghimi, even a pronounced loss of visual function (MD reached −19 dB) did not result in the "floor effect" of VD [126]. Similar results were obtained by Rao [127] who demonstrated that the floor effect for the specified parameter did not occur at MD -15 dB. Other authors reported that the floor effect in the peripapillary retinal VD occurs somewhat earlier, which is observed at MP < −14.0 dB, but at the same time later than for such morphometric parameters as RGC thickness and RNFL [79, 128]. According to Hood et al., this effect for RNFL is already visible at MD of −10 dB [79]. Other authors have also noted the advantages of studying GCC thickness compared to RNFL [129]. Furthermore, the importance of assessing peripapillary VD in the late glaucoma stages has been described in the recent studies [130]. It has been revealed that the detection of glaucoma progression at early stages is more reliable with the use of SD-OCT, while functional deterioration is more visible in the middle and late stages. In our previous studies we reported that the structural parameters (in particular, retinal GCC) have priority over functional ones in early glaucoma compared to advanced stage of the disease [89]. However, peripapillary VD had the highest diagnostic accuracy to distinguish between early, middle and late stages, while parafoveal VD in the surface layer had the highest diagnostic accuracy to distinguish between early glaucoma and healthy eyes. In general, the diagnostic ability of the OCTA parameters in early glaucoma was higher compared to GCC and RNFL thickness.

According to some studies, a decrease in macula VD, OHN, and the peripapillary retina is associated with a higher rate of progression of RNFL loss in mild and moderate glaucoma, suggesting that a VD decrease may be a predictor of progression risk [126]. Their results have shown that vessel density measures tend to be more strongly associated with severity of visual field damage than thickness measures and may be an additional tool to monitor progression in advanced disease. These data are consistent with our results, according to which OCTA parameters serve as predictors of glaucoma progression [121].

There is a lack of information on the influence of lowering IOP on retinal microcirculation. The experimental studies have reported that microcirculation in the retina, choriocapillaris, sclera, and lattice plate remains unchanged even with significant IOP fluctuations [91]. On the other hand, according to some clinical studies, OCTA vessel density strongly correlates with IOP [131–133].

In conclusion, OCTA may significantly improve the early detection of glaucoma progression, as formerly OCT has provided more precise diagnostics in regard to this detection.

References

1. Balendra SI, Zollet P, Casasca GCADGE, Cordeiro MF (2020) Personalized approaches for the management of glaucoma. Exp Rev Precis Med Drug Dev 5(3):145–164. https://doi.org/10.1080/23808993.2020.1756770
2. Nathan M. Radcliffe; Jason Bacharach, Murray Fingeret, Lorraine M Provencher. Glaucoma treatments in 2021: personalizing patient needs 2021
3. Flammer J, Konieczka K, Bruno RM, Virdis A, Flammer AJ, Taddei S (2013) The eye and the heart. Eur Heart J 34(17):1270–1278. https://doi.org/10.1093/eurheartj/eht023
4. Nicolela MT, Ferrier SN, Morrison CA et al (2003) Effects of cold-induced vasospasm in glaucoma: the role of endothelin-1. Invest Ophthalmol Vis Sci 44(6):2565–2572. https://doi.org/10.1167/iovs.02-0913
5. Golubnitschaja O (2019) Flammer syndrome: from phenotype to associated pathologies, prediction, prevention and personalisation. Flammer Syndrome
6. Neves VJ, Moura MJ, Almeida BS et al (2012) Chronic stress, but not hypercaloric diet, impairs vascular function in rats. Stress 15(2):138–148. https://doi.org/10.3109/10253890.2011.601369
7. Konieczka K, Ritch R, Traverso CE et al (2014) Flammer syndrome. EPMA J 5(1):11. Published 2014 Jul 8. https://doi.org/10.1186/1878-5085-5-11
8. Konieczka K, Flammer J, Sternbuch J, Binggeli T, Fraenkl S (2017) Leber's hereditary optic neuropathy, Normal tension glaucoma, and Flammer syndrome: long term follow-up of a patient. Lebersche hereditäre Optikusneuropathie, Normaldruckglaukom und Flammer-Syndrom—eine langzeitige Beobachtung eines Patienten. Klin Monbl Augenheilkd 234(4):584–587. https://doi.org/10.1055/s-0042-119564
9. Schmidl D, Boltz A, Kaya S et al (2012) Comparison of choroidal and optic nerve head blood flow regulation during changes in ocular perfusion pressure. Invest Ophthalmol Vis Sci 53(8):4337–4346. Published 2012 Jul 1. https://doi.org/10.1167/iovs.11-9055
10. Grieshaber MC, Flammer J (2005) Blood flow in glaucoma. Curr Opin Ophthalmol 16(2):79–83. https://doi.org/10.1097/01.icu.0000156134.38495.0b
11. Hayreh SS (2001) Blood flow in the optic nerve head and factors that may influence it. Prog Retin Eye Res 20(5):595–624. https://doi.org/10.1016/s1350-9462(01)00005-2
12. Hwang JC, Konduru R, Zhang X et al (2012) Relationship among visual field, blood flow, and neural structure measurements in glaucoma. Invest Ophthalmol Vis Sci 53(6):3020–3026. Published 2012 May 17. https://doi.org/10.1167/iovs.11-8552

13. Jia Y, Tan O, Tokayer J et al (2012) Split-spectrum amplitude-decorrelation angiography with optical coherence tomography. Opt Express 20(4):4710–4725. https://doi.org/10.1364/OE.20.004710
14. Rusia D, Harris A, Pernic A et al (2011) Feasibility of creating a normative database of colour Doppler imaging parameters in glaucomatous eyes and controls. Br J Ophthalmol 95(9):1193–1198. https://doi.org/10.1136/bjo.2010.188219
15. Weinreb RN, Harris A (2007) Ocular blood flow in glaucoma: consensus series 6. Kugler Publications, Dordrecht
16. Yaoeda K, Shirakashi M, Fukushima A et al (2003) Relationship between optic nerve head microcirculation and visual field loss in glaucoma. Acta Ophthalmol Scand 81(3):253–259. https://doi.org/10.1034/j.1600-0420.2003.00073.x
17. Ben-Zion I, Harris A, Weizman Y, Ehrlich R, Rechtman E (2008) An updated review of methods for human retinal oximetry measurements and current applications. Harefuah 147(10):812–817. 836. Hebrew
18. Jonas JB, Harazny J, Budde WM, Mardin CY, Papastathopoulos KI, Michelson G (2003) Optic disc morphometry correlated with confocal laser scanning Doppler flowmetry measurements in normal-pressure glaucoma. J Glaucoma 12(3):260–265. https://doi.org/10.1097/00061198-200306000-00014
19. Kawasaki R, Wang JJ, Rochtchina E, Lee AJ, Wong TY, Mitchell P (2013) Retinal vessel caliber is associated with the 10-year incidence of glaucoma: the Blue Mountains Eye Study. Ophthalmology 120(1):84–90. https://doi.org/10.1016/j.ophtha.2012.07.007
20. Stalmans I, Vandewalle E, Anderson DR et al (2011) Use of colour Doppler imaging in ocular blood flow research. Acta Ophthalmol 89(8):e609–e630. https://doi.org/10.1111/j.1755-3768.2011.02178.x
21. Wang Y, Bower BA, Izatt JA, Tan O, Huang D (2008) Retinal blood flow measurement by circumpapillary Fourier domain Doppler optical coherence tomography. J Biomed Opt 13(6):064003. https://doi.org/10.1117/1.2998480
22. Chan TCW, Bala C, Siu A, Wan F, White A (2017) Risk factors for rapid glaucoma disease progression. Am J Ophthalmol 180:151–157. https://doi.org/10.1016/j.ajo.2017.06.003
23. Flammer J, Konieczka K, Flammer AJ (2013) The primary vascular dysregulation syndrome: implications for eye diseases. EPMA J 4(1):14. Published 2013 Jun 7. https://doi.org/10.1186/1878-5085-4-14
24. Galassi F, Sodi A, Ucci F, Renieri G, Pieri B, Baccini M (2003) Ocular hemodynamics and glaucoma prognosis: a color Doppler imaging study. Arch Ophthalmol 121(12):1711–1715. https://doi.org/10.1001/archopht.121.12.1711
25. Flammer J, Orgül S, Costa VP et al (2002) The impact of ocular blood flow in glaucoma. Prog Retin Eye Res 21(4):359–393. https://doi.org/10.1016/s1350-9462(02)00008-3
26. Park HY, Park SH, Park CK (2014) Central visual field progression in normal-tension glaucoma patients with autonomic dysfunction. Invest Ophthalmol Vis Sci 55(4):2557–2563. Published 2014 Apr 21. https://doi.org/10.1167/iovs.13-13742
27. Drance S, Anderson DR, Schulzer M, Collaborative Normal-Tension Glaucoma Study Group (2001) Risk factors for progression of visual field abnormalities in normal-tension glaucoma. Am J Ophthalmol 131(6):699–708. https://doi.org/10.1016/s0002-9394(01)00964-3
28. Satilmis M, Orgül S, Doubler B, Flammer J (2003) Rate of progression of glaucoma correlates with retrobulbar circulation and intraocular pressure. Am J Ophthalmol 135(5):664–669. https://doi.org/10.1016/s0002-9394(02)02156-6
29. Phelps CD, Corbett JJ (1985) Migraine and low-tension glaucoma. A case-control study. Invest Ophthalmol Vis Sci 26(8):1105–1108
30. Zhou W, Sabel B (2023) Vascular dysregulation in glaucoma: retinal vasoconstriction and normal neurovascular coupling in altitudinal visual field defects. EPMA J 14(1):87–99. https://doi.org/10.1007/s13167-023-00316-6
31. Gherghel D, Hosking SL, Cunliffe IA (2004) Abnormal systemic and ocular vascular response to temperature provocation in primary open-angle glaucoma patients: a case for autonomic failure? Invest Ophthalmol Vis Sci 45(10):3546–3554. https://doi.org/10.1167/iovs.04-0290

32. Kurysheva NI, Ryabova TY, Shlapak VN (2018) Heart rate variability: the comparison between high tension and normal tension glaucoma. EPMA J 9(1):35–45. https://doi.org/10.1007/s13167-017-0124-4
33. Feke GT, Pasquale LR (2008) Retinal blood flow response to posture change in glaucoma patients compared with healthy subjects. Ophthalmology 115(2):246–252. https://doi.org/10.1016/j.ophtha.2007.04.055
34. Wierzbowska J, Wierzbowski R, Stankiewicz A, Siesky B, Harris A (2012) Cardiac autonomic dysfunction in patients with normal tension glaucoma: 24-h heart rate and blood pressure variability analysis. Br J Ophthalmol 96(5):624–628. https://doi.org/10.1136/bjophthalmol-2011-300945
35. Gherghel D, Hosking SL, Cunliffe IA, Heitmar R (2010) Transient cardiac ischaemia and abnormal variations in systemic blood pressure in unselected primary open angle glaucoma patients. Ophthalmic Physiol Opt 30(2):175–181. https://doi.org/10.1111/j.1475-1313.2009.00704.x
36. Chai E, Goldberg I, Chia A, Chen J (1999) Visual field responses to a hand vibration stimulus. Surv Ophthalmol 43(Suppl 1):S79–S86. https://doi.org/10.1016/s0039-6257(99)00051-x
37. Liu B, Zhao Y, Zhang H (2022) The effect of autonomic nervous system dysfunction on the progression of primary open-angle glaucoma. Int J Gen Med 15:4565–4573. Published 2022 May 2. https://doi.org/10.2147/IJGM.S362275
38. Na KS, Lee NY, Park SH, Park CK (2010) Autonomic dysfunction in normal tension glaucoma: the short-term heart rate variability analysis. J Glaucoma 19(6):377–381. https://doi.org/10.1097/IJG.0b013e3181c4ae58
39. Riccadonna M, Covi G, Pancera P et al (2003) Autonomic system activity and 24-hour blood pressure variations in subjects with normal- and high-tension glaucoma. J Glaucoma 12(2):156–163. https://doi.org/10.1097/00061198-200304000-00011
40. Brown CM, Dütsch M, Michelson G, Neundörfer B, Hilz MJ (2002) Impaired cardiovascular responses to baroreflex stimulation in open-angle and normal-pressure glaucoma. Clin Sci (Lond) 102(6):623–630. https://doi.org/10.1042/cs1020623
41. Mroczkowska S, Benavente-Perez A, Negi A, Sung V, Patel SR, Gherghel D (2013) Primary open-angle glaucoma vs normal-tension glaucoma: the vascular perspective. JAMA Ophthalmol 131(1):36–43. https://doi.org/10.1001/2013.jamaophthalmol.1
42. Bossuyt J, Vandekerckhove G, De Backer TLM et al (2015) Vascular dysregulation in normal-tension glaucoma is not affected by structure and function of the microcirculation or macrocirculation at rest: a case-control study. Medicine (Baltimore) 94(2):e425. https://doi.org/10.1097/MD.0000000000000425
43. Ahrlich KG, De Moraes CG, Teng CC et al (2010) Visual field progression differences between normal-tension and exfoliative high-tension glaucoma. Invest Ophthalmol Vis Sci 51(3):1458–1463. https://doi.org/10.1167/iovs.09-3806
44. Choi J, Jeong J, Cho HS, Kook MS (2006) Effect of nocturnal blood pressure reduction on circadian fluctuation of mean ocular perfusion pressure: a risk factor for normal tension glaucoma. Invest Ophthalmol Vis Sci 47(3):831–836. https://doi.org/10.1167/iovs.05-1053
45. Thonginnetra O, Greenstein VC, Chu D, Liebmann JM, Ritch R, Hood DC (2010) Normal versus high tension glaucoma: a comparison of functional and structural defects. J Glaucoma 19(3):151–157. https://doi.org/10.1097/IJG.0b013e318193c45c
46. Kaiser HJ, Schoetzau A, Stümpfig D, Flammer J (1997) Blood-flow velocities of the extraocular vessels in patients with high-tension and normal-tension primary open-angle glaucoma. Am J Ophthalmol 123(3):320–327. https://doi.org/10.1016/s0002-9394(14)70127-8
47. Kurysheva N, Kiseleva T, Irtegova E, Parshunina O (2015) Venous ocular blood flow in primary open angle glaucoma. Int J Ophthalmol Eye Res 3:1–7
48. Gasser P, Flammer J (1991) Blood-cell velocity in the nailfold capillaries of patients with normal-tension and high-tension glaucoma. Am J Ophthalmol 111(5):585–588. https://doi.org/10.1016/s0002-9394(14)73703-1
49. Grunwald JE, Piltz J, Hariprasad SM, DuPont J (1998) Optic nerve and choroidal circulation in glaucoma. Invest Ophthalmol Vis Sci 39(12):2329–2336

50. Koch EC, Staab J, Fuest M, Witt K, Voss A, Plange N (2015) Blood pressure and heart rate variability to detect vascular dysregulation in glaucoma. J Ophthalmol 2015:798958. https://doi.org/10.1155/2015/798958
51. Drance SM, Douglas GR, Wijsman K, Schulzer M, Britton RJ (1988) Response of blood flow to warm and cold in normal and low-tension glaucoma patients. Am J Ophthalmol 105(1):35–39. https://doi.org/10.1016/0002-9394(88)90118-3
52. Hood DC, Anderson SC, Wall M, Raza AS, Kardon RH (2009) A test of a linear model of glaucomatous structure-function loss reveals sources of variability in retinal nerve fiber and visual field measurements. Invest Ophthalmol Vis Sci 50(9):4254–4266. https://doi.org/10.1167/iovs.08-2697
53. Ojima T, Tanabe T, Hangai M, Yu S, Morishita S, Yoshimura N (2007) Measurement of retinal nerve fiber layer thickness and macular volume for glaucoma detection using optical coherence tomography. Jpn J Ophthalmol 51(3):197–203. https://doi.org/10.1007/s10384-006-0433-y
54. Nakatani Y, Higashide T, Ohkubo S, Takeda H, Sugiyama K (2011) Evaluation of macular thickness and peripapillary retinal nerve fiber layer thickness for detection of early glaucoma using spectral domain optical coherence tomography. J Glaucoma 20(4):252–259. https://doi.org/10.1097/IJG.0b013e3181e079ed
55. Kurysheva NI, Parshunina OA, Shatalova EO, Kiseleva TN, Lagutin MB, Fomin AV (2017) Value of structural and hemodynamic parameters for the early detection of primary open-angle glaucoma. Curr Eye Res 42(3):411–417. https://doi.org/10.1080/02713683.2016.1184281
56. Kurysheva NI, Kiseleva TN, Hodak NA (2012) The study of bioelectricactivity and regional hemodynamics in glaucoma. Klinicheskaya oftalmologiya 3:91–94
57. Flammer J, Orgül S (1998) Optic nerve blood-flow abnormalities in glaucoma. Prog Retin Eye Res 17(2):267–289. https://doi.org/10.1016/s1350-9462(97)00006-2
58. Tobe LA, Harris A, Hussain RM et al (2015) The role of retrobulbar and retinal circulation on optic nerve head and retinal nerve fibre layer structure in patients with open-angle glaucoma over an 18-month period. Br J Ophthalmol 99(5):609–612. https://doi.org/10.1136/bjophthalmol-2014-305780
59. Martínez A, Sánchez M (2005) Predictive value of colour Doppler imaging in a prospective study of visual field progression in primary open-angle glaucoma. Acta Ophthalmol Scand 83(6):716–722. https://doi.org/10.1111/j.1600-0420.2005.00567.x
60. Mokbel TH, Ghanem AA (2011) Diagnostic value of color Doppler imaging and pattern visual evoked potential in primary open-angle glaucoma. J Clin Exp Ophthalmol 2(1). https://doi.org/10.4172/2155-9570.1000127
61. Jia Y, Wei E, Wang X et al (2014) Optical coherence tomography angiography of optic disc perfusion in glaucoma. Ophthalmology 121(7):1322–1332. https://doi.org/10.1016/j.ophtha.2014.01.021
62. Manalastas PIC, Zangwill LM, Saunders LJ et al (2017) Reproducibility of optical coherence tomography angiography macular and optic nerve head vascular density in glaucoma and healthy eyes. J Glaucoma 26(10):851–859. https://doi.org/10.1097/IJG.0000000000000768
63. Chen HS, Liu CH, Wu WC, Tseng HJ, Lee YS (2017) Optical coherence tomography angiography of the superficial microvasculature in the macular and Peripapillary areas in glaucomatous and healthy eyes. Invest Ophthalmol Vis Sci 58(9):3637–3645. https://doi.org/10.1167/iovs.17-21846
64. Kurysheva NI (2016) Macula in glaucoma: vascularity evaluated by OCT angiography. Res J Pharm, Biol Chem Sci 7(5):651–662
65. Xu H, Yu J, Kong X, Sun X, Jiang C (2016) Macular microvasculature alterations in patients with primary open-angle glaucoma: a cross-sectional study. Medicine (Baltimore) 95(33):e4341. https://doi.org/10.1097/MD.0000000000004341
66. Akil H, Chopra V, Al-Sheikh M et al (2017. bjophthalmol-2016-309816) Swept-source OCT angiography imaging of the macular capillary network in glaucoma [published online ahead of print, 2017 Aug 9]. Br J Ophthalmol. https://doi.org/10.1136/bjophthalmol-2016-309816

67. Shoji T, Zangwill LM, Akagi T et al (2017) Progressive macula vessel density loss in primary open-angle glaucoma: a longitudinal study. Am J Ophthalmol 182:107–117. https://doi.org/10.1016/j.ajo.2017.07.011
68. Holló G (2016) Intrasession and Between-Visit Variability of Sector Peripapillary Angioflow Vessel Density Values Measured with the Angiovue Optical Coherence Tomograph in Different Retinal Layers in Ocular Hypertension and Glaucoma [published correction appears in PLoS One. 2016 Dec 9;11(12):e0168231]. PloS One 11(8):e0161631. Published 2016 Aug 18. https://doi.org/10.1371/journal.pone.0161631
69. Park HL, Kim JW, Park CK (2018) Choroidal microvasculature dropout is associated with progressive retinal nerve fiber layer thinning in glaucoma with disc hemorrhage. Ophthalmology 125(7):1003–1013. https://doi.org/10.1016/j.ophtha.2018.01.016
70. Moghimi S, Zangwill LM, Penteado RC et al (2018) Macular and optic nerve head vessel density and progressive retinal nerve fiber layer loss in glaucoma. Ophthalmology 125(11):1720–1728. https://doi.org/10.1016/j.ophtha.2018.05.006
71. Yarmohammadi A, Zangwill LM, Diniz-Filho A et al (2016) Relationship between optical coherence tomography angiography vessel density and severity of visual field loss in glaucoma. Ophthalmology 123(12):2498–2508. https://doi.org/10.1016/j.ophtha.2016.08.041
72. Jia Y, Morrison JC, Tokayer J et al (2012) Quantitative OCT angiography of optic nerve head blood flow. Biomed Opt Express 3(12):3127–3137. https://doi.org/10.1364/BOE.3.003127
73. Wang X, Jiang C, Ko T et al (2015) Correlation between optic disc perfusion and glaucomatous severity in patients with open-angle glaucoma: an optical coherence tomography angiography study. Graefes Arch Clin Exp Ophthalmol 253(9):1557–1564. https://doi.org/10.1007/s00417-015-3095-y
74. Liu L, Jia Y, Takusagawa HL et al (2015) Optical coherence tomography angiography of the peripapillary retina in glaucoma. JAMA Ophthalmol 133(9):1045–1052. https://doi.org/10.1001/jamaophthalmol.2015.2225
75. Lee EJ, Lee KM, Lee SH, Kim TW (2016) OCT angiography of the peripapillary retina in primary open-angle glaucoma. Invest Ophthalmol Vis Sci 57(14):6265–6270. https://doi.org/10.1167/iovs.16-20287
76. Lévêque PM, Zéboulon P, Brasnu E, Baudouin C, Labbé A (2016) Optic disc vascularization in glaucoma: value of spectral-domain optical coherence tomography angiography. J Ophthalmol 2016:6956717. https://doi.org/10.1155/2016/6956717
77. Yarmohammadi A, Zangwill LM, Diniz-Filho A et al (2016) Optical coherence tomography angiography vessel density in healthy, glaucoma suspect, and glaucoma eyes. Invest Ophthalmol Vis Sci 57(9):OCT451–OCT459. https://doi.org/10.1167/iovs.15-18944
78. Chihara E, Dimitrova G, Amano H, Chihara T (2017) Discriminatory power of superficial vessel density and prelaminar vascular flow index in eyes with glaucoma and ocular hypertension and normal eyes. Invest Ophthalmol Vis Sci 58(1):690–697. https://doi.org/10.1167/iovs.16-20709
79. Hood DC (2017) Improving our understanding, and detection, of glaucomatous damage: an approach based upon optical coherence tomography (OCT). Prog Retin Eye Res 57:46–75. https://doi.org/10.1016/j.preteyeres.2016.12.002
80. Hood DC, Raza AS, de Moraes CG, Johnson CA, Liebmann JM, Ritch R (2012) The nature of macular damage in glaucoma as revealed by averaging optical coherence tomography data. Transl Vis Sci Technol 1(1):3. https://doi.org/10.1167/tvst.1.1.3
81. Bowd C, Tafreshi A, Zangwill LM, Medeiros FA, Sample PA, Weinreb RN (2011) Pattern electroretinogram association with spectral domain-OCT structural measurements in glaucoma. Eye (Lond) 25(2):224–232. https://doi.org/10.1038/eye.2010.203
82. May JG, Ralston JV, Reed JL, Van Dyk HJ (1982) Loss in pattern-elicited electroretinograms in optic nerve dysfunction. Am J Ophthalmol 93(4):418–422. https://doi.org/10.1016/0002-9394(82)90131-3
83. Bobak P, Bodis-Wollner I, Harnois C et al (1983) Pattern electroretinograms and visual-evoked potentials in glaucoma and multiple sclerosis. Am J Ophthalmol 96(1):72–83. https://doi.org/10.1016/0002-9394(83)90457-9

84. Wanger P, Persson HE (1983) Pattern-reversal electroretinograms in unilateral glaucoma. Invest Ophthalmol Vis Sci 24(6):749–753
85. Bach M, Hiss P, Röver J (1988) Check-size specific changes of pattern electroretinogram in patients with early open-angle glaucoma. Doc Ophthalmol 69(3):315–322. https://doi.org/10.1007/BF00154412
86. Parisi V, Miglior S, Manni G, Centofanti M, Bucci MG (2006) Clinical ability of pattern electroretinograms and visual evoked potentials in detecting visual dysfunction in ocular hypertension and glaucoma. Ophthalmology 113(2):216–228. https://doi.org/10.1016/j.ophtha.2005.10.044
87. Rejdak R, Toczołowski J, Kurkowski J et al (2003) Oral citicoline treatment improves visual pathway function in glaucoma. Med Sci Monit 9(3):PI24–PI28
88. Tong Y, Wang P, Xia Z, Xia X, Xu X (2009) Color pattern reversal visual evoked potentials in primary open angle and angle closure glaucoma. Zhong Nan Da Xue Xue Bao Yi Xue Ban 34(8):771–775. Chinese
89. Kurysheva NI, Maslova EV, Zolnikova IV, Fomin AV, Lagutin MB (2018) A comparative study of structural, functional and circulatory parameters in glaucoma diagnostics. PloS One 13(8):e0201599. Published 2018 Aug 23. https://doi.org/10.1371/journal.pone.0201599
90. Kurysheva NI, Maslova EV, Trubilina AV, Fomin AV, Likhvantseva VG, Lagutin MB (2017) OCT angiography and color doppler imaging in glaucoma diagnostics. J Pharm Sci Res 9(5):527–536
91. Investigators AGIS (2002) The advanced glaucoma intervention study (AGIS): 12. Baseline risk factors for sustained loss of visual field and visual acuity in patients with advanced glaucoma. Am J Ophthalmol 134(4):499–512. https://doi.org/10.1016/s0002-9394(02)01659-8
92. Leske MC, Heijl A, Hussein M et al (2003) Factors for glaucoma progression and the effect of treatment: the early manifest glaucoma trial. Arch Ophthalmol 121(1):48–56. https://doi.org/10.1001/archopht.121.1.48
93. Leske MC, Heijl A, Hyman L et al (2007) Predictors of long-term progression in the early manifest glaucoma trial. Ophthalmology 114(11):1965–1972. https://doi.org/10.1016/j.ophtha.2007.03.016
94. Miglior S, Zeyen T, Pfeiffer N et al (2005) Results of the European glaucoma prevention study. Ophthalmology 112(3):366–375. https://doi.org/10.1016/j.ophtha.2004.11.030
95. Chauhan BC, Mikelberg FS, Balaszi AG et al (2008) Canadian glaucoma study: 2. Risk factors for the progression of open-angle glaucoma [published correction appears in arch Ophthalmol. 2008 Oct;126(10):1364]. Arch Ophthalmol 126(8):1030–1036. https://doi.org/10.1001/archopht.126.8.1030
96. Kim SH, Lee EJ, Han JC, Sohn SW, Rhee T, Kee C (2016) the effect of diurnal fluctuation in intraocular pressure on the evaluation of risk factors of progression in normal tension glaucoma. PloS One 11(10):e0164876. Published 2016 Oct 24. https://doi.org/10.1371/journal.pone.0164876
97. De Moraes CG, Juthani VJ, Liebmann JM et al (2011) Risk factors for visual field progression in treated glaucoma [published correction appears in arch Ophthalmol. 2011 Jul;129(7):878]. Arch Ophthalmol 129(5):562–568. https://doi.org/10.1001/archophthalmol.2011.72
98. Musch DC, Gillespie BW, Niziol LM, Lichter PR, Varma R, CIGTS Study Group (2011) Intraocular pressure control and long-term visual field loss in the collaborative initial glaucoma treatment study. Ophthalmology 118(9):1766–1773. https://doi.org/10.1016/j.ophtha.2011.01.047
99. Medeiros FA, Sample PA, Zangwill LM, Bowd C, Aihara M, Weinreb RN (2003) Corneal thickness as a risk factor for visual field loss in patients with preperimetric glaucomatous optic neuropathy. Am J Ophthalmol 136(5):805–813. https://doi.org/10.1016/s0002-9394(03)00484-7
100. De Moraes CV, Hill V, Tello C, Liebmann JM, Ritch R (2012) Lower corneal hysteresis is associated with more rapid glaucomatous visual field progression. J Glaucoma 21(4):209–213. https://doi.org/10.1097/IJG.0b013e3182071b92

101. Bengtsson B, Leske MC, Yang Z, Heijl A, EMGT Group (2008) Disc hemorrhages and treatment in the early manifest glaucoma trial. Ophthalmology 115(11):2044–2048. https://doi.org/10.1016/j.ophtha.2008.05.031
102. Martínez A, Sanchez-Salorio M (2010) Predictors for visual field progression and the effects of treatment with dorzolamide 2% or brinzolamide 1% each added to timolol 0.5% in primary open-angle glaucoma. Acta Ophthalmol 88(5):541–552. https://doi.org/10.1111/j.1755-3768.2009.01595.x
103. Actis AG, Versino E, Brogliatti B, Rolle T (2016) Risk factors for primary open angle glaucoma (POAG) progression: a study ruled in Torino. Open Ophthalmol J 10:129–139. Published 2016 Apr 29. https://doi.org/10.2174/1874364101610010129
104. Leske MC, Wu SY, Nemesure B, Hennis A (2002) Incident open-angle glaucoma and blood pressure. Arch Ophthalmol 120(7):954–959. https://doi.org/10.1001/archopht.120.7.954
105. Gugleta K (2009) Vaskuläre Risikofaktoren beim Glaukom - Diagnostik [Vascular risk factors in glaucoma - diagnostics]. Praxis 98(4):201–207. https://doi.org/10.1024/1661-8157.98.4.201
106. Memarzadeh F, Ying-Lai M, Chung J, Azen SP, Varma R, Los Angeles Latino Eye Study Group (2010) Blood pressure, perfusion pressure, and open-angle glaucoma: the Los Angeles Latino eye study. Invest Ophthalmol Vis Sci 51(6):2872–2877. https://doi.org/10.1167/iovs.08-2956
107. Weinreb RN, Aung T, Medeiros FA (2014) The pathophysiology and treatment of glaucoma: a review. JAMA 311(18):1901–1911. https://doi.org/10.1001/jama.2014.3192
108. Ghahari E, Bowd C, Zangwill LM et al (2019) Association of macular and circumpapillary microvasculature with visual field sensitivity in advanced glaucoma. Am J Ophthalmol 204:51–61. https://doi.org/10.1016/j.ajo.2019.03.004
109. Hou H, Moghimi S, Zangwill LM et al (2020) Association between rates of retinal nerve fiber layer thinning after intraocular pressure-lowering procedures and disc hemorrhage. Ophthalmol Glaucoma 3(1):7–13. https://doi.org/10.1016/j.ogla.2019.11.002
110. Kamalipour A, Moghimi S, Hou H et al (2022) Multilayer macula vessel density and visual field progression in glaucoma. Am J Ophthalmol 237:193–203. https://doi.org/10.1016/j.ajo.2021.11.018
111. Kwon JM, Weinreb RN, Zangwill LM, Suh MH (2019) Parapapillary deep-layer microvasculature dropout and visual field progression in glaucoma. Am J Ophthalmol 200:65–75. https://doi.org/10.1016/j.ajo.2018.12.007
112. Li F, Lin F, Gao K et al (2022) Association of foveal avascular zone area with structural and functional progression in glaucoma patients. Br J Ophthalmol 106(9):1245–1251. https://doi.org/10.1136/bjophthalmol-2020-318065
113. Alm A, Bill A (1973) Ocular and optic nerve blood flow at normal and increased intraocular pressures in monkeys (Macaca irus): a study with radioactively labelled microspheres including flow determinations in brain and some other tissues. Exp Eye Res 15(1):15–29. https://doi.org/10.1016/0014-4835(73)90185-1
114. Lejoyeux, R., Benillouche, J., Ong, J., , et al. Choriocapillaris: fundamentals and advancements. Prog Retin Eye Res 2022;87:100997. https://doi.org/10.1016/j.preteyeres.2021.100997
115. Suh MH, Zangwill LM, Manalastas PI et al (2016) Deep retinal layer microvasculature dropout detected by the optical coherence tomography angiography in glaucoma. Ophthalmology 123(12):2509–2518. https://doi.org/10.1016/j.ophtha.2016.09.002
116. Lee SH, Kim TW, Lee EJ, Girard MJA, Mari JM (2020) Focal lamina cribrosa defects are not associated with steep lamina cribrosa curvature but with choroidal microvascular dropout. Sci Rep 10:6761. Published 2020 Apr 21. https://doi.org/10.1038/s41598-020-63681-6
117. Lee EJ, Kim TW, Kim JA et al (2019) Elucidation of the strongest factors influencing rapid retinal nerve fiber layer thinning in glaucoma. Invest Ophthalmol Vis Sci 60(10):3343–3351. https://doi.org/10.1167/iovs.18-26519
118. Jo YH, Shin JW, Song MK, Won HJ, Kook MS (2021) Baseline choroidal microvasculature dropout as a predictor of subsequent visual field progression in open-angle glaucoma. J Glaucoma 30(8):672–681. https://doi.org/10.1097/IJG.0000000000001853

119. Lee EJ, Kim TW, Kim JA, Lee SH, Kim H (2022) Predictive modeling of long-term glaucoma progression based on initial ophthalmic data and optic nerve head characteristics. Transl Vis Sci Technol 11(10):24. https://doi.org/10.1167/tvst.11.10.24
120. Kim SH, Park KH (2006) The relationship between recurrent optic disc hemorrhage and glaucoma progression. Ophthalmology 113(4):598–602. https://doi.org/10.1016/j.ophtha.2005.12.018
121. Kurysheva NI, Shatalova EO (2022) Parafoveal vessel density dropout may predict glaucoma progression in the long-term follow up. J Ophthalmol Res 5:150–166
122. Janulevičiene I, Ehrlich R, Siesky B, Nedzelskienė I, Harris A (2011) Evaluation of hemodynamic parameters as predictors of glaucoma progression. J Ophthalmol 2011:164320. https://doi.org/10.1155/2011/164320
123. Chen CL, Zhang A, Bojikian KD et al (2016) Peripapillary retinal nerve fiber layer vascular microcirculation in glaucoma using optical coherence tomography-based microangiography. Invest Ophthalmol Vis Sci 57(9):OCT475–OCT485. https://doi.org/10.1167/iovs.15-18909
124. Yarmohammadi A, Zangwill LM, Diniz-Filho A et al (2017) Peripapillary and macular vessel density in patients with glaucoma and single-Hemifield visual field defect. Ophthalmology 124(5):709–719. https://doi.org/10.1016/j.ophtha.2017.01.004
125. Lommatzsch C, Rothaus K, Koch JM, Heinz C, Grisanti S (2018) OCTA vessel density changes in the macular zone in glaucomatous eyes. Graefes Arch Clin Exp Ophthalmol 256(8):1499–1508. https://doi.org/10.1007/s00417-018-3965-1
126. Moghimi S, Bowd C, Zangwill LM et al (2019) Measurement floors and dynamic ranges of OCT and OCT angiography in glaucoma. Ophthalmology 126(7):980–988. https://doi.org/10.1016/j.ophtha.2019.03.003
127. Rao HL, Pradhan ZS, Weinreb RN et al (2017) Relationship of optic nerve structure and function to peripapillary vessel density measurements of optical coherence tomography angiography in glaucoma. J Glaucoma 26(6):548–554. https://doi.org/10.1097/IJG.0000000000000670
128. Mwanza JC, Budenz DL, Warren JL et al (2015) Retinal nerve fibre layer thickness floor and corresponding functional loss in glaucoma. Br J Ophthalmol 99(6):732–737. https://doi.org/10.1136/bjophthalmol-2014-305745
129. Belghith A, Medeiros FA, Bowd C et al (2016) Structural change can be detected in advanced-glaucoma eyes. Invest Ophthalmol Vis Sci 57(9):OCT511–OCT518. https://doi.org/10.1167/iovs.15-18929
130. Holló G (2019) Peripapillary capillary vessel density progression in advanced glaucoma: a case report. BMC Ophthalmol 19(1):2. Published 2019 Jan 5. https://doi.org/10.1186/s12886-018-1021-x
131. In JH, Lee SY, Cho SH, Hong YJ (2018) Peripapillary vessel density reversal after trabeculectomy in glaucoma. J Ophthalmol 2018:8909714. Published 2018 Jun 26. https://doi.org/10.1155/2018/8909714
132. Shin JW, Sung KR, Uhm KB et al (2017) Peripapillary microvascular improvement and lamina Cribrosa depth reduction after trabeculectomy in primary open-angle glaucoma. Invest Ophthalmol Vis Sci 58(13):5993–5999. https://doi.org/10.1167/iovs.17-22787
133. Holló G (2017) Influence of large intraocular pressure reduction on peripapillary OCT vessel density in ocular hypertensive and glaucoma eyes. J Glaucoma 26:e7

Wearable Revolution: Predictive, Preventive, Personalized Medicine (PPPM) Par Excellence

Russell J. Andrews

Abbreviations

AF	atrial fibrillation
AHS	Apple Heart Study
AI	Artificial intelligence
AW	Apple Watch
BP	Blood pressure
CES-D	Center for Epidemiologic Studies Depression Scale
cryoMN	Cryomicroneedle
CT	Computerized tomography
CTTI	Clinical Trials Transformation Initiative
DCT	Digital clinical trial
ECG	Electrocardiogram
GI	Gastrointestinal
LED	Light-emitting diode
MN	Microneedle
MRI	Magnetic resonance imaging
NASA	National Aeronautics and Space Administration (USA)

R. J. Andrews (✉)
NASA Ames Research Center, Moffett Field, CA, USA

World Federation of Neurosurgical Societies, Brussels, Belgium
e-mail: rja@russelljandrews.org

H. Podbielska, M. Kapalla (eds.), *Predictive, Preventive, and Personalised Medicine: From Bench to Bedside*, Advances in Predictive, Preventive and Personalised Medicine 17, https://doi.org/10.1007/978-3-031-34884-6_19

NBA	National Basketball Association (USA)
PD	Parkinson's disease
PFA	Perfluoroalkoxy alkane
PGLA	Poly D,L-lactide-co-glycolide
PPPM	Predictive, preventive, personalized medicine
RT-PCR	Reverse transcription polymerase chain reaction
USA	United States of America

1 Introduction

Revolutions are common. At present electric and self-driving vehicles are revolutionizing personal transportation. Less than two decades ago the iPhone revolutionized personal communication: audio, video, texting. Four to five decades ago computerized tomography (CT), then magnetic resonance imaging (MRI), revolutionized personal medical imaging. The 2020 decade is the wearable revolution decade.

This brief chapter has two goals:

1. Provide representative examples of wearables for predictive, preventive, personalized medicine (PPPM) diagnosis and treatment.
2. Provide representative examples of the techniques and technologies involved so the creative reader may conceive and implement innovative wearable applications.

2 What Are "Wearables"?

"Wearables" can be defined in either a limited or an inclusive manner. A limited definition would be wearables as devices such as smart wrist watches, wrist and ankle bracelets, and smart rings (Fig. 1). A somewhat more inclusive definition would include smart clothing. More inclusive still would be smart skin patches. Temporarily worn devices such as smart masks (e.g., breathalyzers) can be included. Broader still would be including smart ingestibles—devices that are swallowed and collect information as they transit the gastrointestinal (GI) tract or attach to the wall of the GI tract for longer term monitoring or treatment. The broadest definition includes implantable devices—under the skin, in the bloodstream, or in specific organs (e.g., joints, heart, brain).

Since this review is primarily concerned with the gamut of current and prospective personalized diagnostic and therapeutic devices as well as the technologies involved, we will consider "wearables" as follows:

> *"Wearables" are devices, in close contact with the individual, that provide personalized information to guide and optimize prediction, prevention, diagnosis, and treatment of conditions affecting the individual's healthcare and quality of life.*

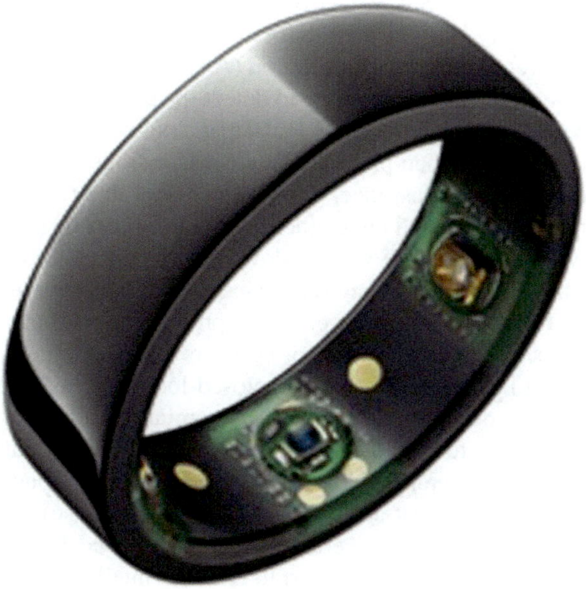

Fig. 1 Multisensory sleep and activity tracker by Oura Health, Oulu, Finland. (The image was taken from the open access article in [13])

3 Wearables Are Becoming an Essential Component of PPPM

Wearables have become a major factor in the evolution of digital clinical trials (DCTs) [1]. DCTs offer the advantages of (1) large numbers of participants, (2) passive data collection (reducing the need/personnel for in-person follow-up assessments), (3) voluminous longitudinal data collection [2]. The design and implementation of DCTs has become formalized thanks to the Clinical Trials Transformation Initiative (CTTI), an organization composed of academia, government, industry, and patient advocate representatives [3]. The development of mobile health applications (apps) for smartphones has made DCTs practical for large numbers of study participants over the past 7 years [4].

4 Examples of Wearables for PPPM

One traditional "wearable device" would be the thermometer; another would be the sphygmomanometer (blood pressure cuff). However, we are interested in **devices with more autonomous and continuous capabilities**: both the thermometer and the sphygmomanometer provide only an instant "snapshot" and lack the interconnectivity attributed to "smart" devices.

Some of the earliest wearables include **wristband physical monitors** (e.g., Fitbit) and smart watches (e.g., Apple Watch—AW). One of the early large studies of a wearable device (and an example of industry-academic partnership) was the

Apple Heart Study (AHS), a collaboration between Apple Inc. and Stanford University [2]. The AHS built upon CTTI's recommendations for a DCT to collect data regarding atrial fibrillation (AF) digitally from over 400,000 participants. The AW uses an optical sensor to detect the pulse waveform to measure heart rate, thus enabling detection of AF. Participants who demonstrated (through the AW) probable AF were then provided an electrocardiogram (ECG) patch to confirm the presence of AF. In essence, one fulltime wearable (the AW) provided continuous data that was validated by another temporary wearable (the ECG patch). All participants with suspected AF were followed by a telehealth doctor, i.e., the AHS DCT was "site-less" and used **smart devices and telemedicine** for continuous PPPM.

Diabetes, a disorder of global proportion, has been a topic of personalized diagnosis and treatment for over 60 years [5]. The term "**artificial pancreas**" has been used to describe personalized closed-loop systems to monitor the need for, and provide the delivery of, insulin. Commercially available systems for diabetes at present are limited to hybrid closed-loop systems: although automated for the most part, one needs to program additional insulin for meals. Conditions requiring manual input include those that are temporary (meals, exercise) as well as those that are longer term (pregnancy). The era of **completely closed-loop diabetes systems** will soon be upon us, thanks in large part to artificial intelligence (AI). Algorithms following the rate of change of blood glucose levels can detect the effect of meals; coordination with another "wearable" such as a smart watch can provide heart rate data essential for quantifying exercise. An additional refinement is a system that incorporates not only insulin but also glucagon to counteract hypoglycemic episodes. Such a system is complicated by issues such as (1) the need for a form of glucagon that is biochemically stable for an implanted system and (2) the differing pharmacokinetics of insulin and glucagon (the latter being much more rapid in onset of its effect).

Parkinson's disease (PD) is another disorder amenable to wearables for PPPM. The smartphone itself can collect much of the relevant individual information in this disorder of movement, thanks to the smartphone's accelerometer and other sensing capabilities. One early pilot study of 20 individuals (10 PD patients and 10 controls) demonstrated that five smartphone tests (voice, gait, posture, finger tapping, response time) could distinguish those with PD from controls [6]. More recently, findings from the mPower observational study of PD (using smartphone data from tests of voice, gait, balance, finger tapping, memory) have been reported [7]. This report is notable for the thoughtful, detailed discussion of the potential limitations of smartphone collection of study data. A particular benefit of the smartphone technology for PPPM is the ability for the PD patient to assess the effects of medication changes on objective performance measures.

Early diagnosis of the more than one in ten infants who have **neurodevelopmental abnormalities** is a universal healthcare challenge: assessment by trained professionals who administer standardized neurodevelopmental tests in an office or clinic setting is impractical for many reasons. Objective measurement of spontaneous infant motor behavior at home is a practical alternative [8]. An **infant jumpsuit** incorporating a sensor (linear acceleration and angular velocity) for each of the infant's four limbs allows Bluetooth streaming of data (Fig. 2); video recordings of

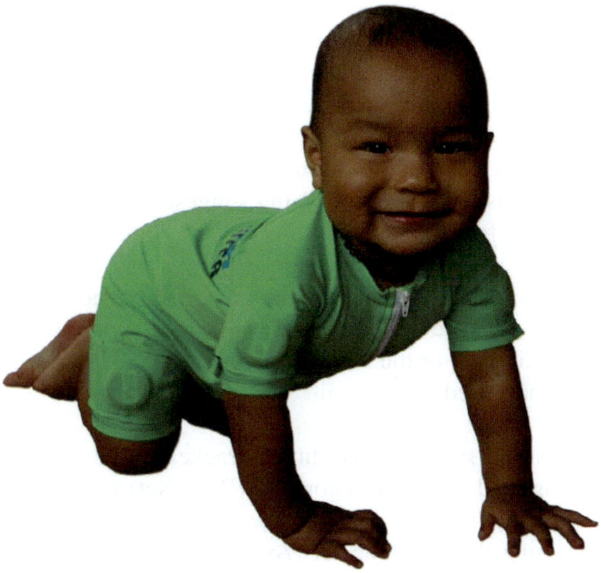

Fig. 2 A 10-month-old subject crawling at home with the MAIJU (Motor ability Assessment of Infants with a Jumpsuit) jumpsuit, equipped with movement sensors in the proximal pockets of each limb. (The image was taken from the open access article in [8])

infant activity scored by independent annotators and sensor data were mapped by convolutional neural network techniques. The very detailed description of the methodology and the challenges faced by the group in Finland is informative; the potential for wearable sensor-based technology to advance the diagnosis and treatment of **disorders of motor function** (e.g., neurodevelopmental, PD, stroke) personally, cost-effectively, and globally is demonstrated.

The potential of wearables to enhance PPPM for more population-wide conditions is just beginning to be appreciated:

1. **Weight management** is becoming a universal concern, particularly in countries where obesity rates are increasing rapidly, and pharmaceutical companies are developing "blockbuster" drugs to combat this global epidemic [9]. Wearables for weight management are going beyond activity monitors (e.g., Fitbit) and smartphone apps to bite counters as another approach to weight reduction [10];
2. For women planning to become pregnant, the **Ava bracelet** (Ava AG, Zurich) has been used to measure seven parameters (including wrist skin temperature, heart rate, heart rate variability, respiratory rate, skin perfusion) plus machine learning to develop an algorithm **to predict the "fertile window"** [11];
3. **A nametag-like device** that records both **face-to-face interactions** (infrared sensor) and **body activity** (accelerometer) has been used to correlate the group interaction and individual body activity data with the results of the Center for Epidemiologic Studies Depression Scale (CES-D). Data were gathered from 449 employees at ten companies in Japan. Evidence of depression on the CES-D was negatively correlated with more robust interactions as well as more animated body activity (more individual body movements, e.g., gesticulations) [12].

4. A minimally-invasive biometric ring allows lifestyle modification through feedback of sleep and exercise behaviors [13]. The Oura ring (Fig. 1) supplied data on pulse rate, amplitude and variability, motion, and skin temperature that underwent extensive machine learning-based analyses to yield information on sleep status and physical activity. This information was in turn provided to each subject as text messages providing information (e.g., number of steps the previous day) as well as encouraging suggestions on how to improve sleep and activity going forward.

COVID-19 has fostered wearables for diagnosis (ideally in the pre-symptomatic stage), with the advantages of (1) privacy (home-based), (2) logistics (no need for the individual or the sample to travel to the lab), (3) cost. Several techniques have been proposed:

1. Using a smartwatch or fitness tracker to follow resting heart rate plus deep learning to develop an algorithm (PCovNet) to identify COVID-19 patients in the pre-symptomatic stage [14];
2. Using the Ava bracelet (Ava AG, Zurich)—parameters measured given in the previous paragraph—worn at night plus a machine learning algorithm to identify 68% of COVID-19 patients up to 2 days before symptom onset [15];
3. Using breath analysis with a mask and mass spectroscopy for COVID-19 diagnosis [16].

5 Examples of Wearables Technology

A primary advance in wearables technology is making the wearable as unobtrusive as possible. Possibilities are (1) miniaturization and (2) incorporation of the wearable sensors into existing customs (watches, bracelets, clothing). One example of miniaturization and incorporation into existing customs—a step beyond smart watches—is the Oura ring (Fig. 1) [17, 18]. The Oura ring, monitoring heart rate, blood oxygenation, temperature using LED sensors, temperature sensors, a 3D accelerometer, and a gyroscope, has been used by professional sports organizations such as the National Basketball Association (NBA) in the USA for, e.g., optimizing sleep to enhance athletic performance [17, 18].

A crucial issue for wearable sensors is durability matching that of the clothes harboring the sensor, one major aspect being the ability to communicate the data acquired with an external device (typically a smartphone). Traditional electronics—even at the micro-scale—are inflexible. One proposed solution is a **liquid metal fiber**: perfluoroalkoxy alkane (PFA) tubing infused with galinstan (a liquid metal) [19]. The liquid metal fiber is digitally embroidered onto the existing fabric/garment (Fig. 3); an axillary temperature monitoring garment has been illustrated (Fig. 4).

A very different approach to wearable sensors—an approach appropriate for detecting small molecules (e.g., environmental toxins) as well as bacteria and viruses (e.g., COVID-19)—involves **freeze-dried cell-free genetic detectors and**

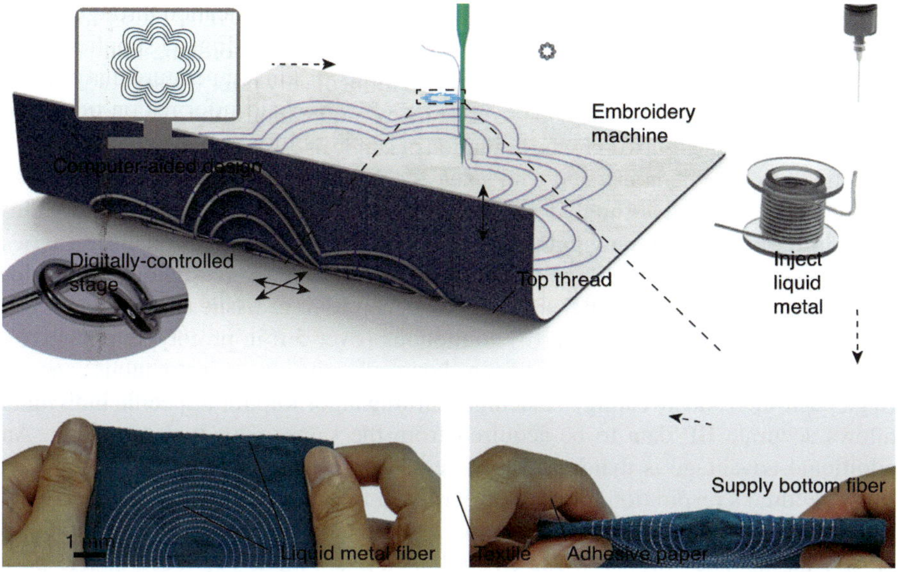

Fig. 3 Illustration of the digital embroidery process. Liquid metal fibers consist of perfluoroalkoxy alkane tubing infiltrated with galinstan. (The image was taken from the open access article in [19])

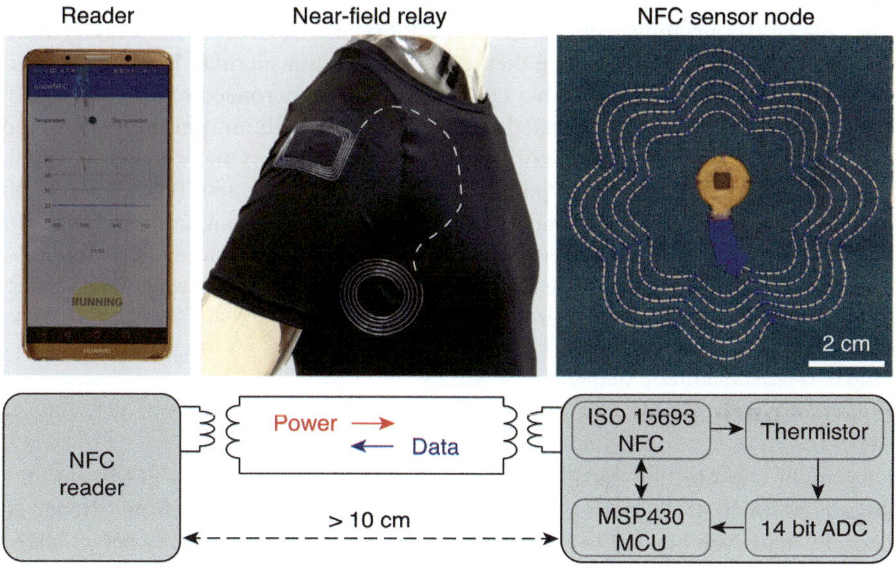

Fig. 4 Textile thermal monitoring system comprising a sensor node connected with a smart-phone reader via a near-field relay integrated on a shirt. The top row shows images of the system components; the bottom row shows the block diagram. The distance between the reader and sensor node is more than 10 cm apart. (The image was taken from the open access article in [19])

colorimetric or fluorescent outputs (much like current COVID-19 tests for home use) [20, 21]. Cell-free genetic templates are freeze-dried for long-term storage, embedded in textiles or masks, then rehydrated immediately prior to use; colorimetric response occurs within an hour or so. For many applications, the simplicity of not requiring electronics outweighs the limitation of single use. A face mask for COVID-19 detection has been demonstrated with a detection rate similar to RT-PCR assays [20].

Another technique—suitable for blood pressure (BP) monitoring–utilizes **bio-impedance and a graphene patch** or tattoo placed over the radial and ulnar arteries at the distal forearm/wrist area [22]. Major advantages of **graphene patch bio-impedance monitoring of BP** are (1) deep penetration of tissue (20 mm or more); (2) ultrathin (down to 200 nm); (3) continuous (over 5 h in prototype, potentially much longer). Such a BP patch has been shown effective through strenuous exercise (e.g., push-ups) and sweating; a machine learning algorithm for a specific individual allows accurate BP data to be acquired from the same individual days later. An additional advantage is that by post-processing (including fast Fourier transform) the individual's respiration rate can be extracted from the BP data acquired [22].

Microneedle (MN) patches are being 3D fabricated to allow transdermal delivery for therapeutic purposes. One example is a patch made of biodegradable poly (D,L-lactide-co-glycolide) (PGLA) 1 × 1 cm in size with approximately 200 MNs [23]. Each MN consists of a PGLA shell with a core or payload of drug or vaccine. The PGLA can be formulated to release at a specific time (from a few days up to 48 days); patches with differing release times can be applied to the skin to provide multiple release times (mimicking multiple drug or vaccine injections over time). The role of 3D printing technology in the fabrication of MNs has recently been reviewed [24]. A variation on the theme of MNs for transdermal delivery—a technique capable of delivering viable cells—is the cryomicroneedle (cryoMN) [25]. The therapeutic cells are suspended in the cryogenic medium (phosphate-buffered saline plus 2.5% dimethyl sulfoxide and 100 mM sucrose) and cast into a mold. Over several hours the **cyroMN patch** is cooled from −20 °C to −196 °C. Although the cryoMNs are clearly biodegradable, they suffer the same limitation as COVID-19 mRNA vaccines in that they require ultracold shipping and storage conditions—plus very rapid application to the skin. However, the ability to deliver cells transdermally is a crucial advantage of cryoMNs.

6 Conclusions

One might consider the decade 2010–2020 the initial decade of PPPM—and the decade 2020–2030 the decade of wearables to implement PPPM from "Bench to bedside" and even beyond to be capable of early prediction, and very personalized prevention. Thanks to advances in data gathering technology such as patches down to the nano level, spectroscopy, and bioimpedance—and advances in data analytical technology such as AI—the health and wellbeing applications of wearables will increase exponentially in the years until 2030 thus increasing the potential for practical application of PPPM in the future healthcare.

References

1. Inan OT, Tenaerts P, Prindiville SA, Reynolds HR, Dizon DS, Cooper-Arnold K et al (2020) Digitizing clinical trials. NPJ Digit Med 3:1–7. https://doi.org/10.1038/s41746-020-0302-y
2. Garcia A, Balasubramanian V, Lee J, Gardner R, Gummidipundi S, Hung G et al (2022) Lessons learned in the apple heart study and implications for the data management of future digital clinical trials. J Biopharm Stat 32:496. https://doi.org/10.1080/10543406.2022.2080698
3. Clinical Trials Transformation Initiative (CTTI). Digital health trials. CTTI website: https://ctti-clinicaltrials.org. Accessed 8 Aug 2022
4. Dorsey ER, Chen YF, McConnell MV, Shaw SY, Trister AD, Friend SH (2017) The use of smartphones for health research. Acad Med 92:157–160
5. Templer S (2022) Closed-loop insulin delivery systems: past, present, and future directions. Front Endocrinol 13:919942. https://doi.org/10.3389/fendo.2022.919942
6. Arora S, Venkataraman V, Zhan A, Donohue S, Biglan KM, Dorsey ER et al (2015) Detecting and monitoring the symptoms of Parkinson's disease using smartphones: a pilot study. Parkinsonism Relat Disord 21:650–653
7. Omberg L, Neto EC, Perumal TM, Pratap A, Tediarjo A, Adams J et al (2022) Remote smartphone monitoring of Parkinson's disease and individual response to therapy. Nat Biotechnol 40:480–487
8. Airaksinen M, Gallen A, Kivi A, Vijayakrishnan P, Häyrinen T, Ilén E et al (2022) Intelligent wearable allows out-of-the-lab tracking of developing motor abilities in infants. Comms Med 2:69. https://doi.org/10.1038/s43856-022-00131-6
9. Alpert B (2022) Finally, weight-loss drugs that work. Barrons:18–20. Accessed 15 Aug 2022
10. Carpenter CA, Ugwoaba UA, Cardel MI, Ross KM (2022) Using self-monitoring technology for nutritional counseling and weight management. Digit Health 8:1–9. https://doi.org/10.1177/20552076221102774
11. Goodale BM, Shilaih M, Falco L et al (2019) Wearable sensors reveal menses-driven changes in physiology and enable prediction of the fertile window: observational study. J Med Internet Res 21:e13404. https://doi.org/10.2196/13404
12. Lee JH, Sato N, Yano K, Miyake Y (2022) Universal association between depressive symptoms and social-network structures in the workplace. Sci Rep 12:10170. https://doi.org/10.1038/s41598-022-14366-9
13. Browne JD, Boland DM, Baum JT, Ikemiya K, Harris Q, Phillips M et al (2021) Lifestyle modification using a wearable biometric ring and guided feedback improve sleep and exercise behaviors: a 12-month randomized, placebo-controlled study. Front Physiol 12:777874. https://doi.org/10.3389/fphys.2021.777874
14. Abir FF, Alyafei K, Chowdhury MEH, Khandakar A, Ahmed R, Hossain MM et al (2022) PCovNet: a presymptomatic COVID-19 detection framework using deep learning model using wearables data. Comput Biol Med 147:105682. https://doi.org/10.1016/j.compbiomed.2022.105682
15. Risch M, Grossmann K, Aeschbacher S, Weideli OC, Kovac M, Pereira F et al (2022) Investigation of the use of a sensor bracelet for the presymptomatic detection of changes in physiological parameters related to COVID-19: an interim analysis of a prospective cohort study (COVI-GAPP). BMJ Open 12:e058274. https://doi.org/10.1136/bmjopen-2021-058274
16. Shekhawat JK, Banerjee M (2022) Role of breath biopsy in COVID-19. J Appl Lab Med 7:1175. https://doi.org/10.1093/jalm/jfac040/6611531
17. So A (2020) Review: Oura ring. Wired. www.wired.com/review/oura-ring. Accessed 6 Sep 2020
18. Crocombe R (2022) The ever-shrinking optical spectrometer enhances consumer goods. Photonics Spectra 56:36–41
19. Lin R, Kim HJ, Achavananthadith S, Xiong Z, Lee JKW, Kong YL et al (2022) Digitally-embroidered liquid metal electronic textiles for wearable wireless systems. Nat Commun 13:2190. https://doi.org/10.1038/s41467-022-29859-4

20. Nguyen PQ, Soenksen LR, Donghia NM, Angenent-Mari NM, de Puig H, Huang A et al (2021) Wearable materials with embedded synthetic biology sensors for biomolecule detection. Nat Biotechnol 39:1366–1374
21. Lu Y (2022) Textile-embedded cell-free biosensors. Nat Biomed Eng 6:225–226
22. Kireev D, Sel K, Ibrahim B, Kumar N, Akbari A, Jafari R et al (2022) Continuous cuffless monitoring of arterial blood pressure via graphene bioimpedance tattoos. Nat Nanotechnol 17:864. https://doi.org/10.1038/s42565-022-01145-w
23. Tran KTM, Gavitt TD, Farrell NJ, Curry EJ, Mara AB, Patel A et al (2021) Transdermal microneedles for the programmable burst release of multiple vaccine payloads. Nat Biomed Eng 5:998–1007
24. Detamornrat U, McAlister E, Hutton RJ, Larraneta E, Donnelly RF (2022) The role of 3D printing technology in microengineering of microneedles. Small 18:2106392. https://doi.org/10.1002/smll.202106392
25. Chang H, Chew SWT, Zheng M, Lio DCS, Wiraja C, Mei Y et al (2021) Cryomicroneedles for transdermal cell delivery. Nat Biomed Eng 5:1008–1018

GPSR Compliance

The European Union's (EU) General Product Safety Regulation (GPSR) is a set of rules that requires consumer products to be safe and our obligations to ensure this.

If you have any concerns about our products, you can contact us on ProductSafety@springernature.com

In case Publisher is established outside the EU, the EU authorized representative is:

Springer Nature Customer Service Center GmbH
Europaplatz 3
69115 Heidelberg, Germany

Batch number: 10732044

Printed by Printforce, the Netherlands